Ration
A (

MW01140761

Rationale of Drug of Choice
A Comparative Analysis

P Nirmala MD PhD (Pharmacology)
Professor and Head
Department of Pharmacology
Rajah Muthiah Medical College
Annamalai University
Chidambaram, Tamil Nadu, India

N Chidambaram MD FRCP (Glasg) FACC
Professor and Head
Department of Cardiology
Dean
Faculty of Medicine
Rajah Muthiah Medical College
Annamalai University
Chidambaram, Tamil Nadu, India

Forewords
S Vembar MBBS MSc (Pharmacology)
TR Muralidharan MD DM FACC FESC

The Health Sciences Publisher
New Delhi | London | Panama

Jaypee Brothers Medical Publishers (P) Ltd

Headquarters

Jaypee Brothers Medical Publishers (P) Ltd
4838/24, Ansari Road, Daryaganj
New Delhi 110 002, India
Phone: +91-11-43574357
Fax: +91-11-43574314
Email: jaypee@jaypeebrothers.com

Overseas Offices

J.P. Medical Ltd
83 Victoria Street, London
SW1H 0HW (UK)
Phone: +44 20 3170 8910
Fax: +44 (0)20 3008 6180
Email: info@jpmedpub.com

Jaypee-Highlights Medical Publishers Inc
City of Knowledge, Bld. 235, 2nd Floor, Clayton
Panama City, Panama
Phone: +1 507-301-0496
Fax: +1 507-301-0499
Email: cservice@jphmedical.com

Jaypee Brothers Medical Publishers (P) Ltd
17/1-B Babar Road, Block-B, Shaymali
Mohammadpur, Dhaka-1207
Bangladesh
Mobile: +08801912003485
Email: jaypeedhaka@gmail.com

Jaypee Brothers Medical Publishers (P) Ltd
Bhotahity, Kathmandu, Nepal
Phone +977-9741283608
Email: kathmandu@jaypeebrothers.com

Website: www.jaypeebrothers.com
Website: www.jaypeedigital.com

Inquiries for bulk sales may be solicited at: jaypee@jaypeebrothers.com

Rationale of Drug of Choice—A Comparative Analysis

First Edition: **2018**

ISBN: 978-93-5270-134-6

Printed at Rajkamal Electric Press, Plot No. 2, Phase-IV, Kundli, Haryana.

Foreword

I feel privileged to be asked to write the foreword for the book *Rationale of Drug of Choice—A Comparative Analysis*, authored by two of my former colleagues at Rajah Muthiah Medical College, Annamalai University, Chidambaram, Tamil Nadu, India. Both the authors are loved and respected by the students for their erudition, experience in the chosen fields of their specialisation and their teaching prowess.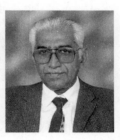
I had the privilege of seeing Dr P Nirmala, a young and dynamic postgraduate student, grow into a full-fledged pharmacologist and become an acknowledged leader in the field. Likewise, I also had the privilege of observing Dr Chidambaram, a young Reader in Medicine, become a leader in the field and it is no wonder that several academic and administrative responsibilities came knocking to him because of the sheer merit he had acquired. So, it was a joy for me to go through the manuscript of their book and I found it to be a masterpiece and path-breaking title in the field of Therapeutics, which has been orphaned by Pharmacology as well as Medicine. Hence, I am sure their book will hit the medical book world with a big bang and would be found desirable by all the students—be they postgraduates in Pharmacology/Medicine or be they graduates/postgraduates in Pharmacy—who wish to get some clarity about 'drugs of choice' in Therapeutics. Besides, I feel the young graduates in Medicine, who set feet in the practice of Medicine as CRRIs, will also find easier access to decision-making in their choice of drugs in different clinical situations.

I commend the authors for their excellent work and wish them all the success.

S Vembar MBBS MSc (Pharmacology)
Director and Professor (Rtd)
Department of Pharmacology
Madras Medical College
Former Dean
Rajah Muthiah Medical College
Annamalai University
Chidambaram, Tamil Nadu, India

Foreword

I am immensely pleased to write the foreword to this book authored by Dr (Mrs) P Nirmala, and co-authored by Dr N Chidambaram. I am thoroughly impressed with the extraordinary efforts put in by the author Dr P Nirmala and the co-author Dr N Chidambaram, which specifically address the need for the clinical choice of a drug for an ideal prescription.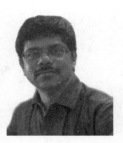

This compilation on *Rationale of Drug of Choice—A Comparative Analysis* proves just how much learning and wisdom are hidden there in bringing out this book on the basis of 'Evidence-based medicine'.

This book would be a great source of information for students, medical officers and practitioners, who would like to excel in their rational thinking in selecting the right medications in the clinical scenarios they encounter during their practice. The author's work is evident in segregation of the choice of drugs for treatment based on its efficacy, safety, its mechanism and the adverse effects.

"You can teach a student a lesson for a day, but if you can teach him to learn by creating curiosity, he will continue the learning process as long as he lives."

I am sure this book will serve that purpose. I strongly recommend this concise book, which will be of great value and interest to all the clinicians as well as trainees at all levels, who wish to gain an understanding of contemporary therapeutics and apply this information effectively to their patients

I would like to congratulate the authors for this endeavor of providing ideal choice in practical situations by a rational approach.

TR Muralidharan MD DM FACC FESC
Professor and Head
Department of Cardiology
Sri Ramachandra University
Chennai, Tamil Nadu, India

Preface

In the ever-widening field of Pharmacology, learning the basis behind rational prescription of drugs is of utmost importance. Several drugs are available for therapy of any given clinical condition and this creates confusion in choosing the best available drug even if they belong to the same group. Drugs are generally classified according to their mechanism of action and may have similar pharmacodynamic profile but their inherent biological differences determine their efficacy, safety and degree of potency. Their affordability also plays an important role.

Rational prescription of drugs through available information from clinical trials forms the basis of 'Evidence-based Medicine'. Constant changes in medical science compounded by development of drug resistance necessitate the pragmatic use of drugs with more focus on the application of pharmacological principles. Since Pharmacology forms the backbone of Medicine, a rational prescription narrows down the gap between the good and poor patient compliance, that directly influences the outcome of treatment. Basic understanding of pharmacodynamic, pharmacokinetic details and safety profile of a drug often helps to improve its therapeutic efficacy. Hence, this book deals with the selection of a rational drug from the current list of approved drugs. Such a selection of drug is suitably justified through analysis with references from standard textbooks and publications in indexed journals and explains the reason for the selection of a drug based on the principles of pharmacology.

The main objective of this book is to specifically address the clinical choice of a drug for an ideal prescription, so as to maximize the therapeutic benefits and to minimise adverse effects. An ideal prescription improves the compliance of a patient and boosts the success rate of therapy. Rational prescription using right medication at right dose, through proper route of administration with adequate frequency and duration is the ultimate objective of this book. This facilitates a comprehensive outlook with therapeutic modalities for easy understanding and attempts to improve the knowledge of a reader.

The sequence of topics is based on the main division with the underlying subheadings. Recent topics like ocular, dermatological, obstetric and gynecological pharmacology are also included. The discussion eloborates on the drugs used in various clinical situations.

The choice of two drugs discussed in each situation was made as follows:

1. Both the drugs are indicated as the first-line drugs in a particular clinical condition but one drug is superior to the other by virtue of its pharmacodynamic and kinetic properties, and its toxicity profile

   OR

2. Both the drugs are approved for use in a given clinical condition but one drug is absolutely contraindicated in the associated comorbid condition

   OR

3. Of the two drugs discussed, one is a first-line and the other is a second-line drug

   OR

4. Of the two drugs mentioned, one is indicated and the other is contraindicated.

By comparing efficacy, safety, mechanism of action and adverse effects between the two best available drugs (in some clinical conditions, drugs that are contraindicated are also being discussed), this book will help the readers understand the choice of the best drug for any given clinical condition and clearly defines the logic behind such a selection through justification. It also explains the reason for not using a particular drug in certain clinical conditions. Moreover, this book also provides a clear-cut and logical explanation and aims to teach the correct prescription practice to the undergraduates, CRRIs and postgraduate students in their early formative stage itself. Besides, this book can be used as a ready-reckoner by the general practitioners, and specialists even during their busy practice schedules.

P Nirmala
N Chidambaram

Acknowledgments

Foremost, I am extremely grateful to our honorable Vice Chancellor Professor S Manian, our respected Registrar Professor K Arumugam for acknowledging and permitting the publication of this book.

I wish to profoundly thank Dr S Vembar MBBS, MSc (Pharmacology), former Dean, Rajah Muthiah Medical College, Annamalai University, Chidambaram, Tamil Nadu, India for his continuous guidance from the inception of this project, for his patience, immense knowledge, for his help in language edition of this book and for writing the foreword.

My special thanks to Dr PSRK Haranath MD, DSc, former DME, AP, and first Head of the Department of Pharmacology, Rajah Muthiah Medical College, Annamalai University, Chidambaram, Tamil Nadu, India for his continuous support and motivation.

I would like to express my sincere gratitude to Dr TR Muralidharan MD, DM (Cardiology), FACC, FESC, Professor and Head of Cardiology, Sri Ramachandra Medical Institute, Chennai, Tamil Nadu, India for writing the foreword of this book.

I sincerely thank Dr N Chidambaram MD, FRCP (Glasg), FACC, Professor and Head, Department of Cardiology, and Dean, Faculty of Medicine, Rajah Muthiah Medical College, Annamalai University, Chidambaram, Tamil Nadu, India for coauthoring this book.

Thanks to my colleagues Dr Vanitha Samuel, Dr M Sekkizhar, Dr Sylvia Santhakumari, Dr Swadin Ranjan Behera, and Dr M Selvaraju for their moral support and for providing valuable help in the time of need.

I wish to immensely thank Ms Sheetal Arora Kapoor, Senior Development Editor, Jaypee Brothers Medical Publishers and her team for their patience, prompt response and the excellent support provided towards proofreading and typesetting.

I profoundly thank Shri Jitendar P Vij (Group Chairman), Mr Ankit Vij (Group President), and Ms Chetna Malhotra Vohra (Associate Director–Content Strategy) of Jaypee Brothers Medical

Publishers (P) Ltd, New Delhi, India for enabling us to publish this book. I further thank Mr R Jayanandan, Senior Commissioning Editor, Chennai Branch for being instrumental in publishing this book.

P Nirmala

Contents

SECTION 1

Autonomic Nervous System and Autacoids

Section Outline

1. Adrenergic Drugs
2. Alpha Blockers
3. Beta Blockers
4. Cholinergic Drugs
5. Anticholinergic Drugs
6. Skeletal Muscle Relaxants
7. Local Anesthetics
8. Histamine, Antihistamines and Leukotrienes
9. Serotonin Agonists and Antagonists
10. Prostaglandins

Adrenergic Drugs

1. *Apraclonidine/Brimonidine as adjunct in therapy of glaucoma.*

BACKGROUND

The main goal in treatment of glaucoma is reduction of intraocular pressure. The drugs either reduce aqueous humor production or increase its drainage. Apraclonidine and brimonidine are α_2 adrenergic agonists. They are mainly used as adjuncts in glaucoma. Both drugs bind to postsynaptic α_2 autoreceptors. They decrease synthesis of aqueous humor by inhibiting production of cyclic AMP and the intraocular pressure is reduced by facilitating uveoscleral outflow. The intraocular pressure is reduced by about 25%. These drugs are used as topical agents.

BRIMONIDINE

Brimonidine is a highly selective α_2 agonist. It is highly lipophilic and penetrates cornea more effectively. Being lipophilic, it crosses blood brain barrier causing hypotension and sedation. Brimonidine should therefore be avoided in patients with cardiac conditions. Brimonidine is effective for both short and long-term therapy. It is better tolerated and causes minimal allergic reactions as it has weaker α_1 agonist action. Brimonidine is more effective than apraclonidine as an adjunct in therapy.

APRACLONIDINE

Apraclonidine, a selective α_2 agonist is highly ionized at physiological pH. It does not cross blood brain barrier, so does not affect the systemic cardiovascular parameters. It can be used only for short-term therapy as it causes many allergic reactions such as itching and follicular conjunctivitis. It also results in retraction of eyelids and mydriasis.

Drug of Choice: Brimonidine

RATIONALE

α_2 agonists are used only as **adjuncts** in glaucoma. **Apraclonidine** is a **relatively less selective** α_2 **agonist** and **brimonidine** is a **more selective** α_2 **agonist**. **Brimonidine** is **lipophilic** and penetrates cornea easily but **apraclonidine** is **not lipophilic**. They are both **equally effective** in reducing the intraocular pressure but apraclonidine causes frequent allergic reactions that **limit** its use to short-term therapy. Brimonidine needs to be avoided in cardiac patients otherwise it is well-tolerated, causes minimal allergic reactions. Brimonidine is therefore preferred to apraclonidine.

2. *Atomoxetine/Methylphenidate for treatment of attention deficit/hyperactivity disorder (ADHD) in children and adolescents.*

BACKGROUND

ADHD is characterized by inattention, hyperactivity and impulsivity. At cortical level, these actions are modulated by catecholamines. Therefore, psychostimulants are the first line drugs for ADHD in children and adolescents.

METHYLPHENIDATE

Methylphenidate is a CNS stimulant and structurally similar to amphetamine. It is also a psychostimulant like amphetamine. Methylphenidate reduces inattention, impulsivity and hyperactivity. It acts centrally causing release of norepinephrine and dopamine. It has more prolonged central, than peripheral action. It is started at 5 mg twice daily orally and then increased gradually. The dose of methylphenidate should not exceed 60 mg/day. Methylphenidate reduces appetite and causes loss of weight. Other side effects are insomnia and abdominal pain. It is contraindicated in patients with cardiac problems. Methylphenidate has the potential for abuse liability but it has greater efficacy and safety hence preferred to atomoxetine.

ATOMOXETINE

Atomoxetine is a selective norepinephrine reuptake inhibitor (SNRI). Unlike methylphenidate, atomoxetine is not a CNS stimulant. Atomoxetine is reserved for use as a second line drug. It is used as an alternative in patients who cannot tolerate methylphenidate. Like methylphenidate it is also contraindicated in patients with cardiac abnormalities. Atomoxetine increases the risk of seizures and suicidal tendencies. Although atomoxetine has no abuse potential, it does not have long-term safety.

Drug of Choice: Methylphenidate

RATIONALE

Psychostimulants are more effective in the treatment of ADHD than nonstimulants. **Methylphenidate** has **more central** than peripheral action, reduces symptoms of inattention, hyperactivity and impulsivity more effectively than atomoxetine. Although it has a potential to cause **addiction**, it is very effective[1] and **confers long-term safety**[2] when compared to atomoxetine, so it is preferred. **Atomoxetine** is only a **second line drug** with no long-term safety record and it increases the risk of seizures as well as suicidal tendencies. Hence, atomoxetine is not preferred.

3. *Midodrine/Phenylephrine for orthostatic hypotension in autonomic neuropathy.*

BACKGROUND

During standing posture, peripheral venous pooling decreases venous return thereby reducing the blood pressure. Such a fall in BP should normally result in reflex sympathetic stimulation and compensatory peripheral vasoconstriction, but due to impaired autonomic reflexes, orthostatic hypotension and fainting attacks occur in patients with autonomic neuropathy. Diabetes mellitus is one of the major causes of autonomic neuropathy and induces orthostatic hypotension. Imipramine, diuretics and tricyclic anti-depressants can cause orthostatic hypotension.

MIDODRINE

Midodrine is a prodrug and orally effective, selective α_1 agonist used in the treatment of orthostatic hypotension. It achieves peak plasma concentration within an hour and has a plasma half-life of about 25 minutes. Its metabolite, desglymidodrine is pharmacologically active with a half-life of 3 hours. Therefore, the duration of action of midodrine is 4 to 6 hours. It causes α_1 mediated contraction of both arterial and venous smooth muscles. Such a potent vasoconstriction increases the blood pressure but leads to supine hypertension as an adverse effect. Midodrine should preferably be given 4 hours prior to bed time and patient should avoid lying down to avoid supine hypertension.

PHENYLEPHRINE

Phenylephrine is also a directly acting relatively pure α_1 agonist but it has no selectivity and stimulates beta receptors at a higher dosage. It is not available as oral formulation. It is not metabolized by catechol-o-methyltransferase, so has a longer duration of action resulting in sustained increase in blood pressure. Since phenylephrine can cause sustained hypertension, it is not suitable for the management of orthostatic hypotension.

Drug of Choice: Midodrine

RATIONALE

Selective α_1 agonists are potent vasoconstrictors and increase blood pressure by causing intense peripheral vasoconstriction. Midodrine is a prodrug, orally effective, is converted to its active metabolite **desglymidodrine**, causes direct α_1 stimulation and increases blood pressure **immediately.** It can induce hypertension as an extension of its pharmacological action. **Phenylephrine** is a relatively **selective α₁ agonist** but **not used** in the management of orthostatic hypotension as it results in prolonged action and leads to **sustained hypertension**.

4. *Epinephrine/Phenylephrine for subcutaneous administration along with local anesthetics.*

BACKGROUND

Local anesthetics are combined with alpha agonists to prolong their duration of action. When given as subcutaneous injection, alpha agonist causes local vasoconstriction reducing the rate of absorption of coadministered drug and prolonging its duration of action. The effect of local anesthetic is directly proportional to its contact time with nerves. Hence, vasoconstrictors prolong the duration of anesthesia by local anesthetics.

EPINEPHRINE

Epinephrine is combined with local anesthetics at the concentration of 1:20,000. Local anesthetic is a weak base but its hydrochloride salt is mildly acidic, a property that enhances not only its stability but the stability of coadministered drug epinephrine as well. When administered subcutaneously epinephrine causes local vasoconstriction. Epinephrine has dual action when combined with local anesthetics. It modulates the rate of absorption of local anesthetic concentrating it at the site of administration, equilibrating the amount absorbed with the amount metabolized. Vasoconstriction induced by epinephrine reduces its self-absorption into systemic circulation thus preventing its adverse reactions. Further, it prevents the systemic toxicity of coadministered local anesthetics. The degree of vasoconstriction induced by epinephrine is not so intense due to vasodilatation mediated by β_2 receptors. Hence, it does not reduce blood supply at the site of injection.

PHENYLEPHRINE

Phenylephrine is a selective α_1 agonist and stimulates beta receptors only at higher concentration. It is a potent vasoconstrictor and causes intense vasoconstriction. The vasoconstrictor effect persists for a long period of time and such prolonged effect may interfere with absorption of adequate amount of local anesthetic. Besides, phenylephrine is devoid of beta receptor mediated vasodilatation. Hence, it may reduce the local blood supply at the site of injection. So, it is not preferred as a vasoconstrictor for subcutaneous formulations.

Drug of Choice: Epinephrine

RATIONALE

Epinephrine is combined with local anesthetics to **prolong** its duration of action by delaying its rate of absorption and by resulting in **proportionate metabolism**. It also **reduces the systemic toxicity** of local anesthetics by delaying its entry into systemic circulation. Since it causes **vasodilatation** mediated through β_2 **receptors**, gangrene does not occur at the site of injection. **Phenylephrine** is a selective α_1 **agonist**, causes **intense vasoconstriction** for **a prolonged period** and decreases the absorption of local anesthetics. However, it can **interfere** with **local blood supply** and so not preferred to epinephrine.

5. *Epinephrine/Phenylephrine along with local anesthetics for topical anesthesia.*

BACKGROUND

Sympathomimetics are added with local anesthetics for their synergistic action. By causing vasoconstriction, they reduce the rate of absorption of coadministered local anesthetics prolonging their duration of action. Lower rate of absorption reduces the systemic toxicity of local anesthetics.

PHENYLEPHRINE

Phenylephrine is preferred to epinephrine for topical anesthesia. Phenylephrine at a low concentration of 0.005% achieves good vasoconstriction and it is absorbed when sprayed on mucosal membranes. This local mucosal vasoconstriction helps in procedures such as endoscopies. Hence, it is more suitable for topical applications in ENT procedures when combined with local anesthetics.

EPINEPHRINE

Epinephrine is used frequently with local anesthetics for infiltration, spinal, epidural and nerve block anesthesia, but it should never be infiltrated into tissues with 'end on' arteries because the resultant vasoconstriction may potentiate the occurrence of gangrene. If applied topically, the capacity of epinephrine to penetrate the surface is poor because epinephrine is not absorbed from the mucosa directly. Hence, epinephrine is not preferred for local application in topical sprays. It is not suitable for ENT procedures such as endoscopies as it does not prolong the action of coadministered anesthetic when applied topically.

Drug of Choice: Phenylephrine

RATIONALE

Epinephrine is generally preferred for coadministration with local anesthetics. Although it is never infiltrated into tissues with 'end on' arteries to prevent the risk of gangrene, it is routinely used for infiltration, nerve block and spinal anesthesia. But it has a very poor penetrating capacity when applied topically and so is not useful for coadministration with local anesthetics. Even a low dose of phenylephrine causes potent vasoconstriction when applied topically. Hence, phenylephrine is preferred.

6. *Phenylephrine/Cocaine for localizing the postganglionic lesion in Horner's syndrome.*

BACKGROUND

Horner's syndrome occurs due to unilateral interruption of facial sympathetic nerves. It causes ptosis, miosis, loss of sweating and vasodilatation on the affected side. Degeneration distal to the site of nerve lesion is the primary pathophysiology. It causes demyelination of nerves without affecting the neurons. Hence, a preganglionic lesion does not affect postganglionic nerve fiber. It does not interfere with the storage of catecholamines in postganglionic nerve. Cocaine and phenylephrine elicits normal response in preganglionic lesion. However in a postganglionic lesion, their responses are different.

PHENYLEPHRINE

Phenylephrine stimulates the alpha receptors of the smooth muscle of iris. Contraction of the smooth muscles of iris causes mydriasis. Mydriasis occurs in both pre and postganglionic type of lesion. Phenylephrine is effective irrespective of the site of lesion. So, it is preferred for localizing the type of lesion in Horner's syndrome.

COCAINE

Cocaine is an indirectly acting sympathomimetic drug and acts by preventing the reuptake of catecholamines. Hence, in postganglionic lesions, it does not elicit the normal response. It does not dilate the constricted pupil in postganglionic lesion.

Drug of Choice: Phenylephrine

RATIONALE

The symptoms of Horner's syndrome are ptosis, miosis, absence of sweating and vasodilatation on the affected side. **Cocaine** is an

indirectly acting sympathomimetic drug, **does not dilate** the constricted pupil in postganglionic type of lesion as there is already depletion of catecholamines due to denervation of nerve terminals. On the contrary, **phenylephrine** acts directly on **alpha receptors** of smooth muscle of iris and causes **mydriasis** even, if the lesion is postganglionic. Hence, it is preferred to localize the lesion in Horner's syndrome.

7. *Phenylephrine/Cyclopentolate as eye drops for fundoscopy examination in elderly individuals.*

BACKGROUND

Cycloplegia is required for accurate measurement of refractive errors, but it causes paralysis of accommodation and interferes with accommodation reflex. The need for cycloplegia does not arise in fundoscopy examination. Therefore, a drug causing prolonged mydriasis is sufficient.

PHENYLEPHRINE

Phenylephrine decreases aqueous humor production and therefore reduces the intraocular pressure. It is a sympathomimetic drug causing prolonged mydriasis through contraction of radial smooth muscles of iris and phenylephrine does not produce cycloplegia. It can be safely used in elders as it does not precipitate glaucoma.

CYCLOPENTOLATE

Cyclopentolate is an atropine substitute available as eye drops for ophthalmic use. It causes mydriasis through stimulation of parasympathetic nerves. In addition, it also causes paralysis of ciliary muscles resulting in cycloplegia. The duration of action of cyclopentolate is around 24 hours. It is available as 0.5 to 2% solution. In persons with narrow iridocorneal angle, anticholinergic drugs are not preferred because they increase the intraocular pressure. In elders, cyclopentolate increases the risk of inducing or aggravating glaucoma. Hence, cyclopentolate is contraindicated as mydriatic in elders.

Drug of Choice: Phenylephrine

RATIONALE

Atropine substitute **cyclopentolate** causes mydriasis and **cycloplegia**. For fundoscopy, prolonged mydriasis alone is essential and cycloplegia is not required. Cyclopentolate **induces and aggravates** the **risk of glaucoma** in elders. Hence, cyclopentolate is **contraindicated** in older age group. **Phenylephrine** causes **prolonged mydriasis**, reduces intraocular pressure and preferred as eye drops for fundoscopy examination in elders.

Alpha Blockers

1. *Nonselective alpha blockers/Selective alpha blockers as anti-hypertensive agents.*

BACKGROUND

Physiological functions of endogenous catecholamines are mediated through α_1 and α_2 receptors. α_2 receptors are autoreceptors and are present in preganglionic neurons. On stimulation, they inhibit the release of neurotransmitter norepinephrine. They also facilitate lipolysis, platelet aggregation and inhibit insulin secretion. α_1 receptors mediate contraction of smooth muscles of arteries as well as veins and modulate blood pressure. Stimulation of α_1 receptor also leads to contraction of the visceral smooth muscles. Hence, α-receptor blockers reduce blood pressure by inhibiting α receptors-mediated vasoconstriction.

SELECTIVE ALPHA BLOCKERS

Selective α_1 receptor blockers inhibit α_1 receptors specifically but not α_2 receptors and reduce blood pressure through peripheral vasodilatation. They also suppress centrally mediated sympathetic outflow and reduce the venous return, preload and cardiac output. These drugs do not cause compensatory reflex tachycardia.

NONSELECTIVE ALPHA BLOCKERS

Nonselective alpha blockers block both α_1 and α_2 receptors. They are 'classic' alpha blockers and cause intense peripheral vasodilatation. On account of this, they decrease preload but generally increase the cardiac output due to blockade of presynaptic α_2 receptors and enhance norepinephrine release. They cause severe postural hypotension as well as reflex tachycardia. This limits their therapeutic benefit in hypertension.

Drug of Choice: Selective Alpha Blockers

RATIONALE

Nonselective alpha blockers cause peripheral vasodilatation, decrease preload but increase cardiac output due to blockade of α_2 receptors. They cause severe **postural hypotension** and **reflex tachycardia** hence not preferred. **Selective α_1 receptor blockers** inhibit preload, decrease cardiac output and **do not result in reflex tachycardia**. So, their use is safe in hypertension. They have **higher efficacy** than classic alpha blockers but should be **started** at **minimal dose initially** and then gradually increased.

2. *Phentolamine/Phenoxybenzamine in preoperative preparation of pheochromocytoma.*

BACKGROUND

Pheochromocytoma is a catecholamine secreting tumor of adrenal medulla that releases enormous amount of catecholamines into circulation causing severe hypertension. Phentolamine and phenoxybenzamine are both classic nonselective α blockers. They act by blocking both α_1 and α_2 receptors.

PHENOXYBENZAMINE

Phenoxybenzamine is a noncompetitive, irreversible antagonist. It is preferred for preoperative preparation of patients with pheochromocytoma because it has a prolonged duration of action leading to sustained fall in blood pressure augmenting its therapeutic benefit. It is started at a dose of 10 mg twice daily. The dose is gradually increased till the required therapeutic benefit is achieved. It is given for a period of 1 to 3 weeks prior to surgery but can lead to severe postural hypotension, reflex tachycardia and nasal stuffiness.

PHENTOLAMINE

Phentolamine is a competitive antagonist and does not offer long-term benefit. Its action is short lived and it causes postural hypotension. It enhances gastric acid secretion and should be avoided in patients with peptic ulcer.

Drug of Choice: Phenoxybenzamine

RATIONALE

Catecholamines released from pheochromocytoma result in severe hypertension which needs to be controlled by an **effective, long acting alpha blocker**. **Phenoxybenzamine** is an **irreversible** long acting **nonselective** alpha blocker and controls **episodic hypertension** more effectively than the competitive antagonist phentolamine. So, phenoxybenzamine is preferred for preoperative preparation of patients in pheochromocytoma but it can cause postural hypotension, cardiac arrhythmias and nasal stuffiness.

3. *Phentolamine/Phenoxybenzamine for reversing soft tissue anesthesia.*

BACKGROUND

Local anesthetics are generally combined with epinephrine, a sympathomimetic agent and such a combination prolongs the duration of action of local anesthetics. Sympathomimetics delay the absorption of local anesthetics as they cause vasoconstriction at the site of injection. Nonselective α blockers are used to reverse the action of sympathomimetics. Such reversal is required when the action of local anesthetics needs to be terminated. They are effective as they antagonize the alpha receptor mediated vasoconstriction.

PHENTOLAMINE

The nonselective α blocker phentolamine is preferred for reversal as it is a competitive antagonist. Phentolamine has a shorter duration of action hence the chances of its systemic action are less.

Inadvertent extravasation of sympathomimetics can cause tissue sloughing. Phentolamine prevents such sympathomimetic mediated dermal necrosis.

PHENOXYBENZAMINE

Phenoxybenzamine is an irreversible long acting α blocker. It enhances the chances of local edema due to prolonged vasodilatation. Sustained vasodilatation increases the chances of its absorption potentiating the systemic side effects. Therefore, it is not preferred as a drug for reversal of sympathomimetics.

Drug of Choice: Phentolamine

RATIONALE

Prolonged action of sympathomimetics combined with local anesthetics can be reversed by **classical** alpha blockers. Since alpha blockers antagonize the alpha receptors mediated vasoconstriction, they are used in reversal. **Phentolamine** is a **competitive** antagonist with a relatively **shorter duration** of action compared to phenoxybenzamine. Phentolamine causes **more selective local** than **systemic** action and so preferred. It may also be useful in preventing the dermal necrosis in case of extravasation of sympathomimetics. **Phenoxybenzamine** is an **irreversible** agent, with **prolonged** action, causing longer local and systemic action. Hence, phenoxybenzamine is not preferred.

4. *Prazosin/Terazosin as an antihypertensive drug.*

BACKGROUND

Prazosin and terazosin are selective α_1 receptor blockers. They cause vasodilatation of arteries as well as veins. They reduce peripheral resistance, venous return and preload. Being selective alpha blockers, they decrease cardiac output but do not cause reflex tachycardia. They also suppress the centrally mediated sympathetic outflow. They reduce total cholesterol, triglycerides, LDL-C, VLDL-C and increase HDL-C. Dizziness, headache, asthenia and nasal congestion are few of the side effects caused by these drugs. They should be started at a low dose of 1 mg and the dose increased gradually. The maximum dose is around 20 mg per day.

TERAZOSIN

Terazosin has higher oral bioavailability and food does not interfere with its absorption. It has a bioavailability of around 90%. Since it has a longer duration of action for about 18 hours, it controls the blood pressure effectively, even when administered once daily.

PRAZOSIN

Prazosin has 1000 fold higher affinity for α_1 than α_2 receptors and blocks all three subtypes of α receptors such as α_{1A}, α_{1B} and α_{1D} equally. It also acts by inhibiting the cyclic nucleotide phosphodiesterase enzyme. Bioavailability of prazosin is around 50% and it reaches peak plasma concentration within 1 to 3 hours. The duration of action is 7 to 10 hours, so it has to be administered more than once daily. It should be started initially at bed time to prevent the incidence of syncopal attacks or 'first dose effect.'

Drug of Choice: Terazosin

RATIONALE

Prazosin and terazosin are α_1 adrenoceptor antagonists and they have **similar pharmacodynamic profile**. They result in significant reduction of blood pressure with minimal influence on heart rate. **Terazosin** differs from prazosin in having **longer duration** of action and can be conveniently given in **once daily dosage**. Its **bioavailability** is **90%** as its absorption is more predictable. The magnitude of other side effects is also low. Hence, terazosin is preferred to prazosin as an antihypertensive agent.

5. *Terazosin/Doxazosin in the treatment of benign prostatic hypertrophy (BPH).*

BACKGROUND

Terazosin and doxazosin are prazosin analogs and antagonize all three subtypes of α_1 adrenergic receptors. They are quinazoline derivatives used in the treatment of hypertension and benign prostatic hypertrophy. Terazosin and doxazosin are more effective than finasteride in BPH. Therapy is started at a low dose initially and increased gradually up to maximum therapeutic dose in long-term management of BPH. They have longer duration of action and are given once daily. They inhibit cellular proliferation and induce apoptosis in prostatic smooth muscle cells. The capacity to induce selective apoptosis is related to their quinazoline moiety.

DOXAZOSIN

Postural hypotension and syncope occurring after administration of the first dose of an antihypertensive drug is called 'first dose effect'. Doxazosin has longer half-life and causes minimal postural hypotension or syncope after first dose. It is also well tolerated. Hence, it is preferred in BPH.

TERAZOSIN

Terazosin causes postural hypotension and syncope more commonly after the first dose. Hence, though it is cost effective, it is less preferred than doxazosin in the treatment of BPH.

Drug of Choice: Doxazosin

RATIONALE

Terazosin and doxazosin are both **quinazoline** derivatives. They inhibit cellular proliferation and **induce apoptosis** in prostate. They have **similar pharmacodynamic profile** and have long duration of action and administered once daily but **terazosin causes higher incidence of first dose effect**. Although terazosin is cost effective, it is not preferred. Doxazosin is well tolerated by elders hence preferred to terazosin in BPH, a condition occurring commonly in elders.

6. *Tamsulosin/Silodosin in the treatment of BPH.*

BACKGROUND

Benign prostatic hypertrophy (BPH) is the frequent cause of urethral obstruction in elderly men. The symptoms of BPH are due to mechanical pressure and increased smooth muscle tone. While increased muscle tone is due to stimulation of α_1 receptors, mechanical pressure is caused by increased muscle mass due to cellular proliferation. Tamsulosin and silodosin are both selective blockers of α_{1A} receptor subtype in prostate and preferred for the treatment of BPH but not indicated for the treatment of hypertension.

TAMSULOSIN

Abnormal ejaculation occurs only in patients taking higher dose of tamsulosin. It can be started at a very low dose of 0.4 mg daily. The dose can be increased up to 0.8 mg. Tamsulosin is very effective even at a low dose and such low doses do not cause orthostatic hypotension.

SILODOSIN

Even at therapeutic dose, silodosin causes retrograde ejaculation and results in higher incidence of dizziness and orthostatic hypotension.

Drug of Choice: Tamsulosin

RATIONALE

The symptoms of BPH are due to mechanical pressure and increased muscle tone. Increased muscle tone is mediated through α_1 receptors. Tamsulosin and silodosin are both **selective α_{1A} blockers** and they **block** the α_{1A} **receptors** present in **prostate**. They are indicated for the treatment of BPH but not preferred for hypertension. At **therapeutic dose, tamsulosin does not cause orthostatic hypotension** but silodosin is effective only at higher doses which can cause retrograde ejaculation, orthostatic hypotension and dizziness. Hence, silodosin is not preferred.[3]

Beta Blockers

1. *Propranolol/Atenolol for treatment of hypertension in patients with bronchial asthma.*

BACKGROUND

Beta blockers are commonly used in the treatment of hypertension. In patients with bronchial asthma, the drug used should not increase bronchial resistance as it is already compromised and not interfere with bronchial function. Atenolol and propranolol reduce blood pressure and are effective in the treatment of hypertension. In addition to blocking cardiac actions they also inhibit renin secretion mediated through β_1 receptors.

ATENOLOL

Atenolol is classified under second generation selective beta blockers and is a selective β blocker. It has higher selectivity towards β_1 than β_2 receptors and antagonizes only β_1 receptors. Atenolol has neither intrinsic sympathomimetic nor membrane stabilizing property. Since atenolol does not block β_2 receptors, it is less likely to cause bronchoconstriction. Hence, it is relatively safe in patients with bronchial asthma but still should be used cautiously.

PROPRANOLOL

Propranolol is a competitive, nonselective first generation beta receptor antagonist. It has equal affinity to β_1 and β_2 receptors and blocks both receptors. Propranolol has membrane stabilizing property but does not have intrinsic sympathomimetic activity. It reduces blood pressure through centrally mediated action.

Long-term therapy reduces total peripheral resistance. Propranolol also blocks β_2 receptors causing life-threatening bronchoconstriction in patients with bronchial asthma hence, it is contraindicated in this condition.

Drug of Choice: Atenolol

RATIONALE

Propranolol, nonselective beta blocker and atenolol, cardioselective β_1 blocker are used in the treatment of hypertension. They inhibit the heart rate, cardiac contraction and renin release by blocking β_1 receptors. Propranolol has other additional actions as antihypertensive agent. Propranolol blocks the β_2 mediated bronchodilatation and causes life-threatening bronchoconstriction. Atenolol does not produce bronchoconstriction as it does not block β_2 receptors. In view of the above atenolol is preferred.

2. *Timolol/Betaxolol in the treatment of chronic open angle glaucoma.*

BACKGROUND

Beta blockers are not the first line drugs in treatment of glaucoma. Betaxolol and levobetaxolol are selective β_1 receptor blockers effective in chronic, open angle glaucoma. Timolol, levobunolol, carteolol and metipranolol are nonselective beta blockers effective in glaucoma. Timolol and betaxolol are devoid of intrinsic sympathomimetic and membrane stabilizing properties. They inhibit cyclic AMP mediated production of aqueous humor and decrease the intraocular pressure (IOP). They are lipophilic, well tolerated and do not produce miosis, blurred vision or night blindness. Action starts within 30 minutes of instillation of eye drops and lasts for 12 to 24 hours. They do not cause frequent fluctuations in IOP since they are long acting but cause redness, stinging, dryness and sometimes allergic conjunctivitis. They are not membrane stabilizers and do not cause corneal anesthesia and browache. Increased IOP poses a higher risk of damage to retinal neurons. Timolol and betaxolol reduce the neuronal influx of calcium and sodium offering greater protection to retinal neurons.

BETAXOLOL

Betaxolol has superior neuroprotective action as it has much higher efficiency in controlling calcium and sodium entry. Its isomer levobetaxolol is safer than timolol if absorbed into systemic circulation as it does not result in severe bronchoconstriction. It has lower efficacy but better safety profile hence, preferred.

TIMOLOL

Since ocular beta receptors are predominantly of β_2 subtype, the nonselective beta blocker timolol reduces IOP better than betaxolol but if absorbed into systemic circulation, it can cause bronchoconstriction by blocking β_2 receptors. Its neuroprotective activity is inferior to betaxolol.

Drug of Choice: Betaxolol

RATIONALE

Beta blockers are not the first line drugs in the treatment of glaucoma. Betaxolol is a β_1 selective blocker while timolol is a nonselective beta blocker. Both drugs are effective in the treatment of chronic open angle glaucoma. The capacity of timolol to reduce IOP is far superior to betaxolol as the ocular receptors are mainly of β_2 subtype. Although drugs are instilled as eye drops they can get absorbed into systemic circulation through nasolacrimal duct. Betaxolol is relatively safer than timolol even if absorbed, as it rarely results in bronchoconstriction. They are both neuropretectives and prevent retinal neuronal damage. Betaxolol has more efficient neuroprotective activity than timolol. Hence, betaxolol is preferred to timolol.

3. *Propranolol/Atenolol for short-term administration in symptomatic treatment of thyrotoxicosis.*

BACKGROUND

Excessive synthesis and release of thyroid hormone occurs in patients with thyrotoxicosis. Hyperthyroidism causes tachycardia and increased stroke volume. The cardiac index increases due to increased myocardial contractility. Patients also suffer from anxiety, tremors and nervousness due to increased sensitivity to endogenous catecholamines. Increased plasma tri-iodothyronine level stimulates myocardial contractility. T_3 induced fall in peripheral resistance increases risk of high output cardiac failure. Beta blockers are effective in thyrotoxicosis as they reduce tachycardia, tremor, palpitations, anxiety, restlessness and tension.

PROPRANOLOL

The dose of propranolol is 20 to 40 mg four times daily. Propranolol controls cardiac symptoms mediated through T_3 and has additional peripheral actions that are beneficial in thyrotoxicosis. It suppresses iodothyronine-deiodinase type-I enzyme responsible for the conversion of T_4 to T_3 inhibiting peripheral conversion of thyroxine to triiodothyronine and shunting thyroxine to iodothyronine-deiodinase type-III enzyme pathway resulting in the synthesis of 'reverse' T_3 which is metabolically inactive. Therefore, propranolol reduces excessive level of biologically potent T_3 in thyrotoxicosis. Short-term administration of propranolol also reverses the fall in peripheral resistance preventing the patients from vasodilatation induced high-risk cardiac failure. In view of the above advantages propranolol is preferred but should be used judiciously in cardiac patients.

ATENOLOL

The daily dose of atenolol is 50 to 100 mg. It inhibits the T_3-induced cardiac symptoms but lacks other beneficial actions of propranolol.

Drug of Choice: Propranolol

RATIONALE

The cardiac and other symptoms of hyperthyroidism are due to **biologically potent T_3.** The cardiac symptoms are mainly due to **increased sensitivity** to endogenous catecholamines. Atenolol and propranolol are effective in controlling symptoms mediated through sympathetic stimulation such as tachycardia, tremor, anxiety and tension but propranolol **inhibits peripheral conversion of T_4 to**

T_3 by inhibiting iodothyronine-deiodinase type-I and shunting T_4 through type-III enzyme mediated synthesis of biologically inactive **'reverse'T_3**. Propranolol also reverses the fall in peripheral resistance preventing the patient from high risk cardiac failure. Hence, short-term propranolol is preferred to atenolol in symptomatic management of hyperthyroidism.

4. *Propranolol/Celiprolol as antihypertensive agent in patients with diabetes mellitus.*

BACKGROUND

Propranolol is a first generation beta blocker. Celiprolol is a third generation beta blocker.

CELIPROLOL

Celiprolol has β_2 agonist action and nitric oxide mediated vasodilating properties. It is devoid of membrane stabilizing property and causes weak peripheral β_2 blockade. It causes vasodilatation, increases peripheral blood flow, decreases after load and is effective in hypertension. Celiprolol decreases triglycerides and improves serum lipid profile resulting in cardioprotection in patients with diabetes and dyslipidemia. In contrast to propranolol, it inhibits insulin resistance, improves insulin sensitivity and can safely be given in diabetic patients. Since celiprolol is cardioprotective and promotes insulin action, it is preferred.

PROPRANOLOL

Propranolol blocks both β_2 and β_2 receptors lowering blood pressure by reducing heart rate and cardiac contractility. It is most effective in reducing exercise induced cardiac stimulation. By blocking β_1 receptors, it decreases the renin release. On long-term use it reduces peripheral vascular resistance and should not be given in patients with type I diabetes mellitus because it blunts the hypoglycemia induced feedback mechanism by inhibiting the action of counter-regulatory hormones. Hence, it delays the physiological recovery from hypoglycemia. In patients with type-2 diabetes mellitus it impairs insulin action and decreases insulin sensitivity. It inhibits beta receptor mediated activation of hormone sensitive lipoprotein lipase suppressing the influx of free fatty acids into peripheral circulation thereby increasing the level of LDL-C, triglycerides and decreasing HDL-C level.

Drug of Choice: Celiprolol

RATIONALE

Propranolol is an effective antihypertensive agent but seldom used in patients with diabetes mellitus. Propranolol causes lipid abnormalities, increases LDL-C as well as triglycerides and decreases HDL-C. Propranolol potentiates insulin resistance by decreasing insulin sensitivity. It delays the physiological recovery from insulin induced hypoglycemia. **Celiprolol**-induced **nitric oxide production** causes vasodilatation and has β_2 **agonistic** actions. It exerts **cardio-protective** action by improving lipid profile as it reduces the serum triglycerides. It also **inhibits insulin resistance** and **improves insulin sensitivity**. Hence, celiprolol can be safely used in patients with diabetes mellitus.

5. *Propranolol/Pindolol for prophylaxis of migraine.*

BACKGROUND

Prophylaxis is indicated in patients with frequent migraine episodes. It is required if patient gets more than 1 to 2 attacks per week. Recurrent migraine may be disabling and prophylaxis improves the quality of life. Beta blockers are the first line drugs in the prophylaxis of migraine.

PROPRANOLOL

Propranolol at the dose of 80 mg twice a day is effective but needs to be given for a period of at least one year. Being a beta blocker, it should not be stopped abruptly but tapered gradually. The oral bioavailability of propranolol is around 30% but it is highly lipophilic. It probably acts by inhibiting β_2 receptor mediated vasodilatation.

Lethargy, fatigue, insomnia, nightmares and sexual disturbances in men are frequent side effects.

PINDOLOL

Metoprolol and timolol are other beta blockers approved for prophylaxis of migraine. Propranolol and timolol have equal efficacy in migraine prophylaxis. Pindolol is also a nonselective beta antagonist like propranolol, has 100% bioavailability. It is devoid of inter-individual variations but has low lipid solubility and questionable efficacy as a prophylactic. Pindolol has intrinsic sympathomimetic action, so it is not useful in migraine prophylaxis.

Drug of Choice: Propranolol

RATIONALE

Prophylaxis in migraine improves the quality of life and indicated if the patient does not tolerate triptans or show poor response to acute treatment. **Beta blockers** are the **first line** drugs in prophylaxis. They probably **inhibit** β_2 receptor **mediated vasodilatation**. Propranolol and pindolol are both **nonselective** beta receptor antagonists. **Propranolol** is **devoid** of **intrinsic sympathomimetic** action while pindolol has **intrinsic sympathomimetic** activity. **Propranolol** is highly **lipophilic**. Hence, propranolol is very useful in prophylaxis of migraine.

6. *Propranolol/Isosorbide mononitrate in primary prevention of variceal bleeding in portal hypertension.*

BACKGROUND

Around 20% of upper gastrointestinal bleeding is due to portal hypertension. Almost one third of patients with cirrhosis experience acute variceal bleeding within a span of 2 years. In recurrent bleeding, the mortality rate may go up to 80% in 4 years. Esophageal varices due to portal hypertension are the most important cause of upper GIT bleeding. Bleeding occurs whenever the pressure gradient between IVC and portal vein exceeds 12 mm of Hg. The primary site of bleeding is the dilated submucosal esophageal veins.

PROPRANOLOL

Nonselective beta blockers propranolol and nadolol prevent the first occurrence of bleeding as well as recurrent bleeding. The side effects of propranolol such as fatigue and sleep disturbances can be reduced through administration of a long acting propranolol. Long acting preparation helps to reduce the non-compliance due to multiple dosing schedules of short acting preparations. It has a prolonged elimination half-life due to slower GIT absorption and maintains sustained effect. The dose of long-acting propranolol is 60 mg once daily at bed time and significantly reduces the side effects.

ISOSORBIDE MONONITRATE

Isosorbide mononitrate has excellent oral bioavailability. When compared to other nitrate preparations, it has the maximum bio-availability. It does not undergo high first pass metabolism and has longer half-life. Consequently it reduces portal hypertension by dilating arterioles and venules. It is the second line drug in preventing esophageal varices because it has lower efficacy.

Drug of Choice: Propranolol

RATIONALE

Bleeding due to esophageal varices occurs when the **pressure gradient** between portal vein and inferior vena cava **exceeds 12 mm of Hg**. Nonselective beta blocker **propranolol** is very **effective** in preventing the **first time bleeding or recurrent bleeding** in patients with portal hypertension. The **long acting** propranolol given at **bed time**, once daily, reduces side effects significantly. **Isosorbide mononitrate** is a long-acting nitrate with good oral bioavailability but it can be used only as the **second line drug** due to its lower efficacy.

7. *Propranolol/Metoprolol as prophylactic in exertional or exercise-induced angina.*

BACKGROUND

Exercise-induced cardiac stimulation occurs due to catecholamines released during exercise. They increase heart rate, contractility, systolic pressure and myocardial oxygen demand. Beta blockers inhibit the exercise-induced increase in heart rate and myocardial contractility but do not affect cardiac output as it is due to increased stroke volume. Beta blockers increase the myocardial oxygen demand by increasing the end diastolic pressure and systolic ejection period but reduce the oxygen demand by inhibiting cardiac contractility. Therefore, they efficiently balance between cardiac demand and supply improving the exercise tolerance in patients with angina.

METOPROLOL

Metoprolol is a cardioselective beta blocker but does not block the vasodilatory β_2 receptors. Therefore, it does not compromise exercise-induced coronary artery dilatation and blood supply to skeletal muscles.

PROPRANOLOL

The nonselective beta blocker propranolol also blocks the β_2 receptors and decreases the exercise induced vasodilatation in skeletal muscles. Further, it also interferes with coronary vasodilatation induced by exercise.

Drug of Choice: Metoprolol

RATIONALE

Beta blockers are preferred as prophylactic in exertional angina as they reduce heart rate and myocardial contractility without affecting cardiac output. Since they balance between cardiac oxygen demand and supply, they are very effective in preventing exercise-induced angina. As a nonselective beta blocker, propranolol may interfere with exercise-induced dilatation of coronary vessels and blood vessels supplying skeletal muscle. Metoprolol is β_1 selective blocker, devoid of β_2 blocking action and does not interfere with skeletal muscle and coronary vasodilatation. Hence, metoprolol is preferred as a prophylactic in exertional angina.

8. *Propranolol/Sotalol as anti-arrhythmic agent.*

BACKGROUND

Excessive stimulation of beta receptors increases the incidence of *early* and *late after depolarization* mediated arrhythmias. Increased magnitude and decreased inactivation of Ca^{2+} current, as well as increased magnitude of K^+ and Cl^- current mediated repolarization increase the amount of calcium released from sarcoplasmic reticulum. Beta blockers block β_2 mediated catecholamine induced hypokalemia and increase the energy requirement to fibrillate the acutely ischemic tissue. Thus, they confer a protective anti-arrhythmic action and reduce the mortality. Propranolol and sotalol are both nonselective beta blockers and are used in the treatment of ventricular arrhythmias.

PROPRANOLOL

At higher doses, propranolol has additional membrane stabilizing property but this action contributes little to its anti-arrhythmic effect. It inhibits cardiac rhythm, automaticity and is devoid of intrinsic sympathomimetic property. Propranolol does not cause torsades de pointes or prolonged QT syndrome and *early* or *late after depolarizations.*

SOTALOL

Sotalol prolongs the action potential duration (APD) and inhibits the delayed rectifier and possibly other potassium currents. Sotalol tends to cause *early after depolarizations* (EAD) because it does not alter the conduction velocity in fast response tissues. It prolongs QT interval and causes *torsades de pointes.* Hence, it is not preferred.

Drug of Choice: Propranolol

RATIONALE

Stimulation of beta receptors causes EADs and LADs. **Propranolol** blocks beta receptor mediated cardiac action. Although it has an additional membrane stabilizing action at high doses, this property seldom helps in its anti-arrhythmic action. It **inhibits cardiac rhythm** and **automaticity**. It does not cause EADs, LADs and *torsades de pointes*. Sotalol is class III anti-arrhythmic agent, acts mainly by **inhibiting** the **delayed rectifier potassium currents**. **It does not reduce** the **conduction velocity** in **fast response tissues and causes EAD**. It also prolongs QT interval and **causes** *torsades de pointes*. Hence, propranolol is preferred to sotalol as an anti-arrhythmic agent.

CHAPTER

4

Cholinergic Drugs

1. *Carbachol/Bethanechol in postoperative paralytic ileus and atony of bladder.*

BACKGROUND

Cholinergics increase GIT muscular tone, amplitude, peristalsis and secretions. They cause contraction of detrusor, relaxation of trigone and external sphincter. The responses are mediated through M_3 receptors in GIT and M_2 receptors in bladder. Postoperative paralytic ileus and atony of bladder are due to compromised cholinergic activity. In paralytic ileus, intestinal motility is decreased. Reduced bladder capacity and increased voiding pressure are features of bladder atony. Stimulation of cholinergic receptors promotes motility of bowel and emptying of bladder.

BETHANECHOL

Bethanechol is beta-methyl analog of carbachol, is resistant to cholinesterases and has long duration of action. It also has predominant action on smooth muscles of GIT and urinary bladder. Bethanechol is devoid of unwanted nicotinic action on autonomic ganglia, hence preferred to carbachol. The dose of bethanechol is 10 to 50 mg three to four times a day and should be administered in empty stomach to minimize nausea and vomiting.

CARBACHOL

Carbachol is an unsubstituted carbamoyl ester, resistant to hydrolysis by cholinesterases hence has longer duration of action. It has a predominant action on smooth muscles of GIT and urinary bladder and has additional nicotinic action that cannot be antagonized completely by atropine.

Drug of Choice: Bethanechol

RATIONALE

The choline esters carbachol and bethanechol are **long acting** drugs as they are completely resistant to inactivation by cholinesterases. They have **equal propensity** for smooth muscles and effectively stimulate GIT and bladder smooth muscles. They are therefore effective in the treatment of postoperative paralytic ileus and atony of bladder. **Carbachol** can stimulate autonomic ganglia as it **has substantial nicotinic action** but bethanechol does not stimulate nicotinic receptors. Hence, bethanechol is preferred.

2. *Neostigmine/Pyridostigmine in myasthenia gravis.*

BACKGROUND

Myasthenia gravis is an autoimmune disease, characterized by muscular weakness and fatigue. The defect lies in synaptic junction of neuromuscular transmission. Cholinergic receptors in postjunctional motor end plate are involved. Development of antireceptor antibodies to nicotinic cholinergic receptors is the most common immunological cause seen in myasthenia gravis. It may be congenital in 10% of patients due to mutations in acetylcholine receptors. Although subjective improvement is more prominent in autoimmune type, drugs effectively alleviate the symptoms in congenital type. Anticholinesterases are effective and improve skeletal muscle weakness. Neostigmine and pyridostigmine are used for symptomatic treatment in myasthenia gravis. They prolong the presence of acetylcholine in neuromuscular junction.

PYRIDOSTIGMINE

The duration of action of pyridostigmine is 3 to 6 hours but it is available as sustained release preparation containing 180 mg as tablets. Of the 180 mg, 60 mg is released immediately and the remaining 120 mg is released slowly. Sustained release preparation improves the compliance of patients and also reduces muscle fatigue for a longer period.

NEOSTIGMINE

The duration of action of neostigmine is only 2 to 4 hours so it needs to be administered every 6 hours for effective relief. It improves symptoms due to muscle fatigability only when administered four times a day but frequent dosage results in plasma fluctuations. Since it has to be frequently administered it is not preferred.

Drug of Choice: Pyridostigmine

RATIONALE

Myasthenia gravis, the **autoimmune disorder** is characterized by muscle weakness and fatigue. Anticholinesterases lead to the accumulation of acetylcholine in neuromuscular junction. When compared to neostigmine, **pyridostigmine** has **longer** duration of **action**. Neostigmine has to be given four times a day which results in plasma level fluctuations. Pyridostigmine is available as **sustained release** preparation and **once daily dose will suffice**. It alleviates symptoms of myasthenia gravis and improves the compliance of patients. Hence, pyridostigmine is preferred.

3. *Edrophonium/Neostigmine for diagnosis of myasthenia gravis.*

BACKGROUND

History, signs and symptoms may help in the diagnosis of myasthenia gravis but it is necessary to differentiate it from severe muscular weakness of cholinergic crisis. The symptoms of cholinergic crisis are due to excessive cholinergic stimulation causing generalized depolarization of motor end plate.

EDROPHONIUM

Edrophonium is a short acting reversible anticholinesterase drug. A rapid IV infusion of 2 mg of edrophonium improves the symptoms.

If the symptoms do not improve, an additional dose of 8 mg should be administered after 45 seconds. Edrophonium aggravates symptoms due to cholinergic crises and results in predominant lingual fasciculation. Muscle strength worsens but it does not cause respiratory paralysis as it is short acting. Improvement in muscle strength indicates the diagnosis of myasthenia gravis.

NEOSTIGMINE

Although a reversible anticholinesterase agent, neostigmine is longer acting than edrophonium so should not be used for diagnosis of myasthenia gravis. In cholinergic crisis, neostigmine may exaggerate the symptoms and may result in respiratory paralysis since it has long duration of action.

Drug of Choice: Edrophonium

RATIONALE

Muscular weakness can occur either due to myasthenia gravis or cholinergic crisis. In case of myasthenia gravis, it is due to defective neuromuscular transmission while the symptoms of cholinergic crisis are due to excessive cholinergic stimulation. Since the pathophysiology is diagonally opposite, the treatment also differs. Myasthenia gravis requires administration of anticholinesterases while cholinergic crisis requires withholding of anticholinesterases. **Neostigmine** is longer acting than edrophonium and **worsens** the symptoms in **cholinergic crisis**, potentiating life-threatening **respiratory paralysis**. Hence, neostigmine should not be used. **Edrophonium** is **short acting**, will **improve** symptoms in myasthenia gravis and it **will not aggravate** the symptoms in cholinergic crisis. So edrophonium is the drug of choice for definitive diagnosis.

4. *Physostigmine/Neostigmine in the treatment of atropine poisoning with central symptoms.*

BACKGROUND

Atropine poisoning is characterized by both central and peripheral symptoms. Peripheral symptoms are dryness of secretions, redness, fever and blurring of vision. Central symptoms are excitement, ataxia, delirium, restlessness and irritability. Physostigmine and neostigmine are reversible anticholinesterase drugs and are competitive antagonists of atropine. Reversible anticholinesterases antagonize the binding of atropine at muscarinic receptors.

PHYSOSTIGMINE

Physostigmine is a tertiary amine which crosses the blood brain barrier. It counteracts the central symptoms but causes undesirable CNS side effects in their absence. Therefore, it is reserved only for counteracting the central symptoms of atropine overdose.

NEOSTIGMINE

Neostigmine is a quaternary ammonium compound. It does not cross the blood brain barrier due to its bigger molecular size. Hence, neostigmine is not effective in antagonizing the central symptoms but it can block the peripheral symptoms of atropine poisoning.

Drug of Choice: Physostigmine

RATIONALE

In severe atropine poisoning with central symptoms, **physostigmine** is the specific antidote. Physostigmine is a **tertiary amine**, **crosses blood brain barrier** and antagonizes the central effects of atropine. **Neostigmine** is a quaternary ammonium compound, **does not enter CNS** hence not useful in blocking central symptoms though effective in the treatment of peripheral symptoms. However, physostigmine should be reserved for use only in case of central excitatory symptoms since it can cause undesirable centrally mediated side effects in the absence of central symptoms of atropine poisoning.

5. *Physostigmine/Neostigmine in the treatment of glaucoma.*

BACKGROUND

Anticholinesterase drugs are not the first line drugs in the treatment of glaucoma. Glaucoma can cause irreversible blindness, if left untreated. Increased intraocular pressure can damage optic nerve. The three types of glaucoma are primary, secondary and congenital glaucoma. Anticholinesterases are used to manage primary glaucoma and in some secondary types such as glaucoma after cataract surgery or aphakic glaucoma. Chronic wide angle glaucoma has a gradual or insidious onset. It is managed by other drugs and anticholinesterases are reserve drugs. Reversible anticholinesterases are mainly indicated for those with chronic wide angle glaucoma, resistant to first line drugs.

PHYSOSTIGMINE

Physostigmine is effective in the treatment of glaucoma. It is a tertiary amine administered topically as eye drops. It is highly lipophilic, achieves high ocular concentration and is useful in glaucoma. It increases ciliary muscle tone and trabecular patency facilitating effective drainage of aqueous humor resulting in reduction of intraocular pressure. It causes miosis, minimal visual acuity and brow pain due to persistent spasm of iris and ciliary muscles.

NEOSTIGMINE

Neostigmine is a quaternary ammonium compound and does not penetrate through corneal membrane. Neostigmine is not used as it is not effective.

Drug of Choice: Physostigmine

RATIONALE

Anticholinesterases are miotics and used as **reserve drugs** in the management of chronic wide angle glaucoma. Physostigmine and neostigmine are **reversible** anticholinesterases. Physostigmine is **lipophilic**, a tertiary amine, achieves **higher ocular concentration**, increases tone of ciliary muscle, increases trabecular patency, facilitates effective drainage of aqueous humor and reduces intraocular pressure. It can cause brow ache, minimal visual acuity and miosis. **Neostigmine** is not effective as it **does not penetrate** corneal membrane due to its particle size. Hence, physostigmine is preferred to neostigmine in the treatment of glaucoma.

6. *Neostigmine/Physostigmine in postoperative decurarization.*

BACKGROUND

D-tubocurarine is a competitive neuromuscular blocker used during surgery. It results in persistent postoperative curarization as it is long acting. Reversible anticholinesterases antagonize the actions of d-tubocurarine.

NEOSTIGMINE

Neostigmine is a reversible anticholinesterase and effectively antagonizes the symptoms of curarization. It blocks the actions of the competitive blocker, d-tubocurarine by displacing it from its binding site at N_M receptors. Neostigmine has higher affinity to nicotinic receptors than physostigmine and prolongs the presence of acetylcholine at motor end plates. It has additional direct action at neuromuscular junction and reverses the blockade but may induce muscarinic side effects. Either atropine or glycopyrrolate can be co-administered with neostigmine to prevent such side effects. Neostigmine is also effective in cobra bite as it reverses the curarimimetic effects of the venom.

PHYSOSTIGMINE

Physostigmine is not used in d-tubocurarine overdose and is less effective in antagonizing the blockade because it does not act directly on nicotinic cholinergic receptors. Its affinity to nicotinic N_M receptors is inferior to neostigmine.

Drug of Choice: Neostigmine

RATIONALE

D-tubocurarine is a long acting skeletal muscle relaxant and its actions need to be reversed by a cholinergic agonist. Neostigmine is a reversible anticholinesterase that potentiates the action of acetylcholine at nicotinic cholinergic receptors. It also acts directly on the nicotinic receptors. It is co-administered with a muscarinic antagonist like atropine or glycopyrrolate for preventing muscarinic actions and side effects. Physostigmine cannot be used as it does not act directly on nicotinic receptors and neostigmine is a better choice.

5

Anticholinergic Drugs

1. *Atropine/Scopolamine for prevention of motion sickness.*

BACKGROUND

Motion sickness occurs as a consequence of vestibular system stimulation. Vestibular system is rich in histaminergic and cholinergic receptors. The receptors are mainly of H_1 and muscarinic type. Hence, muscarinic blockers and H_1 blockers are effective in motion sickness.

SCOPOLAMINE

Scopolamine crosses blood brain barrier more effectively than atropine. The CNS actions are prominent even at low therapeutic doses. Drowsiness, fatigue, amnesia, xerostomia euphoria and dreamless sleep are a few side effects. At therapeutic doses, it depresses the vestibular apparatus in inner ear thereby blocking the neural pathways to brainstem emetic center. It is the first line drug for the prevention of motion sickness. However, it is not effective if given after the onset of nausea and vomiting. Transdermal preparation of scopolamine delivers the drug for 72 hours. It is applied on postauricular mastoid region to improve its absorption. Mydriasis, cycloplegia and blurred vision can occur due to unintentional transfer of the drug from hand to eye following its application.

ATROPINE

Atropine does not have selective action but acts indiscriminately on all systems hence atropine induces many systemic side effects.

While therapeutic concentration of atropine causes only mild CNS stimulation, higher doses stimulate CNS resulting in restlessness, delirium and disorientation. CNS depression occurs only at toxic doses of atropine and such high doses can cause circulatory collapse.

Drug of Choice: Scopolamine

RATIONALE

Scopolamine, at therapeutic doses **crosses BBB** more than atropine. Atropine inhibits vestibular system only at very high doses so not used as a prophylactic agent in motion sickness. **Low dose scopolamine depresses vestibular apparatus** in the inner ear and so is the drug of choice in motion sickness. It is available as **transdermal application** to be applied on the postauricular mastoid region to accelerate its absorption. It is useful as a **prophylactic** only and **not after the onset of emesis**. Drowsiness, fatigue, amnesia, xerostomia and dreamless sleep occur due to antagonism of muscarinic receptors.

2. *Solifenacin/Darifenacin in overactive urinary bladder.*

BACKGROUND

Muscarinic antagonists relax detrusor muscles, contract trigone and external sphincter thereby increasing bladder capacity, promoting retention and reducing the intravesicular as well as voiding pressure. They reduce the frequency of micturition and therefore are effective in overactive urinary bladder. Darifenacin and solifenacin act selectively on M_3 receptors in bladder. Since M_1 receptors in CNS mediate cognition and memory, blockade of M_1 receptors interferes with these abilities. They have minimal effects on central M_1 receptors so devoid of central side effects. When compared to other vesicoselective agents these agents have better benefit toxicity ratio.

DARIFENACIN

Darifenacin acts for 13 hours so given as extended release preparations. Daily dose is 7.5 to 15 mg and it is metabolized by CYP3A4 as well as CYP2D6, the subtypes of CytP450 enzyme responsible for metabolism of more than 50% of drugs. Hence, darifenacin is prone for extensive drug interactions with coadministered drugs. Generally overactive bladder is more common in older age group who are already on polytherapy so darifenacin is not preferred as it may interact with many coadministered drugs.

SOLIFENACIN

Solifenacin has long duration of action and immediate release preparation of 5 to 10 mg of solifenacin is effective for 55 hours. Solifenacin is metabolized by CYP3A4 and prone for interactions with enzyme substrates. It requires dose reduction if coadminis-tered with drugs metabolized by CYP3A4. Since solifenacin causes fewer drug interactions, it is more suitable for the treatment of over-active bladder.

Drug of Choice: Solifenacin

RATIONALE

M_3 receptors present in bladder play a role in decreasing intravesicu-lar pressure and in reducing the frequency of micturition. Darifenacin and solifenacin selectively inhibit M_3 receptors and are effective in overactive bladder. They do not cause any systemic side effects. Since they do not interact with central M_1 receptors, they are devoid of central side effects such as impairment of cognition and memory and can be administered safely in older age group. Solifenacin has longer duration of action and prone for fewer drug interactions than darifenacin. Hence, solifenacin is preferred to darifenacin.

3. *Atropine/Glycopyrrolate as preanesthetic medication.*

BACKGROUND

Muscarinic antagonists reduce the bronchial and salivary secre-tions hence can be used in preanesthetic medication.

GLYCOPYRROLATE

M_3 subtype receptors mediate salivary and bronchial secretions. Glycopyrrolate is a selective blocker of M_3 receptors. It is a synthetic compound and structurally dissimilar to atropine and facilitates smooth endotracheal intubation during anesthesia. Being a quaternary ammonium compound it does not cross the blood brain barrier. It has minimal tendency to cause tachycardia.

ATROPINE

Atropine is a nonselective muscarinic antagonist. It does not abolish laryngospasm but prevents its development. It should be given at least 30 minutes before administration of general anesthetics. When administered with nonirritant anesthetics, it causes dryness of throat that manifests as sore throat in postoperative period due to its long duration of action. Atropine reduces bronchial secretion causing inspissation of mucus plugs. Either tachycardia or tachyarrhythmia occurs due its vagolytic action.

Drug of Choice: Glycopyrrolate

RATIONALE

Anticholinergics are given with nonirritant general anesthetics, to reduce salivary and bronchial secretions to facilitate smooth endotracheal intubation. **Atropine** is **nonspecific**, causes predictable side effects due to **blockade** of **muscarinic** receptors. Endotracheal intubation is difficult as atropine causes dryness of secretions and inspissations of mucus plugs. Atropine causes **sore throat** during postoperative period, tachycardia, tachyarrhythmia and CNS stimulation. **Glycopyrrolate selectively** blocks M_3 **receptors** responsible for salivary and bronchial secretions. Therefore, it helps in smooth endotracheal intubation. It neither causes CNS mediated side effects nor promotes cardiac stimulation. Hence, glycopyrrolate is preferred to atropine for preanesthetic medication.

4. *Dicyclomine/Glycopyrrolate as antispasmodic in irritable bowel syndrome (IBS).*

BACKGROUND

Anticholinergic drugs inhibit gastrointestinal smooth muscles. They reduce smooth muscle tone, amplitude and contraction of the smooth muscles. M_3 muscarinic receptors mediate cholinergic actions of GIT smooth muscles. Antispasmodic anticholinergics are indicated in IBS but have limited tolerability. Glycopyrrolate and dicyclomine act by inhibiting M_3 mediated cholinergic actions. They reduce salivary as well as bronchial secretions and cause urinary retention because these pharmacological effects are also mediated through M_3 receptors.

GLYCOPYRROLATE

Glycopyrrolate is a quaternary ammonium compound so almost devoid of centrally mediated anticholinergic side effects. It is available as immediate release tablets and administered as 1 to 2 mg, two to three times a day. It is more potent and has better safety profile.

DICYCLOMINE

Dicyclomine is a tertiary amine and inhibits M_3 receptors. Dicyclomine is a weak muscarinic antagonist compared to glycopyrrolate and also has a direct antispasmodic action. The action is nonspecific, not mediated through any mechanism, but this nonspecific action is responsible for its therapeutic benefit. Being a tertiary amine dicyclomine can cross blood-brain barrier resulting in central nervous system side effects. Dose of dicyclomine is 20 to 40 mg four times a day but only the maximum dose of 160 mg is clinically effective thus increasing the incidence of side effects. Hence, dicyclomine is not preferred.

Drug of Choice: Glycopyrrolate

RATIONALE

Anticholinergic drugs are used as antispasmodics in IBS to reduce pain as well as fecal urgency and administered only if required as they have limited tolerability. **Dicyclomine** is a **nonspecific** agent with direct actions on GIT smooth muscles and minimal antimuscarinic activity, usually effective only at **maximum dose** range thereby increasing its liability to cause central side effects like drowsiness, nervousness or light-headedness. **Glycopyrrolate**, a **selective M₃ antagonist**, is **more potent**, blocks cholinergic mediated GIT stimulation, effective in small doses, does not lead to centrally mediated side effects. Hence, glycopyrrolate is the drug of choice.

5. *Atropine/Scopolamine in organophosphorus compound (OPC) poisoning.*

BACKGROUND

The symptoms of OPC poisoning are due to excessive stimulation of muscarinic and nicotinic receptors by irreversible anticholinesterases. Muscarinic symptoms are rhinorrhea, tightness of chest, urination, bradycardia, excessive salivation, involuntary defecation, hypotension and bronchoconstriction. Nicotinic symptoms manifest as involuntary twitching, fasciculation, weakness and paralysis of respiratory muscles. OPCs are highly lipophilic and cause CNS symptoms such as ataxia, confusion, convulsions, hypotension and respiratory paralysis.

ATROPINE

Atropine is the first line drug in the treatment of OPC poisoning. Cholinesterase reactivators are only supplementary to the action of atropine. At therapeutic doses atropine blocks mainly the peripheral effects but at a higher dose it can block the central effects of OPCs. Initial intravenous dose of atropine is 2 to 4 mg. It should be repeated every 5 to 10 minutes, if administered intramuscularly until the disappearance of muscarinic symptoms.

SCOPOLAMINE

Scopolamine has more central actions and limited peripheral actions so not preferred. If given to patients in pain scopolamine induces drowsiness, fatigue, restlessness, amnesia, dreamless sleep, hallucinations and aggravates delirium.

Drug of Choice: Atropine

RATIONALE

Peripheral and central symptoms are both prominent in OPC poisoning. **Scopolamine** crosses blood-brain barrier even at therapeutic doses but it is a **CNS depressant** and has **minimal peripheral blockade** so not suitable in OPC poisoning. **Atropine** causes **intense peripheral blockade**, enters CNS at higher doses, **blocks centrally mediated actions** and is the first line drug in preventing respiratory paralysis, bradycardia, hypotension and excessive secretions due to OPC poisoning. So, atropine is preferred to scopolamine in OPC poisoning.

6. *Pralidoxime/Obidoxime as enzyme reactivators in OPC poisoning.*

BACKGROUND

Oximes reactivate acetylcholinesterase inhibited by organophosphorus compounds. They are effective only as an adjunct to atropine in OPC poisoning and are not effective as monotherapy agents. The esteratic site of cholinesterase is phosphorylated in OPC poisoning. Hydrolytic regeneration of the phosphorylated site is usually slow but spontaneous. Oximes are enzyme reactivators and reactivate cholinesterase at a much more rapid rate than physiological regeneration. Enzyme reactivators are ineffective if acetylcholinesterase is carbamylated, so they are not useful in neostigmine or physostigmine overdose. Oximes are ineffective if phosphorylated acetyl cholinesterase enzyme undergoes 'aging' due to loss of an alkoxy group as this forms a more stable monoalkoxy-phosphoryl-acetylcholinesterase. They are effective in diethyl pesticide (parathion) but less effective in dimethyl pesticide (monocrotophos) poisoning and not effective if the poisoning is due to S-alkyl linked compounds.[4] The difference is due to the rate of 'aging' and diethyl pesticides undergo gradual aging.

OBIDOXIME

Obidoxime is more potent, much faster and more effective than pralidoxime.[5] It has superior clinical efficacy when combined with atropine and so preferred to pralidoxime.

PRALIDOXIME

Pralidoxime or pyridine-2-aldoxime methyl chloride reactivates cholinesterase. It is one of the widely used but least effective oxime although its rate of reactivation is million times faster.

Drug of Choice: Obidoxime

RATIONALE

Oximes are used as **adjuvants** to atropine in the treatment of OPC poisoning. They are **effective** only if given **before** the process of **'aging'** of phosphorylated acetyl cholinesterase enzyme. Oximes are not effective in carbamylated acetylcholinesterase overdose. The capacity to **reactivate** cholinesterase by oximes depends on the rate at which 'aging' occurs. They are ineffective against compounds that undergo rapid aging. **Pralidoxime** is widely used but it is **less effective**. **Obidoxime** is **more potent** and **very effective** hence preferred to pralidoxime.

7. *Valethamate bromide/Drotaverine hydrochloride for cervical dilatation during delivery.*

BACKGROUND

Cervical ripening and dilatation facilitate labor. Prostaglandins are commonly used for cervical ripening. Drotaverine and valethamate facilitate cervical dilatation, decreasing the time spent in first stage of labor, shortening the duration and augmenting the progress of labor. Valethamate and drotaverine do not affect the second and third stages of labor.

DROTAVERINE HYDROCHLORIDE

Drotaverine hydrochloride is a non-anticholinergic smooth muscle relaxant. It acts by selectively inhibiting the enzyme phosphodiesterase type IV (PDE-4), in smooth muscles increasing cyclic AMP and cyclic GMP. Drotaverine is used to enhance cervical dilatation during childbirth. Drotaverine induces mild headache and other minimal side effects.

VALETHAMATE BROMIDE

Valethamate bromide is a tertiary amine anticholinergic. It is a semisynthetic derivative of atropine and widely used for inducing cervical dilatation. It is very effective when given during first stage of labor but causes side effects such as dryness of mouth, facial flushing, tachycardia in fetus and mothers. Valethamate is one of the widely used drugs during labor but is an unlisted drug in Indian Pharmacopoeia.[6] It has no individual IP number indicating questionable safety profile, so should be less preferred as its safety is not well established.

Drug of Choice: Drotaverine Hydrochloride

RATIONALE

Drotaverine is a nonanticholinergic drug, acts by **inhibiting phosphodiesterase type IV** enzyme specific for smooth muscles. It is used to augment first stage of labor as it causes cervical dilatation. **Valethamate bromide** is an anticholinergic drug with **no IP number** indicating **questionable safety and efficacy**. It is widely and commonly used for facilitating cervical dilatation during first stage of labor. Although these drugs are found to be equally effective,[7] valethamate causes more side effects and its safety index is not established hence should be less preferred.

8. *Cyclopentolate/Tropicamide as mydriatic for testing refractory error.*

BACKGROUND

Atropine substitutes are preferred to atropine because they have a shorter duration of action. Antimuscarinic agents should not be used unless prolonged cycloplegia is required. Cycloplegia results in loss of accommodation due to paralysis of ciliary muscle and it is necessary for testing the refractory error. Shorter acting antimuscarinic agent is used as mydriatic for this purpose.

TROPICAMIDE

Tropicamide has a very quick onset of action but the action persists only for a short period of six hours. It is an effective mydriatic and is also a cycloplegic. It does not interfere with accommodation for long time as it produces cycloplegia only for 6 hours. Hence, it is used for testing refractory error as cycloplegia is required.

CYCLOPENTOLATE

Mydriasis and cycloplegia occur within an hour after instillation of cyclopentolate and pharmacological effects of cyclopentolate last for 24 hours. It produces clinically satisfactory cycloplegia as it is very potent but gets absorbed through nasolacrimal duct resulting in unwanted antimuscarinic side effects.

Drug of Choice: Tropicamide

RATIONALE

Atropine substitutes are used only when cycloplegia is required as for testing errors of refraction. Cyclopentolate causes both **mydriasis** and **cycloplegia**. Although it is a very **potent** drug, its effect lasts for about a day. **Tropicamide** is very **short acting** and its **cycloplegic** action does not extend beyond 6 hours and so **it is suitable** for testing refractive error as cycloplegia is required.

6

Skeletal Muscle Relaxants

1. *Rocuronium/Succinylcholine for endotracheal intubation in patients with cardiovascular disease.*

BACKGROUND

Endotracheal intubation in patients with CVS disease is a high-risk procedure. It potentiates the risk of hypoxia and cardiovascular collapse in such patients hence the intubation should be rapid known as rapid sequence intubation (RSI). Depolarizing blockers such as succinylcholine depolarizes the motor end plate but makes it refractory for further stimulation. Nondepolarizing blockers such as rocuronium block nicotinic cholinergic neurotransmission as they antagonize N_M receptors causing relaxation of skeletal muscles. Rocuronium and succinylcholine facilitates RSI as they are short acting and are given as single/multiple intravenous injections. Frequency of administration depends upon the required depth of blockade.

ROCURONIUM

Rocuronium is a competitive or non-depolarizing type of skeletal muscle relaxant. It directly competes with acetylcholine for binding at nicotinic receptors. Rocuronium has quick onset with intermediate duration of action. The action starts within 2 minutes and persists for approximately 70 minutes. It is relatively safe and does not cause histamine release. It does not induce tachycardia mediated by vagal blockade and does not result in hyperkalemia. Therefore, it is more cardiac friendly than succinylcholine.

SUCCINYLCHOLINE

Succinylcholine is ultra short acting depolarizing skeletal muscle relaxant. The onset is around 1 minute and the duration is for 11 minutes. It causes potassium release and can lead to life threatening hyperkalemia potentiating pre-existing cardiac abnormality. It can lead to ventricular arrhythmia and cardiac arrest. Hence, it is absolutely contraindicated in patients with cardiovascular disease.

Drug of Choice: Rocuronium

RATIONALE

Endotracheal intubation in patients with cardiac dysfunction is a high-risk procedure and should be done quickly to avoid hypoxia and cardiovascular collapse. **Succinylcholine** is an **ultra short acting** skeletal muscle relaxant. **Rocuronium** has **quick onset** but **intermediate** duration of action. Although succinylcholine can facilitate **rapid intubation**, it cannot be used as it results in **life-threatening hyperkalemia**, potentiating cardiac damage.[8] **Rocuronium** is relatively **safe**, more **cardiac friendly** and **does not cause histamine release** or vagal blockade. So, it is preferred in cardiac patients for tracheal intubation.

2. *Vecuronium/Succinylcholine for tracheal intubation.*

BACKGROUND

Neuromuscular blockers are commonly used as adjuvants to general anesthetics for providing adequate muscular relaxation. They are also used during endotracheal intubation and for diagnostic scopies. The choice of neuromuscular agents depends on their safety profile, onset and duration of action. For short-term procedures, a short acting drug with rapid recovery rate is preferred as it reduces the risk of complications and accelerates postanesthetic recovery.

SUCCINYLCHOLINE

Succinylcholine causes persistent depolarization followed by skeletal muscle paralysis. It has the advantage of quick onset and short duration of action as it undergoes rapid hydrolysis by hepatic and plasma butyrylcholinesterases (pseudocholinesterase). Although it is short acting, it produces adequate muscular relaxation for tracheal intubation and has quick recovery rate so that the patient begins to breathe spontaneously. Prolonged action is common in patients with high 'dibucaine number', a factor that determines the patient's metabolizing capacity. Succinylcholine increases intraocular pressure, intragastric pressure and muscle pain.

VECURONIUM

Vecuronium is a competitive skeletal muscle relaxant and acts by blocking nicotinic cholinergic receptors. It has quick onset within 2 to 3 minutes and intermediate duration of 45 minutes. Recovery is generally spontaneous but sometimes requires reversal for termination of action. Neostigmine competes with vecuronium for nicotinic receptors binding sites terminating its action. Vecuronium is devoid of vagolytic action, does not cause histamine release but still not preferred as the recovery takes longer time.

Drug of Choice: Succinylcholine

RATIONALE

For brief procedures such as tracheal intubation, a drug with quick onset and recovery is preferred. **Succinylcholine** is a depolarizing blocker with an onset of action within 1 minute and duration of 11 minutes due to its rapid hydrolysis by hepatic and plasma pseudocholinesterases. The main advantage of succinylcholine is its **immediate recovery rate** and the patient starts breathing spontaneously. **Vecuronium** results in **quick onset** but **recovery** may **not** be always **spontaneous** and may require neostigmine reversal. Therefore, succinylcholine is preferred for brief procedures like tracheal intubation.

3. *Cisatracurium/Pancuronium as muscle relaxant in patients with hepatic or renal dysfunction.*

BACKGROUND

Cisatracurium and pancuronium are nondepolarizing or competitive blockers. Pancuronium is an ammonio steroid with long duration of action. Cisatracurium is a potent stereoisomer of atracurium, the benzylisoquinoline with intermediate duration of action. The clinical action of both muscle relaxants starts within 3 to 4 minutes.

CISATRACURIUM

The action of cisatracurium lasts up to 90 minutes. It is inactivated by spontaneous molecular rearrangement known as "Hoffmann elimination". Cisatracurium causes minimal histamine release so the chances of hypotension are minimal. It undergoes organ independent spontaneous metabolism and can be safely used in liver and kidney disease, hence preferred in patients with hepatic or renal dysfunction.

PANCURONIUM

The action of pancuronium persists roughly for around 2 hours. The redistribution of drug reduces its clinical action but the residual action persists until its plasma level remains high. Such persistent blockade causes difficulty in immediate and complete reversal. Pancuronium does not release histamine and does not cause hypotension or bronchospasm but has vagolytic action and causes intense tachycardia. Pancuronium is mainly metabolized in liver and excreted through kidney so should not be administered in patients with hepatic or renal insufficiency.

Drug of Choice: Cisatracurium

RATIONALE

Pancuronium causes **persistent blockade** with prolonged action. It is mainly metabolized by liver and excreted through kidney. It can also cause **intense tachycardia**. **Cisatracurium** has **intermediate duration** of action and has **minimal tendency** to cause **histamine induced hypotension**. It is deactivated through **Hoffmann elimination**. Since it undergoes organ independent spontaneous chemodegradative metabolism, it is safe in patients with hepatic and renal insufficiency. Hence, it is preferred for patients with hepatic or renal dysfunction.

4. *Dantrolene/Succinylcholine for treatment of malignant hyperthermia.*

BACKGROUND

Malignant hyperthermia is characterized by severe hyperthermia, muscle contracture as well as rigidity and vulnerability which are determined by autosomal dominant trait that causes mutation of gene. Mutation of ryanodine receptor-1(RyR1) gene is the main causative factor which increases the susceptibility. Increased muscular metabolism stimulates the muscle contracture triggered by excessive release of calcium from muscular sarcoplasmic reticulum causing hyperthermia. The temperature increases at the rate of 1°C every five minutes. Administration of 100% oxygen and rapid cooling are the adjuvant measures while intravenous sodium bicarbonate counters the acidosis.

DANTROLENE

Dantrolene is a directly acting skeletal muscle relaxant and effective in controlling malignant hyperthermia. It inhibits the release of calcium from sarcoplasmic reticulum as it binds to and blocks the opening of to RyR-1 channel. Sedation, dizziness and dose dependent liver toxicity are its main adverse effects.

SUCCINYLCHOLINE

Coadministration of fluorinated anesthetics such as halothane and neuromuscular blockers such as succinylcholine cause malignant hyperthermia. Halothane mediates the release of calcium from sarcoplasmic reticulum and succinylcholine potentiates the calcium release induced by halothane. Succinylcholine is the causative agent, potentiates the risk of hyperthermia as it stimulates calcium release, it is better avoided.

Drug of Choice: Dantrolene

RATIONALE

Coadministration of succinylcholine along with fluorinated anesthetics such as halothane, isoflurane or sevoflurane is responsible for inducing malignant hyperthermia in susceptible patients. Patients with mutations in ryanodine receptor-1 gene are susceptible for malignant hyperthermia. It occurs due to excessive intracellular release of calcium from sarcoplasmic reticulum. **Dantrolene** is a **directly acting** skeletal muscle relaxant, effective in the management of malignant hyperthermia. It acts by preventing the **release of calcium**. **Succinylcholine** may **cause hyperthermia**. Hence, dantrolene is preferred.

5. *Sugammadex/Neostigmine for reversal of rocuronium.*

BACKGROUND

Rocuronium is an intermediate acting nondepolarizing skeletal muscle relaxant. It has quick onset of action but its effect persists for approximately 70 minutes. Prolonged action is due to elevated plasma concentration. Recovery from rocuronium is most often spontaneous but sometimes it may need 'reversal' by reversible anticholinesterases.

SUGAMMADEX

Rocuronium is a competitive neuromuscular blocker. Sugammadex is a cyclodextrin used in 'reversal' of rocuronium. It reverses rocuronium induced muscle relaxation effectively and causes rapid dose dependent reversal of the neuromuscular blockade. Muscular relaxation induced by very high dose of rocuronium can also be reversed. Each molecule of sugammadex engulfs a molecule of rocuronium forming an inactive complex that gets excreted quickly thereby reducing its plasma concentration. So, rocuronium rapidly dissociates from its binding sites as its plasma concentration falls accelerating the rate of recovery. Sugammadex helps in rapid and complete reversal without residual blockade. It causes minimal side effects such as dysgeusia and hypersensitivity with greater therapeutic benefit.

NEOSTIGMINE

Neostigmine or pyridostigmine are most often used in reversal of rocuronium. They antagonize the effect by stimulating nicotinic cholinergic receptors. Neostigmine prevents the occurrence of 'residual block' and is effective even if the blockade is intense but can also cause muscarinic side effects potentiating bronchospasm, intestinal colic and hypotension. Prior administration of atropine is required for preventing muscarinic side effects.

Drug of Choice: Sugammadex

RATIONALE

Rocuronium most often results in persistent muscular relaxation requiring 'reversal'. **Neostigmine** causes effective 'reversal' without residual blockade but it requires prior administration of atropine for prevention of muscarinic side effects. Besides, it **may not induce quick reversal**. **Sugammadex** forms inactive complex with rocuronium that is quickly excreted causing dissociation of rocuronium from its binding sites at the neuromuscular junction hence the **reversal is more complete**. Sugammadex causes complete absence of residual blockade so preferred to neostigmine.

Local Anesthetics

1. *Bupivacaine/Ropivacaine as anesthetic during labor.*

BACKGROUND

Labor pain is due to visceral dilatation originating from rhythmic uterine contractions. Progressive cervical dilatation adds to the pain caused during first stage of labor. Pain in second stage of labor is principally somatic in nature. Bupivacaine and ropivacaine cause higher level of sensory blockade than motor blockade. They confer an added advantage of motor sparing property. Since their motor blockade is minimal, they do not interfere with the progress of labor thereby making them favored local anesthetics during labor.

ROPIVACAINE

Ropivacaine is a long acting local anesthetic. It is little less potent than bupivacaine. In comparison to bupivacaine, it causes relatively less motor blockade but the duration of action is similar to bupivacaine. Ropivacaine is less cardiotoxic than bupivacaine. Hence, it is preferred as anesthetic during labor or postoperative period.

BUPIVACAINE

Bupivacaine is an amide type of local anesthetic. It is highly potent, long acting anesthetic that offers prolonged anesthesia. It rapidly blocks the cardiac sodium channels but has a very slow rate of dissociation precipitating its cardiac toxicity which manifests as severe ventricular arrhythmias and myocardial depression. Bupivacaine induced cardiac toxicity is difficult to treat since such toxicity is cumulative and very severe. Besides, pregnancy increases the risk of cardiotoxicity of bupivacaine due to its rapid vascular uptake through epidural route. The level of toxicity is reduced with lower concentrations of bupivacaine. 0.25%, 0.125% or 0.0625% of bupivacaine with fentanyl may reduce its toxicity.

Drug of Choice: Ropivacaine

RATIONALE

Bupivacaine and ropivacaine are **long acting** local anesthetics. Since they cause more sensory blockade compared to motor blockade, they **do not interfere** with labor but bupivacaine **increases** the risk of **cardiotoxicity** through prolonged blockade of cardiac sodium channels. Cardiotoxicity is due to **cumulative** effect of bupivacaine and **pregnant women** are more **susceptible. Ropivacaine** is **less potent** but **more motor sparing** than bupivacaine and is less cardiotoxic. Hence, it is preferred to bupivacaine.

2. *Cocaine/Lignocaine with 0.005% phenylephrine for topical anesthesia of ear, nose and throat.*

BACKGROUND

Direct application of soluble solutions and poorly soluble suspensions of local anesthetic causes topical anesthesia. Mucous membranes of nose, throat, mouth, esophagus, tracheobronchial tree and genitourinary tract are common sites. The resultant anesthesia occurs only on the surface and never extends to deeper regions.

LIGNOCAINE

Lignocaine causes faster, longer, extensive and profound anesthesia. Combination of lignocaine with phenylephrine is beneficial. Besides, this combination does not induce toxicity. Phenylephrine decreases the absorption of lignocaine, since it causes intense local vasoconstriction. Phenylephrine prolongs the duration and reduces the toxicity of lignocaine. Hence, the combination of lignocaine with phenylephrine is preferred.

COCAINE

Cocaine is applied topically to nose, nasopharynx, mouth and throat. It should only be used as surface anesthetic and should never be injected as it is a protoplasmic poison and often results in tissue necrosis. It inhibits the reuptake of the neurotransmitter norepinephrine causing vasoconstriction at the site of application. Therefore, it shrinks the mucosa and reduces bleeding during surgical procedures. It has good penetrating capacity in mucous membranes but its diffusion rate into deeper tissues is very minimal. It is very often used as a topical anesthetic for ear, nose and throat and should never be combined with phenylephrine because such a combination results in intense vasoconstriction.

Drug of Choice: Lignocaine

RATIONALE

Cocaine is a surface anesthetic. In addition to its local anesthetic action, it also inhibits the reuptake of norepinephrine. It has good penetrating capacity in mucous membrane with minimal diffusion rate. When combined with phenylephrine, it potentiates vasoconstriction which interferes with its pharmacological action. Hence, it is not preferred. Lignocaine results in longer, more effective local anesthesia. Phenylephrine reduces absorption, prolongs duration and reduces the toxicity of lignocaine. Hence, this combination is preferred as topical anesthetic for ear, nose and throat procedures in otorhinolaryngology.

3. *Prilocaine/Bupivacaine for intravenous regional anesthesia.*

BACKGROUND

Intravenous (IV) regional anesthesia is generally used in surgical procedures of forearm and hand. This technique is simple and performed by using elastic bandage and a tourniquet using BP cuff inflated to 150 mm of Hg above systolic BP. The local anesthetic is injected into the previously cannulated vein. The elastic bandage should be removed before the anesthetic is injected but tourniquet should remain for about 15 to 30 minutes to minimize the entry of local anesthetic into circulation. Prolonged inflation of tourniquet potentiates ischemia mediated nerve injury. The anesthesia starts within 5 to 10 minutes, but pain may follow premature deflation of tourniquet.

PRILOCAINE

Prilocaine is preferred as it has higher therapeutic index. It causes minimal vasodilatation and has higher volume of distribution. Hence, it results in minimal central nervous system (CNS) toxicity. Prilocaine has intermediate duration of action.

BUPIVACAINE

Bupivacaine is long acting compared to prilocaine. Since this technique cannot be continued for a very long time, the need for longer acting anesthetic does not arise. Bupivacaine enters into systemic circulation after deflation of tourniquet increasing the cardiotoxic potential of bupivacaine. Even lower concentrations of bupivacaine can cause toxicity probably due to its longer duration of action. Hence, it is not preferred to prilocaine for intravenous regional anesthesia.

Drug of Choice: Prilocaine

RATIONALE

The chances of entry of the local anesthetic into systemic circulation after the removal of tourniquet are high. Hence, a **long acting** local anesthetic is **unsuitable** for this procedure. **Bupivacaine** is a **long acting** drug. Its prolonged action may potentiate its **risk** of **cardiotoxicity**. **Prilocaine** is an **intermediate acting** drug and has **higher volume** of distribution reducing its CNS toxicity. Hence, prilocaine is preferred.

4. *Chloroprocaine/Lignocaine for epidural anesthesia.*

BACKGROUND

Epidural space lies between ligamentum flavum posteriorly and dura mater anteriorly with spinal periosteum laterally on either side.

The catheter is placed in epidural space facilitating continuous or repeated bolus administration of drugs. Epidural anesthesia does not result in differential sympathetic blockade. It causes almost identical level of sensory and motor blockade. Hence, even short acting drugs can be given as epidural anesthetic and their duration can be prolonged by repeated administration. Local anesthetics administered through epidural route act on spinal nerve roots and paravertebral nerves.

LIGNOCAINE

Intermediate acting 2% lignocaine is preferred as epidural anesthetic. It results in faster and prolonged anesthesia. It causes effective and intense anesthesia with limited toxicity profile.

CHLOROPROCAINE

Procaine is the first ester local anesthetic to be introduced but it is not very potent. Onset of action is delayed and its duration of action short. Its chlorinated derivative chloroprocaine is also short acting with rapid onset and minimal toxic profile as it is metabolized quickly with a plasma half-life of just 25 seconds. If given epidurally, it causes prolonged sensory and motor blockade but increases the incidence of back pain due to muscle spasm. The preservative EDTA used in the formulation binds with calcium and potentiates tetany of paraspinal muscles aggravating the back pain. Accidental injection of chloroprocaine into subarachnoid space is risky because it may cause severe neurological problems.

Drug of Choice: Lignocaine

RATIONALE

Sensory blockade following spinal anesthesia is higher than motor blockade by a few spinal segments. Epidural anesthesia is different from spinal anesthesia and causes almost same degree of sensory and motor blockade. **Chloroprocaine** causes **prolonged sensory** and **motor blockade** but induces muscular back pain due to **tetany**. It has a propensity to cause **neurological** complications if administered into subarachnoid space accidentally. Hence, it is not preferred as an epidural anesthetic. **Lignocaine** is an intermediate acting anesthetic causing **intense, quick and effective** anesthesia with good **safety** profile. Hence, lignocaine is preferred.

5. *0.5% of prilocaine/Low dose low concentration (0.125%) bupivacaine along with fentanyl as epidural anesthetic during labor.*

BACKGROUND

Epidural anesthesia provides pain relief during the first and second stages of labor. Afferent pain impulses arise from cervix and fundus of uterus during first stage of labor and transmitted to spinal cord through T_{10} to L_1. Somatic impulses arising during second stage of labor are transmitted through spinal S_2 to S_4 segments. Epidural anesthesia facilitates patient cooperation during labor and delivery. Local anesthetics provide anesthesia for episiotomy or forceps delivery and extension of anesthesia during caesarean section. They can be coadministered with opioids such as fentanyl to reduce the total dose of opioids. They reduce the maternal and neonatal respiratory depression induced by opioids. Epidural anesthesia increases the systemic concentration of local anesthetics and helps in reduction of pain during labor. This can result in higher neonatal concentration of local anesthetics since they cross placenta and enter fetal circulation leading to neonatal toxicity. Dose, concentration and protein binding, placental blood flow and fetal tissue solubility determine their action.

LOW DOSE, LOW CONCENTRATION (0.125%) BUPIVACAINE

Dilute solutions of bupivacaine reduce fetal toxicity as it is highly lipid soluble. Besides, when combined with fentanyl, its dose is further reduced. Low concentration of bupivacaine in blood reduces the cardiotoxicity.

PRILOCAINE

The metabolite of prilocaine (o-toluidine) causes methemoglobinemia in neonates. The fetal hemoglobin is unable to withstand oxidative stress. Its enzymes are immature and are unable to inhibit the conversion of methemoglobin to its ferrous form in neonates. So, prilocaine should never be used as obstetric anesthetic.

Drug of Choice: Low dose low concentration (0.125%) bupivacaine

RATIONALE

Risk of **cardiotoxicity** due to **bupivacaine** is **negligible** if it is given at **lower dose** and **lesser concentration**. If combined with fentanyl, the dose can be reduced even further. Bupivacaine is preferred in obstetric anesthesia through epidural route because it provides **greater sensory than motor blockade**. **Prilocaine** is **contraindicated** as it causes **methemoglobinemia** due to its metabolite o-toluidine. Since neonates are highly susceptible for methemoglobinemia, it is advisable not to administer prilocaine as epidural anesthetic.

6. *Pramoxine/Dibucaine as surface anesthetic for skin and mucous membranes.*

BACKGROUND

Certain local anesthetics can be used only as a surface anesthetic because they are either too irritant or ineffective to be used otherwise. They are used in symptomatic relief of pruritus, rashes, acute and chronic dermatoses.

PRAMOXINE

Pramoxine is useful in patients allergic to other local anesthetics as it does not exhibit cross sensitivity with other local anesthetics. It is not a benzoate ester and has unique chemical structure. It causes low acute and sub acute toxicity. It is well tolerated on skin and mucous membranes and has low sensitizing index. It is potent, blocks both initiation and conduction of nerve impulses as it inhibits the permeability of neuronal membranes to sodium ions.

DIBUCAINE

Dibucaine belongs to amino amide class of local anesthetics and differs from other anesthetics due to its large quinoline ring. This rigid ring imposes restriction on the molecule and modulates its interaction. It is 15 times more potent than procaine but can cause CNS toxicity if absorbed. It causes convulsions, hypoxia, acidosis, bradycardia, arrhythmia and cardiac arrest. Hence, pramoxine is preferred to dibucaine as a surface anesthetic.

Drug of Choice: Pramoxine

RATIONALE

Pramoxine and dibucaine are surface anesthetics. **Dibucaine** is an amino amide, 15 times more potent than procaine but can cause **CNS toxicity**.[9] **Pramoxine** is effective in patients allergic to other local anesthetics as it does not cause cross sensitivity. It causes **minimal toxicity, well tolerated and has low sensitizing index**. Hence, it is preferred as surface anesthetic for skin and mucous membranes. It is an irritant to eye and should be avoided in ocular conditions.

7. *Procaine/Dyclonine for infiltration anesthesia.*

BACKGROUND

Local anesthetic is directly injected into tissues as infiltration anesthetic. It is usually superficial and may include only the skin but may also include deeper intra-abdominal organs. The level of anesthesia produced is adequate through infiltration anesthesia. It provides anesthesia without affecting other systems or their functions but large amount of drug is needed for this type of anesthesia.

PROCAINE

Procaine is the first synthetic ester to be used as a local anesthetic. It is a less potent and short acting drug. It inhibits the action of sulfonamides and can cause hypersensitivity reactions. It can interfere with cholinergic transmission at neuromuscular junction. Although its action starts slowly, it is preferred because it is less toxic when compared to dyclonine. It is not a surface anesthetic and is effective only as an infiltration anesthetic.

DYCLONINE

Dyclonine has quick onset and its duration of action is comparable to procaine. Dyclonine should never be used as infiltration anesthetic as it is toxic when injected. Although it is a potent local anesthetic causing multisynaptic depression of spinal reflexes it causes CNS stimulation leading to convulsions, tremors and emesis. Hence, it should be avoided as an infiltration anesthetic.

Drug of Choice: Procaine

RATIONALE

Procaine is effective only as an infiltration anesthetic. It is never used as surface anesthetic as it does not penetrate skin and mucous membranes. Lignocaine is the most effective infiltrative anesthetic. However, procaine is **preferred** to dyclonine. **Dyclonine** is a **potent** local anesthetic and is **action is comparable** to procaine but it is more **toxic** and causes **CNS stimulation**.[10] When given as infiltration anesthetic, dyclonine results in tremors, convulsion and vomiting. Hence, it is avoided as an infiltration anesthetic.

8. *Benzocaine/Tetracaine as surface anesthetic on wounds.*

BACKGROUND

Systemic absorption of local anesthetics following topical application is risky especially on denuded or inflamed skin. Systemic absorption of local anesthetics potentiates their toxicity.

BENZOCAINE

Solubility of a local anesthetic determines the rate of absorption. Benzocaine is devoid of terminal diethylamino group of procaine. It is poorly soluble in water as it is hydrophobic in nature and slowly absorbed from wounds and ulcerations. Hence, benzocaine does not cause systemic toxicity. Besides, it has sustained local action resulting in prolonged anesthesia. Hence, it is preferred to tetracaine as surface anesthetic on wounds.

TETRACAINE

Tetracaine is an amino ester, highly soluble, very potent and long acting. Its long duration of action is due to its delayed metabolism. It is generally used in conditions that require prolonged anesthesia. Tetracaine results in sustained action when applied on wounds or ulcerated surfaces. It is absorbed systemically from abraded skin and results in toxicity. So, it is not preferred as surface anesthetic for wounds.

Drug of Choice: Benzocaine

RATIONALE

The solubility of a local anesthetic determines its rate of absorption when applied on a surface. **Tetracaine and benzocaine** are **both long acting drugs**. **Poor solubility** of **benzocaine** is responsible for its **prolonged** action. Benzocaine is **devoid of systemic toxicity** as it is absorbed very slowly. Hence, benzocaine is preferred. **Tetracaine** also has **long duration** of action as it is metabolized slowly. Because of high solubility it is easily absorbed from the site of application leading to **sustained action** if the skin is not intact as in wounds or ulcerated areas. Tetracaine is **absorbed** as it is highly soluble and causes systemic toxicity so, not preferred.

9. *Oxethazaine/Benzocaine as anesthetic antacid.*

BACKGROUND

Hydrochloride salts of local anesthetics are water soluble but its unprotonated amine form is less water soluble because hydrochloride salts are mildly acidic. Local anesthetics are weak bases and hydrochloride salts are soluble formulations.

OXETHAZINE

Oxethazaine is a surface anesthetic and is very potent. It is very effective as a 0.2% suspension. It is the only local anesthetic effective even in acidic conditions. Generally all other local anesthetics are effective only at alkaline pH. It is unique and only a very small quantity is ionized at a low acidic pH. Hence, it is effective for anesthetizing acidic gastric medium. So, it is combined with antacids for symptomatic relief of gastritis or gastric ulcer.

BENZOCAINE

Benzocaine is a potent surface anesthetic but is not effective in acidic pH. It is a good surface anesthetic for wounds as it has poor solubility. Its action is more localized as it is not absorbed from wounds and ulcerations. The pH of chronic wounds or ulcers is highly alkaline. The pH of wounds or ulcers determines its angiogenic and protease activity. Acidic environment favors the process of wound healing. The pH of gastric ulcer is acidic and benzocaine is effective only in alkaline pH. Hence, it is not useful for symptomatic relief of gastric ulcer.

Drug of Choice: Oxethazaine

RATIONALE

Benzocaine is an effective surface anesthetic for wounds and chronic ulcers as it is less soluble, not absorbed, stays at the site of application resulting in prolonged effective anesthesia. The pH of chronic wounds is alkaline and ranges above 7.[11] Benzocaine is **effective** mainly in **alkaline pH** and not in acidic pH. The pH of gastric ulcer is acidic. Hence, benzocaine is not effective in gastritis. **Oxethazaine** is the **only local anesthetic** effective in **acidic pH**. Hence, oxethazaine is combined with antacids for symptomatic relief of gastritis or gastric ulcer.

8 Histamine, Antihistamines and Leukotrienes

1. *First generation/Second generation antihistamines in children and elderly.*

BACKGROUND

H_1 antihistamines are used in allergic conditions and prevent the action of histamine by blocking its interaction with H_1 receptors. They are used for symptomatic treatment of rhinitis primarily due to their anticholinergic action. Renal and hepatic functions are usually compromised in elderly. The chances of impaired clearance of these drugs in elderly potentiate their toxicity.

SECOND GENERATION ANTIHISTAMINES

Second generation H_1 antihistamines have higher selectivity to H_1 receptors and are devoid of anticholinergic and central nervous system (CNS) mediated side effects. So, they are preferred. Dosage reduction and constant monitoring is necessary in children and elders and are not recommended for children below four years of age because they can cause gastrointestinal, hematological and hypersensitivity reactions. Their safety in children aged between 2 and 11 years is being reviewed. Loratadine, desloratadine and fexofenadine are some of the second generation agents. They are also available as syrups, mouth dissolving formulations suitable for children.

FIRST GENERATION ANTIHISTAMINES

Diphenhydramine, dimenhydrinate and chlorpheniramine belong to first generation H_1 antihistamine agents. They have additional anticholinergic action resulting in urinary retention, dysuria, dry mouth and cycloplegia. On account of central histamine receptor blockade, they further impair cognition in elders. Sedation and anticholinergic side effects make them unsuitable in elderly. In children their sedative action impairs learning and interferes with their performance in school. In view of the above reasons, these drugs are not preferred in children and elders.

Drug of Choice: Second Generation Antihistamines

RATIONALE

First generation H_1 antihistamines are unsuitable for therapy in both children and elders. The expected renal and hepatic impairment resulting in impaired elimination in elders prolongs the action of these drugs. So, the magnitude of sedation, anticholinergic side effects and cognitive impairment are high in this age group. In children, sedative effect reduces learning skills. Hence, the second generation agents are preferred in children and elderly as they are devoid of these side effects.

2. *Cetirizine/Levocetirizine preferred as antihistamine for therapy.*

BACKGROUND

Cetirizine and levocetirizine are second generation H_1 antihistamines. They are devoid of CNS side effects as well as psychomotor impairment. They do not cause anticholinergic side effects such as cycloplegia, urinary retention and dryness of mouth.

LEVOCETRIZINE

The degree of entry of antihistamines into CNS is variable and this property determines their capacity to induce sedation. Generally, second generation antihistamines do not cause sedation due to their inability to enter CNS as they do not cross blood-brain barrier. Levocetirizine is an isomer of cetirizine. Unlike cetirizine, it has lower tendency to cause sedation. Even at half the dose of cetirizine, levocetirizine is more potent and highly effective.

CETIRIZINE

Cetirizine is a metabolite of hydroxyzine and has a greater tendency to cause sedation. At high doses, it causes sedation and somnolence in some individuals.

Drug of Choice: Levocetirizine

RATIONALE

The **advantage** of **second generation** antihistamines over the first generation agents is that they are **devoid of CNS side effects**. These agents are generally devoid of sedative property as they do not enter CNS but among them **cetirizine** has **more tendency** to cause **sedation** and **somnolence** in many individuals. **Levocetirizine** is an **enantiomer** of cetirizine, is **highly potent, effective at half the dose** of cetirizine and causes minimal sedation. Hence, it is preferred to cetirizine for therapy.

3. *Hydroxyzine/Cetirizine for pruritus in pregnancy.*

BACKGROUND

Pruritus is an extremely troublesome condition during pregnancy and requires therapy with antihistamines. Second generation antihistamines are more potent and are longer acting than first generation drugs. Many H_1 antihistamines can cross placenta resulting in teratogenicity and only few antihistamines can be used safely during pregnancy. Cetirizine and hydroxyzine are more suitable for the treatment of pruritus. They have superior efficacy in pruritus as they accumulate in skin.

CETIRIZINE

Cetirizine is a second generation antihistamine and a metabolite of hydroxyzine. It belongs to category B in pregnancy with no proven risk for fetus. Since the risk of spontaneous abortion, still birth, major or minor fetal anomalies is minimal it can safely be given during pregnancy whenever indicated.

HYDROXYZINE

Hydroxyzine is a first generation antihistamine and has longer duration of action but it is teratogenic and causes fetal malformations. Hence, it is contraindicated during pregnancy.

Drug of Choice: Cetirizine

RATIONALE

Pruritus is an extremely troublesome condition during pregnancy necessitating therapy with antihistamines.[12] **Hydroxyzine** and its metabolite **cetirizine accumulate** in **skin** so are effective in pruritus but **hydroxyzine** is **teratogenic** and should be avoided in pregnant women. **Cetirizine** belongs to **category B** with no proven risk to fetus[13] and does not cause fetal malformations. Hence, cetirizine is preferred for the treatment of pruritus during pregnancy.

4. *Diphenhydramine/Doxylamine with pyridoxine for morning sickness during first trimester of pregnancy.*

BACKGROUND

Morning sickness usually occurs in first trimester starting around 8th or 9th week of pregnancy. It is often mild and self-limiting and managed through conservative measures. If severe and troublesome it requires pharmacotherapy, otherwise not because drugs may cause negative implications to both fetus and mother. Nausea and vomiting may be due to progesterone induced gastrointestinal dysfunction. Pyridoxine reduces the severity but not the frequency of vomiting in pregnancy. It is not teratogenic and combined with antihistamines for morning sickness. Doxylamine and promethazine are first generation sedative antihistamines and are potent antiemetics.

DOXYLAMINE

Combination of doxylamine, dicyclomine and pyridoxine was earlier banned for therapy of morning sickness. Recently Food and Drug Administration (FDA) in 2013 has approved the combination of doxylamine and pyridoxine. Since this combination has been listed under category A indicating no involvement of risks, it can be safely administered during pregnancy. Starting dose of pyridoxine and doxylamine for severe emesis is 10 mg each.

DIPHENHYDRAMINE

Diphenhydramine belongs to category B indicating no proven risks during pregnancy but higher doses given during the term can potentiate uterine contractions. Hence, doxylamine is preferred to diphenhydramine for morning sickness.

Drug of Choice: Doxylamine

RATIONALE

Diphenhydramine and doxylamine are first generation antihistamines and **potent** antiemetics. They are indicated for the treatment of morning sickness during pregnancy. The **safety** of **doxylamine** was **questionable** till **some time back** and was **withdrawn** from market. Recently, in **2013**, **FDA has approved its safety in pregnancy**[14] and has listed it **under category A**. Doxylamine and pyridoxine effectively controls morning sickness.[15] **Diphenhydramine** belongs to **category B**, is reasonably safe but is not the drug of choice during pregnancy.

5. *Fexofenadine HCl/Chlorpheniramine maleate for symptomatic treatment of rhinitis in those driving vehicles.*

BACKGROUND

Impaired alertness caused by antihistamines affects judging skills and response time of drivers. Chlorpheniramine maleate is a very potent first generation antihistamine. Fexofenadine hydrochloride is second generation antihistamine.

FEXOFENADINE HYDROCHLORIDE

Fexofenadine hydrochloride is a metabolite of terfenadine and unlike terfenadine, fexofenadine does not block cardiac potassium channels. Hence, it does not prolong QT interval and does not cause *torsades de pointes*. Its action lasts for 24 hours and it is excreted in feces. It does not cross the blood-brain barrier and does not cause sedation or psychomotor impairment. Hence, fexofenadine HCl is preferred to chlorpheniramine.

CHLORPHENIRAMINE MALEATE

Chlorpheniramine is a highly potent sedative although when compared to other first generation drugs, it is less prone for daytime sedation. Apart from its antihistaminergic action it has additional anticholinergic action causing dryness of secretions and is more effective as symptomatic therapy for rhinitis. It causes somnolence, reduces alertness and slows down the reaction time, so for individuals driving vehicles, it can be given safely only at bed time. It interferes with their driving skills if given during daytime or prior to driving. The most common side effect is CNS stimulation.

Drug of Choice: Fexofenadine

RATIONALE

Chlorpheniramine maleate, like other first generation antihistamines is a **highly potent** sedative. **Fexofenadine** HCl is a **non-sedative** second generation antihistamine. As a first generation antihistamine, **chlorpheniramine** maleate has **additional anticholinergic** action resulting in dryness of secretions which is helpful in the **symptomatic** treatment of rhinitis. It can cause sedation, somnolence, impair alertness and slow the reaction time. Therefore, it **interferes** with the **performance** and driving skills. Fexofenadine HCl is non-sedative, does not interfere with driving skills. Hence, fexofenadine HCl is preferred.

6. *Diphenhydramine HCl/Doxepin HCl as adjuvant in drug induced Parkinsonism.*

BACKGROUND

Certain drugs are capable of inducing extrapyramidal symptoms due to potent D_2 blockade. Phenothiazines, haloperidol and metoclopramide are few such drugs. Antihistamines are adjuvants to anticholinergics in the treatment of drug induced Parkinsonism.

DIPHENHYDRAMINE HYDROCHLORIDE

Diphenhydramine HCl has a very potent anticholinergic action and induces sedation due to its significant antimuscarinic property. It can even reverse the extrapyramidal symptoms induced by phenothiazines if given during very early stages of this condition.

DOXEPIN HYDROCHLORIDE

Doxepin HCl is a highly potent H_1 antihistamine and a tricyclic antidepressant. It has higher efficacy in antagonizing H_1 receptors and also has additional antimuscarinic action. It is well tolerated mainly by people with symptoms of depression but causes disorientation and confusion in others hence cannot be given in patients with no signs of depression.

Drug of Choice: Diphenhydramine HCl

RATIONALE

Antihistamines are only **adjuvants** and not the first line drugs for suppressing the extrapyramidal symptoms induced by dopamine antagonists. **Diphenhydramine** HCl and doxepin HCl are first generation antihistamines with **additional anticholinergic action**. **Doxepin** HCl also has **antidepressant action**. They cause significant drowsiness. Doxepin HCl is better **tolerated mainly** by people with **depression** and causes confusion or disorientation in others. Hence, doxepin HCl is not preferred.

7. *Ebastine/Azelastine HCl for perennial allergic rhinitis.*

BACKGROUND

In sensitive individuals, allergic rhinitis or hay fever is induced by allergens. Pathogenesis involves both cytotoxic and humoral immune responses. The antigen IgE complex binds to mast cell and basophil surfaces resulting in liberation of inflammatory mediators. Allergic response is augmented as the antigen enters local lymph nodes stimulating T cell dependent cell mediated immunity. Release of cytokines and interleukins with specific activation of mast cells, basophils, eosinophils and T cells further aggravates this condition. The patient suffers from persistent rhinitis with seasonal variation. Antihistamines offer immediate relief but, the effect is usually temporary. Since frequent administration is required for control of symptoms, tolerance develops and reduces its clinical benefit. Oral administration may result in xerostomia in some patients, so topical antihistamines are indicated in such patients.

AZELASTINE HYDROCHLORIDE

Azelastine HCl is a good topical agent and available as intranasal preparation. It inhibits release of histamine, leukotrienes and PAF. It also inhibits expression of intracellular adhesion molecule–1 (ICAM-1) in nasal mucosa. It offers relief for up to 24 hours but the action can last much longer. Nasal irritation and stinging sensation can occur due to azelastine.

EBASTINE

Ebastine is converted to its active metabolite carbastine but results in QT prolongation in animals so preferably avoided.

Drug of Choice: Azelastine HCl

RATIONALE

Therapeutic benefit offered by antihistamines in perennial allergic rhinitis is **immediate** but often **temporary**. Development of tolerance further reduces their clinical benefit. Topical antihistamines are given for those who are unable to tolerate orally administered drugs. **Azelastine HCl** is **long acting** and inhibits the release of mediators involved in the pathogenesis of rhinitis. **Ebastine** is also effective but has resulted in development of **arrhythmias** in **animal studies**. Hence, ebastine is not preferred.

8. *Azelastine HCl/Ipratropium bromide in vasomotor rhinitis.*

BACKGROUND

Vasomotor rhinitis is often the cause of rhinorrhea in elders. It is due to increased sensitivity of vidian nerve. Rhinorrhea can occur due to light, odors, cold or warm air. In vasomotor rhinitis due to venous engorgement, mucosa of the nasal turbinate appears pale.

IPRATROPIUM BROMIDE

Ipratropium bromide is an atropine substitute with selective action on bronchial asthma. Its anticholinergic property is useful in the treatment of rhinorrhea. Intranasal ipratropium spray of 0.03%/ 0.06% is effective. It reduces venous engorgement and the symptoms of vasomotor rhinitis.

AZELASTINE HYDROCHLORIDE

Azelastine HCl is not useful in the treatment of vasomotor rhinitis. The pathophysiology of vasomotor rhinitis is not mediated through histamine. Azelastine is not useful in the treatment of vasomotor rhinitis and effective only in the treatment of allergic rhinitis.

Drug of Choice: Ipratropium Bromide

RATIONALE

Vasomotor rhinitis is **not mediated** through allergy and **histamine release** but occurs due to **increased sensitivity of vidian nerve**. Vasodilatation and venous engorgement are causes for rhinorrhea. Since the pathophysiology is not mediated through histamine, Azelastine HCl is not useful in controlling the symptoms. The anticholinergic drug **ipratropium bromide** as intranasal spray is effective for vasomotor rhinitis.

9. *Olopatadine HCl/Azelastine HCl eye drops in allergic conjunctivitis.*

BACKGROUND

Allergic conjunctivitis can either be a severe seasonal or less severe perennial type. It is a type I allergic reaction mediated by

IgE causing degranulation of mast cells. Ocular itching due to allergic inflammation of ocular surfaces occurs with hyperemia and conjunctival congestion. Olopatadine and azelastine are topical nonsedative antihistamines and are available for topical use as eye drops. They have additional mast cell stabilizing action. Therefore, they also have a prophylactic effect as they prevent the release of histamine.

OLOPATADINE HYDROCHLORIDE

In addition to its antihistaminergic property, olopatadine also inhibits the release of other chemical mediators such as tachykinin, TNF-α and prevents eosinophilic infiltration which contributes to its antiallergic action. Olopatadine results in excellent, strong and safe clinical effect. Patients have better tolerability to olopatadine than azelastine eye drops. Olopatadine does not cause disruption of conjunctival cell membrane and so patients using olopatadine eye drops experience only a low level of discomfort.

AZELASTINE HYDROCHLORIDE

Azelastine inhibits the release of leukotrienes and platelet activating factor. Azelastine results in disruption of conjunctival cell membrane and patients experience discomfort during instillation of azelastine eye drops. Hence, azelastine is not preferred.

Drug of Choice: Olopatadine HCl

RATIONALE

Seasonal or perennial allergic conjunctivitis is managed by antihistamines. Azelastine HCl and olopatadine HCl are available as topical preparations. They have mast cell stabilizing action in addition to their antihistaminic action. Olopatadine is more effective, well tolerated and safe resulting in excellent clinical action.[16] Azelastine causes discomfort during instillation due to conjunctival cell membrane disruption. The pharmacodynamic superiority of olopatadine makes it the drug of choice in allergic conjunctivitis.

10. *Montelukast/Zileuton as a prophylactic in allergic rhinitis.*

BACKGROUND

Leukotrienes are end products of lipoxygenase pathway and involved in inflammatory conditions.

MONTELUKAST

Montelukast is a LTD4 receptor antagonist and inhibits the action of leukotriene. Allergic and other inflammatory conditions are treated by montelukast. It is also effective in prophylaxis of bronchial asthma as it inhibits bronchial hyperactivity and reduces airway inflammation. The dose of montelukast is 10 mg and is given once daily but montelukast can induce headache, rashes, vasculitis and occasional hepatotoxicity.

ZILEUTON

Zileuton is a 5-lipoxygenase inhibitor and acts by inhibiting leuko-triene synthesis. It is useful in allergic and inflammatory condi-tions. It is also used as a prophylactic in asthma. It reduces air-way inflammation mediated bronchial hyperactivity. Zileuton is available as sustained release preparation and given twice daily at a dose of 1200 mg. It causes agitation, aggressiveness, halluci-nation, insomnia and irritability. Zileuton can also induce suicidal tendencies and liver toxicity.

Drug of Choice: Montelukast

RATIONALE

Leukotrienes are involved in the pathophysiology of allergy and inflammation. **Zileuton inhibits leukotriene synthesis** and **montelukast antagonizes leukotriene action**. They are effective in allergic rhinitis, allergic conjunctivitis and inflammation. They are also used for the prophylaxis of bronchial asthma. Recently **FDA** has issued a **warning** against the possible **neuropsychiatric** events associated with these drugs. **Zileuton** is required in large doses and has **short duration** of action **necessitating twice daily dose** and its **hepatotoxic** potential are the limitations that restrict its use, hence it is less frequently prescribed.

Serotonin Agonists and Antagonists

1. *Serotonin (5HT$_{1B/1D}$) agonists/Serotonin (5HT$_2$) antagonists in acute migraine headache.*

BACKGROUND

Migraine can manifest in many different forms, primary type manifesting with or without aura. Exact pathogenesis is yet to be characterized but it involves both vascular and neural components. Activation of trigeminovascular system is mainly responsible for pain but cortical spreading depression (CSD) and neuronal sensitization are also involved. Trigeminal ganglionic neurons innervate trigeminocervical complex and neurons arising from upper cervical dorsal roots are also involved. Activation of these neurons stimulates pain sensitive dual vascular structures. CSD mediated depolarization occurs across cerebral cortex depressing neuronal bioelectrical activity. 5HT, substance P, neurokinin A and calcitonin gene related peptide (CGRP) are responsible for inflammation. Expansion of perivascular space and edema occurs due to inflammation which stimulates nerve endings, causing pain. CGRP is also a very potent vasodilator and causes perivascular edema.

SEROTONIN (5HT$_{1B/1D}$) AGONISTS

Serotonin mediated vasodilatation is the main pathophysiology of acute migraine. Agonists of 5HT$_{1B/1D}$ receptors, such as triptans result in selective vasoconstriction of cerebral blood vessels. They are effective in the treatment of acute migraine.

SEROTONIN (5HT$_2$) ANTAGONISTS

These receptors cause depolarization of cortical neurons and such blockade prevents spread of neuronal pain inhibiting further progression of acute migraine and inhibits the conversion of prodromal stage to phases of aura. Methysergide is neither a serotonin agonist nor an antagonist and it blocks 5HT$_{2A}$ and 5HT$_{2C}$ receptors, resulting in hyperpolarization. Therefore, it can be used only as a prophylactic and not effective in acute phase of migraine because it does not cause selective cerebral vasoconstriction.

Drug of Choice: Serotonin (5HT$_{1B/1D}$) Agonists

RATIONALE

Vascular and neuronal mechanisms are involved in the pathogenesis of migraine. Neuronal mechanisms are responsible for prodromal stage as well as aura and vascular mechanisms are involved in acute phase of migraine. Serotonin agonists such as **triptans** cause **selective cerebral vasoconstriction** and therefore are effective in the treatment of acute phase of migraine. **Methysergide**, a serotonin antagonist is more effective in inhibiting the **neuronal phase**. It prevents the progression of migraine to acute phase by increasing potassium conductance and causing hyperpolarization of neurons. Hence, it is effective only as a **prophylactic** agent and not in the treatment of acute migraine.

2. *Triptans/Ergot alkaloids for the treatment of acute migraine headache.*

BACKGROUND

Triptans and ergot alkaloids are serotonin agonists and act on 5HT$_{1B/1D}$ receptors at presynaptic trigeminal nerves. As serotonin agonists, they directly inhibit vasodilatation and reduce the release of vasodilating peptides. They result in vasoconstriction by stimulating 5HT$_{1B/1D}$ receptor and result in selective vasoconstriction of cerebral blood vessels. They inhibit abnormal dilatation of carotid arteriovenous anastamosis which is a prominent feature of acute migraine. This prevents shunting of carotid arterial blood and protects the brain from cerebral ischemia and hypoxia.

TRIPTANS

$5HT_{1B/1D}$ receptors act as autoreceptors at presynaptic terminals. These receptors modulate the release of neurotransmitters. Triptans are very effective in reducing the pain. They do not potentiate nausea or vomiting associated with migraine. They have selectivity towards the serotonin receptors and do not interact with adrenergic, dopaminergic, cholinergic or other receptors. They can be administered orally or as intranasal spray and can also be given subcutaneously in patients with nausea and vomiting. They should not be given to individuals with ischemic coronary disease and are also contraindicated in cerebrovascular or peripheral vascular disease.

ERGOT ALKALOIDS

Ergot alkaloids interact with adrenergic and dopaminergic receptors and also have an additional serotonin agonistic action. Since, they lack selectivity they cannot be used frequently. They should be given only in those with frequent or severe migraine headache. Sublingual ergotamine tartrate can be given immediately after the pain starts. It is a potent emetic and complicates emesis associated with migraine, increasing the frequency and severity of nausea and vomiting. Numbness, tingling, weakness of extremities or precordial pain may occur. It is contraindicated in those with peripheral vascular disease.

Drug of Choice: Triptans

RATIONALE

As vasoconstrictors, serotonin agonists effectively counteract the vasodilatation mediated neuralgic pain induced by neuropeptides in migraine. Ergot alkaloids and triptans are $5HT_{1B/1D}$ agonists and are equally effective in migraine. Triptans act selectively on serotonin receptors while ergot alkaloids act additionally on adrenergic and dopamine receptors. Due to their nonselective action, ergot alkaloids induce severe emesis as dopamine agonists and precordial pain due to vasospastic action mediated through adrenergic α receptors. Triptans are devoid of these side effects and do not induce vomiting hence preferred to ergot alkaloids.

3. *Sumatriptan/Rizatriptan for acute attack of migraine associated with emesis.*

BACKGROUND

Triptans should be reserved for those who do not respond to other drugs and should be tried only after an adequate trial period with a prophylactic agent. They only produce symptomatic relief of acute pain and do not prevent future episodes of migraine and do not have prophylactic action. Triptans also inhibit release of proinflammatory vasodilatory neuropeptides thus preventing the formation of perivascular edema reducing headache mediated through mechanical stretching of perivascular space. They also inhibit the sensory neural pain originating from trigeminal nerve. Most triptans are short acting and have to be administered repeatedly. The safety of frequent administration of triptans is not established and they should not be used for more than 3 to 4 times within a period of one month. Triptans should not be coadministered with ergot alkaloids and should be avoided within 24 hours of ergot administration.

SUMATRIPTAN

The duration of action of sumatriptan extends only for a few hours as its oral bioavailability is only 40%. It is available as tablet, as intranasal spray and injections. Sumatriptan is less potent and cheaper than rizatriptan but does not offer complete relief in the presence of residual headache. It minimizes the recurrence of migraine and incidence of side effects is also infrequent. Since sumatriptan has a better safety profile and low recurrence rate it is preferred.

RIZATRIPTAN

Rizatriptan, the second generation triptan, has a half-life of 3 hours with 45% oral bioavailability. It is available only as tablets and so is difficult for administration in patients with emesis. Dose wise, rizatriptan is 10 times more potent but costlier than sumatriptan and results in almost complete relief from headache within 2 hours. Occurrence of side effects such as chest pain, dizziness, numbness and fatigue are very high. It has good efficacy and results in sustained response but recurrence rate is very high.

Drug of Choice: Sumatriptan

RATIONALE

Triptans are indicated only for those who do not respond to prophylactic therapy. **Rizatriptan**, the second generation triptan, is **10 times more potent**[17] than sumatriptan and provides complete relief from headache within 2 hours. Since it is available **only** as **oral** formulation, the absorption is erratic in patients with emesis, reducing its clinical benefit. It is costlier and has **higher rate of recurrence** and side effects. **Sumatriptan** is **cost effective**, has a **better safety** profile and can be given either subcutaneously or as intranasal spray in patients with emesis.

4. *Flunarizine/Methysergide in prophylaxis of migraine.*

BACKGROUND

Prophylaxis is indicated in patients who get frequent migraine headache, if the incidence is more than two times per month. Prophylaxis is also effective for those who get less frequent but prolonged headache and for those who do not tolerate drugs given for acute therapy. It is preferably started as monotherapy with a low dose and then titrated upwards with a trial period of 2 to 3 months. Prophylaxis should be terminated after 1 year even, if there is no expected outcome.

FLUNARIZINE

Flunarizine is a calcium channel blocker and reduces spasm of smooth muscles. Its efficacy is similar to propranolol, the first line drug[18] in prophylaxis and reduces the frequency of migraine but can cause somnolence and weight gain. Rarely flunarizine can cause depression and extrapyramidal side effects. It is not available in USA and UK but available in many other countries.

METHYSERGIDE

Methysergide, a congener of methylergonovine, blocks $5HT_{2A}$ and $5HT_{2C}$ receptors but, prolonged administration can cause severe adverse effects. It can cause reteropulmonary, endocardial and pleuropulmonary fibrosis, usually reversible but may lead to permanent cardiac valvular fibrosis. Hence, methysergide is not preferred for prophylaxis of migraine.

Drug of Choice: Flunarizine

RATIONALE

Prophylaxis of migraine is essential for those who get more frequent headache or less frequent but prolonged headache. **Methysergide** is an **antagonist** at $5HT_{2A}$ and $5HT_{2C}$ receptor site. Although it is quite effective as a prophylactic drug, it frequently causes reversible pleuropulmonary, reteropulmonary and permanent cardiac valvular fibrosis. **Flunarizine** is **not available in USA and UK** but is available in many other countries. It **reduces spasm** of muscles, has **efficacy equal** to propranolol, the first line drug. It is well tolerated but can **cause somnolence** otherwise, toxicity profile is minimal. Hence, flunarizine is preferred for prophylaxis of migraine.

5. *Ondansetron/Palonosetron in chemotherapy-induced vomiting.*

BACKGROUND

$5HT_3$ receptors of vagus and enterochromaffin cells are mainly responsible for inducing emesis. Vagal and sympathetic afferents stimulate the CTZ in area postrema directly inducing vomiting. Peripherally the serotonergic afferents arising from GIT also induce vomiting by stimulating vomiting center through nucleus tractus solitarius that have high concentration of serotonin receptors. Serotonergic transmission of enteric and myenteric plexus is also involved and they trigger peristaltic contraction increasing the intraluminal pressure causing gastric relaxation, retroperistalsis, retching and vomiting. These symptoms occur due to relaxation of upper esophageal sphincter. Cancer chemotherapy induces serotonin release from enterochromaffin cells in the small intestine stimulating vagal afferents through $5HT_3$ receptors inducing vomiting. Therefore, $5HT_3$ antagonists are very effective in control of chemotherapy induced vomiting as they inhibit the $5HT_3$ receptors in nucleus tractus solitarius and CTZ. $5HT_3$ antagonists result in residual effect even after their elimination hence, once daily administration is adequate to produce the required benefit.

PALONOSETRON

Palonosetron has a long half-life of about 40 hours and has the highest affinity for $5HT_3$ receptors. It is clinically superior to ondansetron and also effective in delayed emesis thereby improving the quality of life in patients. The dose of palonosetron is only about 0.25 mg. It has a better safety profile, causes mainly headache but incidence rate is less than ondansetron. It is costlier than ondansetron but the total cost of therapy is almost similar because ondansetron has to be given in repeated doses.

ONDANSETRON

Ondansetron has a shorter half-life of about 4 hours and has only moderate affinity to $5HT_3$ receptors. It does not inhibit delayed emesis and is effective only in the control of active emesis. The dose of ondansetron is about 0.15 mg/kg and has to be administered more frequently. It has lower safety profile and causes frequent headache.

Drug of Choice: Palonosetron

RATIONALE

Blockade of $5HT_3$ receptor controls emesis through **central** and **peripheral** mechanism. Chemotherapy induced vomiting is mainly triggered by peripheral serotonergic mechanism hence $5HT_3$

receptor antagonists are very effective in treating chemotherapy induced vomiting. **Palonosetron** has **longer duration** of action and **controls delayed emesis also**. It has a **higher affinity** for serotonin receptors, so it is clinically superior to ondansetron.[19] The cost of total therapy is almost similar as it does not require repeated administration. Therefore, palonosetron is preferred to ondansetron for chemotherapy induced vomiting.

6. *Cyproheptadine/Octreotide in carcinoid syndrome.*

BACKGROUND

Carcinoid syndrome is due to excessive secretion of serotonin and kallikrein from carcinoid tumor. Excessive serotonin causes bowel hyper motility and diarrhea. Massive amounts of kallikrein gets converted to bradykinin and results in flushing. Bronchoconstriction occurs due to interaction of serotonin on pulmonary $5HT_2$ receptors. Niacin deficiency can occur due to extensive diversion of tryptophan to serotonin synthesis.

OCTREOTIDE

Octreotide is a synthetic somatostatin analog, long acting and more potent in inhibiting the release of growth hormone, other hormones, growth factors and cytokines thereby reducing the symptoms of carcinoid syndrome. It can be administered subcutaneously or as intramuscular injection and also available as a long acting biodegradable formulation.

CYPROHEPTADINE

Cyproheptadine blocks both histamine and $5HT_{2A}$ receptors and has a weak anticholinergic activity. Although, it blocks histamine receptors it does not interfere with gastric acid secretion. It reduces intestinal motility mediated by both histamine and serotonin and is effective in carcinoid syndrome. Although serotonin is primarily responsible for carcinoid syndrome cyproheptadine is not first line drug in the treatment of carcinoid syndrome.

Drug of Choice: Octreotide

RATIONALE

The symptoms of diarrhea and flushing in carcinoid syndrome are mainly due to serotonin and kallikrein. **Cyproheptadine antagonizes** $5HT_{2A}$ receptors without interfering with the secretion of serotonin. **Octreotide**, the synthetic analog of somatostatin **inhibits the synthesis of serotonin** and controls symptoms of carcinoid syndrome more effectively. Hence, octreotide is preferred.

10

Prostaglandins

1. *Dinoprostone/Misoprostol for induction of labor.*

BACKGROUND

Dinoprostone is a prostaglandin E_2 analog and misoprostol is a prostaglandin E_1 analog. They are approved by Food and Drug Administration (FDA) for induction of labor as they cause uterine contraction. Dinoprostone and misoprostol are very effective in inducing labor and their efficacy is on par with oxytocin. They are available as vaginal inserts or vaginal pessary.

DINOPROSTONE

The dose of dinoprostone is 10 mg as a controlled release preparation but the induction-delivery period is slightly delayed. It neither causes hyperstimulation nor causes uterine rupture and does not result in higher incidence of fetal distress. It has the advantage of safe delivery, so it is preferred.

MISOPROSTOL

The dose of misoprostol ranges between 25 and 100 µg and has higher efficacy compared to dinoprostone. It is cheaper and can be stored at room temperature. Most women deliver within 24 hour period after administration of misoprostol as spontaneous rupture of membranes frequently occurs. It lowers the induction—delivery interval significantly and there is a minimal need for simultaneous augmentation with oxytocin. It is highly potent and causes uterine hyperstimulation leading to higher incidence of uterine rupture and abnormal fetal heart rate. It lowers Apgar score in most of the delivered neonates who do not require resuscitation. It does not result in birth asphyxia. Hyperstimulation of uterus is common at the dose of 50 µg and lower doses of misoprostol can reduce the risk. The advantage of misoprostol is quick delivery.

Drug of Choice: Dinoprostone

RATIONALE

Dinoprostone, PGE_2 analog and misoprostol, PGE_1 analog are both approved drugs for induction of labor. Misoprostol causes spontaneous rupture of membranes, delivery of fetus at a shorter time as it reduces the interval between induction and delivery. This pharmacological action of misoprostol is mainly due to its hyperstimulation of uterus resulting in uterine rupture, fetal distress and abnormal fetal heart rate. The **delivery induced by misoprostol is quick but delivery induced by dinoprostone is safe**.[20] Hence, dinoprostone is preferred.

2. *Carboprost/Dinoprostone for induction of labor in asthmatic pregnant women.*

BACKGROUND

Induction of labor is indicated, if pregnancy is prolonged beyond 41 weeks. It is helpful to prevent maternal and fetal risks and to reduce the perinatal morbidity and mortality. Both prostaglandins E_2 and $F_{2\alpha}$ cause contractions of pregnant uterus as they have potent oxytocic activity but unlike oxytocin, they are devoid of antidiuretic effect and PGE_2 has additional natriuretic effect promoting excretion of sodium.

DINOPROSTONE

Dinoprostone is a synthetic preparation of prostaglandin E_2 (PGE_2) and more potent than carboprost. When applied as intravaginal insert it causes cervical softening and results in greater degree of uterine stimulation. It does not result in any cardiovascular complications. It results in minimal GIT related side effects, so it can be given safely through oral route. Being PGE_2 analog, dinoprostone can be used safely in pregnant women with asthma as it does not result in bronchoconstriction.

CARBOPROST

Carboprost is an analog of prostaglandin $F_{2\alpha}$ $(PGF_{2\alpha})$ and only one tenth as potent as dinoprostone but has equal efficacy, if given intravenously. Carboprost stimulates uterine contraction and also induces cervical ripening. Cardiovascular complications do not occur with carboprost but causes higher GIT toxicity. It causes severe abdominal pain, nausea and vomiting, so can be given only through parenteral route. It is not suitable for oral route of administration. Being a $F_{2\alpha}$ analog it causes potent bronchoconstriction and should be avoided in asthmatic women.

Drug of Choice: Dinoprostone

RATIONALE

Prostaglandins are indicated for induction of labor in post-dated pregnancy. Carboprost and dinoprostone are **equally effective** in inducing labor and are comparable to the efficacy of oxytocin but **carboprost** causes **intense bronchoconstriction** and GIT related side effects. **Dinoprostone** can be applied as vaginal insert and can be **safely administered** in individuals with **asthma**. Hence, dinoprostone is preferred.

3. *Epoprostenol/Treprostinil for the treatment of pulmonary arterial hypertension (PAH).*

BACKGROUND

PGE and PGI are very potent vasodilators that promote vasodilatation by increasing cAMP levels and reducing intracellular calcium of smooth muscles through interaction with IP and EP_4 receptors. Epoprostenol and treprostinil are prostaglandin I_2 analogs and potent vasodilators. Smooth muscle cell and endothelial cell can synthesize PGI_2. These drugs have been used in the treatment of both primary and secondary pulmonary hypertension. Epoprostenol and treprostinil cause vasodilatation of pulmonary arterioles lowering the pulmonary resistance. They improve symptoms, delay progression of disease and improve the survival rate.

TREPROSTINIL

Treprostinil has a longer half-life with duration of clinical action of 4 hours. It is available as inhalational and injectable formulations. The dose ranges from 1 to 10 mg a day given subcutaneously or intravenously otherwise it can be inhaled once in 6 hours when the patient is awake. Treprostinil is preferred to epoprostenol for the treatment of PAH.

EPOPROSTENOL

Epoprostenol has an extremely short half-life of only about 3 to 5 minutes necessitating repeated administration. It is available only as intravenous formulation and has to be given as a continuous infusion creating great inconvenience for the patient which limits its use. Besides, it causes flushing, hypotension, headache, nausea and diarrhea.

Drug of Choice: Treprostinil

RATIONALE

Prostaglandin I$_2$ analogs epoprostenol and treprostinil cause **vasodilatation**, lower pulmonary resistance and are useful in the treatment of PAH. **Epoprostenol** has an **extremely short half-life** of just 3 to 5 minutes. Hence, it has to be administered only as continuous intravenous infusion. So, epoprostenol is not preferred. **Treprostinil** has a **longer half-life** of about 4 hours and can be administered through subcutaneous, intravenous or inhalational route. Hence, treprostinil is preferred to epoprostenol for the treatment of pulmonary arterial hypertension.

4. *Lubiprostone/Prucalopride in constipation dominant irritable bowel syndrome (IBS) in women.*

BACKGROUND

IBS is characterized by recurrent, severe abdominal pain and altered bowel movements. It may involve both visceral afferents of motor or sensory neurons. Visceral dysfunction is usually associated with affective dysfunctions as it is a psychosomatic disorder and may present as diarrhea or constipation dominant form. Increased visceral sensitivity or visceral hyperalgesia due to either a noxious or physiological stimuli causes hyperactivity. Serotonin may have a possible role in increased sensitization.

LUBIPROSTONE

It is a prostanoid activator of chloride channels approved for constipation dominant IBS in women. The chloride channels mediate transport of fluid in intestinal epithelial cells. Lubiprostone activates type 2 chloride channel increasing intestinal fluid secretion facilitating bowel movement, increasing intestinal transit and passage of stools. It improves spontaneous movement of bowels resulting in sustained improvement. Presynaptic receptors of intrinsic primary afferent nerves of GIT contain mainly $5HT_4$ receptors. Lubiprostone also promotes release of calcitonin gene related peptide. Acetylcholine and calcitonin gene related peptide favor the stimulation of peristalsis. It directly stimulates $5HT_4$ receptors and also increases the release of acetyl choline. It is well-tolerated and results in nausea as its main side effect. It is listed under category C and should be avoided in pregnant women.

PRUCALOPRIDE

Prucalopride is a derivative of benzofuran with $5HT_4$ receptor agonistic activity. It facilitates cholinergic neurotransmission selectively increasing bowel motility. It acts throughout the entire length of GIT increasing its transit time but does not interfere with gastric emptying time. When compared to lubiprostone, prucalopride has a lower efficacy. It causes nausea, diarrhea, abdominal pain and headache as frequent adverse effects. It interacts with cardiac pore forming subunits of HERG K^+ channels and has the potential to prolong QT interval and to cause arrhythmias.

Drug of Choice: Lubiprostone

RATIONALE

IBS is a psychosomatic disorder and can present as diarrhea or constipation dominant form. $5HT_3$ receptors are involved in diarrhea dominant type while $5HT_4$ receptors are involved in constipation dominant type. **Lubiprostone** is **a $5HT_4$** receptor **agonist, induces peristalsis and motility**. It activates type 2 chloride channel increasing intestinal fluid secretion facilitating bowel movement. Therefore, it increases intestinal transit and passage of stools. It is **better tolerated** than prucalopride but produces nausea as a side effect. Lubiprostone is approved for constipation dominant IBS in women. **Prucalopride** is a derivative of benzofuran with **$5HT_4$** receptor **agonist** activity. **It facilitates** cholinergic neurotransmission specifically increasing the **motility** but has **a lower efficacy**. It interacts with the cardiac pore forming subunits of HERG K^+ channels so, has a higher risk of causing **cardiac arrhythmias**. Hence, prucalopride is not preferred.

Nonsteroidal Anti-inflammatory Drugs, Gout, Rheumatoid Arthritis and Central Nervous System

CHAPTER
11

Nonsteroidal Anti-inflammatory Drugs

1. *Aspirin/Naproxen in secondary prevention of myocardial infarction and stroke.*

BACKGROUND

Vascular endothelial damage causes release of thromboxane A_2 leading to formation of thrombus. The prostaglandin I_2 synthesized in intima of vessels inhibits the platelet aggregation. Arterial thrombus is different from venous thrombus because it consists of platelets mainly. Therefore, a drug inhibiting platelet aggregation will prevent the formation of arterial thrombus. Cyclooxygenase-1 or COX_1 derived thromboxane A_2 is the dominant prostanoid in platelets, whereas COX_2 derived thromboxane A_2 is the dominant prostanoid in macrophages. Activation of COX_1 leads to synthesis of TXA_2 while COX_2 activation releases PGI_2.

ASPIRIN

Among NSAIDs, aspirin is the only irreversible inhibitor of COX enzyme; all other NSAIDs are reversible inhibitors of cyclooxygenase enzyme. Aspirin at 75 mg/day causes selective, cumulative, irreversible inhibition of COX_1. At higher doses, it causes inhibition of COX_2 mediated PGI_2 synthesis. Since PGI_2 inhibits platelet aggregation, higher dose of aspirin should be avoided as it favors platelet aggregation. Aspirin binds covalently to serine 529 of platelet COX_1 causing permanent acetylation, so synthesis of TXA_2 is inhibited permanently during the life time of platelets. Since anucleated platelet is incapable of synthesizing COX_1 it causes permanent inhibition of thromboxane A_2.

NAPROXEN

Naproxen is a long acting reversible nonselective COX inhibitor and causes persistent platelet inhibition but it is effective only at a high dose of 500 mg b.i.d thereby increasing the possibility of side effects. It causes only 10% risk reduction of myocardial infarction (MI) in contrast to 25% reduction by aspirin. The choice of NSAID is determined by its dose, duration and degree of cyclooxygenase selectivity. Naproxen has to be given at a high dose for longer duration as it is non selective and causes headache, dizziness and ototoxicity.

Drug of Choice: Aspirin

RATIONALE

Low dose aspirin is preferred to naproxen as an antiplatelet agent because it results in a **more selective, cumulative, irreversible inhibition of COX$_1$** while **naproxen** causes **non-selective COX inhibition** and has to be given at a higher dose for a longer period thereby increasing the risk of its adverse effects. Its toxicity is further potentiated by its prolonged half-life. Hence, naproxen is not preferred.

2. *Indomethacin/Ibuprofen in patent ductus arteriosus of premature infants and neonates.*

BACKGROUND

The patency of ductus arteriosus is maintained by prostaglandin E derived from COX$_1$ so a drug causing more selective inhibition of PGE will be more effective. Left to right cardiac shunt in patent ductus arteriosus (PDA) causes higher pulmonary perfusion but reduces the systemic perfusion. Systemic hypoperfusion may result in cerebral intraventricular hemorrhage. Closure of PDA is dependent mainly on the period of gestation and failure of spontaneous closure of PDA may not always require surgical ligation. Intravenous administration of indomethacin and ibuprofen are approved by Food and Drug Administration (FDA) for medical management of PDA. NSAIDs are useful only in premature infants and neonates but not in full term babies. They are both contraindicated in premature infants and neonates with renal failure, hyperbilirubinemia, enterocolitis and thrombocytopenia.

INDOMETHACIN

Indomethacin is more COX_1 selective but ibuprofen is a nonselective COX inhibitor. Hence, indomethacin results in a direct COX dependent vasoconstriction leading to closure of ductus arteriosus and decreases the incidence of cerebral intraventricular hemorrhage. Effective dose is 0.1 to 0.25 mg/kg IV every 12 hours repeated three times but renal output has to be monitored continuously. An additional course of indomethacin therapy may be needed to prevent reopening of ductus arteriosus.

IBUPROFEN

Ibuprofen is a nonselective COX inhibitor and does not decrease the incidence of intraventricular hemorrhage but causes higher incidence of chronic lung disease in due course. Ibuprofen is given at the dose of 10 mg /kg IV bolus, followed by 5 mg/kg/day for two consecutive days.

Drug of Choice: Indomethacin

RATIONALE

Indomethacin is the **standard drug** preferred for closure of patent ductus arteriosus in premature infants and neonates as it is more COX_1 selective and inhibits COX_1 dependent PG-E mediated PDA while **decreasing** the **incidence of intraventricular hemorrhage**, a usual complication seen in PDA. **Ibuprofen** is **equieffective** to indomethacin but **does not decrease the incidence of intraventricular hemorrhage**. Its therapeutic dose is higher than indomethacin and leads to **higher incidence of chronic lung disease** in latter part of life. Hence, ibuprofen is not preferred.

3. *Ketorolac tromethamine 0.5%/Prednisolone acetate 1% eye drops in immediate postoperative period for pain and inflammation following cataract extraction and corneal refractive surgery.*

BACKGROUND

Post-surgical inflammatory response occurs due to accumulation of prostaglandins. This results in complications such as posterior synechiae, uveitis and secondary glaucoma. Prostaglandins cause intense inflammation after surgery and increase the vascular permeability resulting in edema. Swelling of fovea and cystoid macular edema may occur few weeks after surgery. Postoperative pain and photophobia are common complaints after corneal refractive surgery so, it is necessary to inhibit the synthesis of PG to control pain and inflammation. NSAIDs and corticosteroids can inhibit the synthesis of PGs. NSAIDs diclofenac sodium 0.1% and ketorolac tromethamine 0.5% are effective.

KETOROLAC TROMETHAMINE

NSAIDs inhibit hyperemia and pain by suppressing the synthesis of PGs. They also prevent intraoperative miosis[21] during cataract surgery. Administration through systemic route does not achieve sufficient level in ciliary body and iris but topical administration achieves adequate concentration in these target tissues.

PREDNISOLONE ACETATE

Steroids used are prednisolone acetate 1% and betamethasone sodium 0.1%. NSAIDs interfere with the synthesis of PGs by inhibiting cyclooxygenase enzyme, but corticosteroids act at a step higher to NSAIDs. They inhibit phospholipase A_2 necessary for the formation of arachidonic acid. This establishes their supremacy over NSAIDs as anti-inflammatory agents. Steroids are highly potent and have good ocular penetration and they achieve high intraocular concentration, yet they are not the preferred drugs and have only limited benefit because steroids delay wound healing process by inhibiting fibroblast infiltration. They also have the propensity to cause dose dependent increase in IOP.[22] In view of the above they should be avoided during immediate postoperative period.

Drug of Choice: Ketorolac Tromethamine 0.5% Eye Drops

RATIONALE

Although proven to be a **better anti-inflammatory** agent when compared to ketorolac, **prednisolone** acetate as eye drops is **not preferred** as it **delays** postoperative **wound healing** and can cause a **dose dependent increase** in **intraocular pressure**. Hence, corticosteroids should be avoided during the **immediate postoperative period**. **Ketorolac** is preferred[23] because it **prevents intraoperative miosis** in addition to inhibiting PG mediated pain, hyperemia, leucocytic infiltration and inflammation.

4. *Etodolac/Piroxicam as analgesic for acute pain during early postoperative period.*

BACKGROUND

Inflammatory mediators are responsible for postoperative pain and inflammation. Tissue injury releases mediators that cause peripheral sensitization of nociceptors. Central sensitization also contributes to hyperalgesia and allodynia during this period. Centrally acting PGE_2 increases the excitability of peripheral dorsal horn neurons. COX_1 derived PGs play a dominant role during the early phase of inflammation. Generally, major source of proinflammatory PGs are COX_2 and COX_1 which accounts for only 10% of PGs synthesized during inflammation. COX_2 is rapidly inducted in inflamed tissue and cells at sites of inflammation. During early stage of post- operative inflammation there is upregulation of COX_2. This activates dorsal horn neurons contributing to central sensitization and pain. Therefore, a COX_2 selective inhibitor will be more preferable in acute postoperative pain. NSAIDs are organic acids and accumulate at sites of inflammation as the pH is acidic.

ETODOLAC

Etodolac is a COX_2 selective hydrophobic agent that binds freely with the hydrophobic domain of COX_2 and inhibits conversion of arachidonic acid to prostaglandin. A single oral dose of 200 to 400 mg provides good relief for 6 to 8 hours.

PIROXICAM

Piroxicam is nonselective anti-inflammatory agent and provides additional benefit through inhibition of neutrophils activation. Piroxicam undergoes enterohepatic circulation and has a prolonged duration of action. It has a slow onset of action and has a considerable delay in reaching steady state concentration. Hence, piroxicam is not suitable as analgesic in acute conditions.

Drug of Choice: Etodolac

RATIONALE

Etodolac is **preferred** to piroxicam as an analgesic and anti-inflammatory agent in **early stages** of postoperative period because it is a **selective COX_2 inhibitor,** the principal **mediator** of pain and inflammation during this period. Although **piroxicam** offers **additional benefit** in preventing inflammation by inhibiting leucocytic infiltration resulting in prolonged postoperative analgesia, it is **not suitable in early phases** of postoperative period as its **onset of action and the time required for reaching steady state concentration is delayed**.

5. *Tramadol/Diclofenac as postoperative analgesic after colorectal surgeries.*

BACKGROUND

Colorectal surgery is a high risk surgery where colonic blood flow plays a critical role. Adequate blood supply is necessary for early restoration of tissue tensile strength. Colorectal cancer, inflammatory bowel disease, diverticulitis are few conditions that require colorectal surgery. Analgesics relieve pain and help to achieve early mobilization after surgery.

TRAMADOL

Tramadol, a synthetic codeine analog is preferred to other opioids such as morphine. It does not cause drug dependence and respiratory depression. Apart from being μ agonist, tramadol has additional mechanisms. It inhibits reuptake of norepinephrine and serotonin. It results in significant nausea and vomiting, so metoclopramide or ondansetron are given as prophylactic antiemetics. Otherwise, it is generally well-tolerated and devoid of respiratory depression which is the most severe side effect of opioids. SSRIs, MAOIs and tricyclic antidepressants are contraindicated in patients receiving tramadol.

DICLOFENAC

The analgesic action of the NSAID diclofenac is comparable to opioids induced analgesia. It is used either alone or in combination with opioids during postoperative period and reduces the incidence of opioid induced respiratory depression. During early healing process the anastomotic strength of colon tissue depends on colonic blood supply. The balance between production and breakdown of connective tissue plays a vital role in the process of healing. Diclofenac inhibits matrix metalloproteinases involved in the synthesis of collagen needed for formation of connective tissue. Inhibition of collagen results in anastomotic leakage at the site of surgery. As a more selective COX_2 inhibitor diclofenac reduces the blood supply of colon by inhibiting the synthesis of PGI_2, a potent vasodilator. Therefore, diclofenac should not be used as postoperative analgesic for colorectal surgeries.

Drug of Choice: Tramadol

RATIONALE

Tramadol, an opioid analgesic with **additional mechanisms** of action, is **preferred** to diclofenac, a potent, more selective COX_2 inhibitor as it **does not inhibit colonic blood supply** and **synthesis** of **collagen** during post operative period of colorectal surgeries. Tramadol induced nausea and vomiting can be managed by an antiemetic. It can be either given alone in the dose of 50 to 100 mg qid IM or in combination with acetaminophen (paracetamol) (multimodal analgesia). **Diclofenac** should be **avoided**, as it **increases** the **incidence** of **anastomotic leakage**, due to its interference with formation of collagen and colonic blood supply.

6. *Diclofenac/Aectaminophen (Paracetamol) as an anti-inflammatory agent.*

BACKGROUND

Factors promoting inflammation are physical injury, environmental pathogens and infection. Histamine, prostaglandins, leukotrienes, interleukin and TNF-α are some of the mediators involved in promoting and resolving process. Hydrogen peroxide plays a key role as a signaling molecule in inflammation and its concentration is very high at sites of inflammation. COX_1 and COX_2 play an important role in inflammation but COX_2 generates around 80 to 90% of PGs that take part in this process. In the presence of peroxides, a drug with selective COX_2 inhibitor action is preferable as it decreases PG synthesis.

DICLOFENAC

Diclofenac is a highly selective COX_2 inhibitor and potent anti-inflammatory agent. The action of diclofenac is not inhibited by peroxides found at sites of inflammation. It is absorbed rapidly and highly protein bound but has a short half-life of 1 to 2 hours due to high first pass metabolism. It can be administered as a gel or transdermal patch over inflamed surfaces. Such formulations reduce its gastrointestinal and renal side effects.

ACETAMINOPHEN (PARACETAMOL)

Acetaminophen (paracetamol) is a very potent analgesic and antipyretic but it is a weak anti-inflammatory agent. It inhibits only 50% of COX accumulated at sites of inflammation. The action of acetaminophen (paracetamol) is minimal at sites of inflammation due to high level of peroxides.

Drug of Choice: Diclofenac

RATIONALE

Diclofenac is preferred to acetaminophen (paracetamol) as anti-inflammatory agent because it is a **more selective COX$_2$ inhibitor**, a major mediator of PGs synthesis involved in inflammation. **Acetaminophen (paracetamol)** is **incapable** of inhibiting COX in the **presence** of **peroxides** found at the site of **inflammation**. This makes acetaminophen (paracetamol) a weak anti-inflammatory agent, therefore it is not preferred.

7. *Sulindac/Celecoxib in familial adeno polyposis (FAP).*

BACKGROUND

Familial adeno polyposis (FAP) is a rare hereditary disorder during adolescence and is characterized by numerous adenomatous polyps in large intestine. Mutations in autosomal dominant APC gene results in hereditary adenoma syndrome and autosomal recessive FAP is due to mutation of autosomal recessive MUTYH gene. If left untreated, FAP may progress to colorectal cancer. COX$_2$ mediated PGE$_2$ promotes tumor cell proliferation and PGI$_2$ favors angiogenesis and spread of tumor. Among NSAIDs, sulindac and celecoxib reduce polyp burden. They are therefore indicated as adjuncts in medical management of FAP.

SULINDAC

Sulindac is a congener of indomethacin but with lower toxicity profile. It is a prodrug and its metabolite is 500 times more potent than the parent compound. It is a COX inhibitor and inhibits angiogenesis and tumor cell proliferation. Its toxic profile is similar to NSAIDs but does not increase the risk of thrombosis. Sulindac is therefore more suited than Celecoxib. Currently a phase III trial is evaluating the effect of sulindac and eflornithine, an irreversible inhibitor of ornithine decarboxylase.

CELECOXIB

Celecoxib is a selective COX_2 inhibitor and preferentially inhibits angiogenesis. It inhibits proangiogenic PGI_2 and PGE_2, the tumor cell proliferator. It confers a risk of thrombosis and atherogenesis as it inhibits synthesis of PGI_2. Celecoxib is associated with higher incidence of myocardial infarction and stroke and therefore better avoided in medical management of FAP.

Drug of Choice: Sulindac

RATIONALE

Even though celecoxib is a **selective COX_2 inhibitor** and offers protection in FAP by **inhibiting cellular proliferation** and tumor spread, it is still **not preferred** to sulindac on account of its capacity to **induce thrombosis** and **atherogenesis**. **Sulindac** is a congener of indomethacin sharing **similar toxic profile** of nonselective NSAIDs but it inhibits angiogenesis and cellular proliferation **without increasing the risk of thrombosis**. Hence, sulindac is preferred.

8. *Indomethacin/Aspirin in fever due to Hodgkin lymphoma refractory to Acetaminophen (Paracetamol).*

BACKGROUND

Fever is often associated with Hodgkin lymphoma, stroke and advanced pelvic malignancies. Various types of lymphomas and leukemia present most commonly as fever of unknown origin. Hodgkin lymphoma is also known to cause relapsing pyrexia that may present as classical Pal Ebstein fever with intermittent temperature above 38°C. It may be lasting one to two weeks or may be nonclassical. It is usually refractory to common antipyretic like acetaminophen (paracetamol).

INDOMETHACIN

Indomethacin is a much more potent nonselective inhibitor of COX than aspirin and has excellent oral bioavailability. It achieves peak plasma concentration within 2 hours. Although it results in fatal

GIT side effects, acute pancreatitis and frontal headache, it is still the drug of choice for refractory fever associated with Hodgkin's disease because it is very effective for those who are capable of tolerating it.

ASPIRIN

Aspirin is a more potent irreversible inhibitor of COX and inhibits the synthesis of prostaglandins by inhibiting this enzyme. Aspirin is an efficient analgesic and antipyretic but fever associated with Hodgkin's usually fails to respond to aspirin.

Drug of Choice: Indomethacin

RATIONALE

Indomethacin is **not** a **commonly** used agent as an **antipyretic** because of its capacity to cause severe side effects **but** given the severity of fever associated with **Hodgkin's** lymphoma and the fact that it does not usually respond to an irreversible, potent COX inhibitor like aspirin, it is considered to be the drug of choice **provided** it is well **tolerated** by the individual.

9. *Aspirin/Acetaminophen (Paracetamol) as antipyretic in fever of viral origin.*

BACKGROUND

Reye's syndrome is severe complication of type B influenza viral infection. It is rapidly progressive, characterized by hepatic failure and encephalopathy and responsible for 30% mortality rate. Its pathogenesis is unknown and it increases serum prothrombin time and elevates serum transaminases.

ACETAMINOPHEN (PARACETAMOL)

Acetaminophen (Paracetamol) is not associated with Reye's syndrome in children and young adults. It is a nonselective COX inhibitor with disproportionately more central effect. This effect of acetaminophen (paracetamol) forms the basis for its antipyretic action.

It has a quick onset, reaches peak plasma concentrations within 30 minutes. It is very effective, has rapid onset of action, an important property useful in speedy termination of fever.

ASPIRIN

Reye's syndrome is often associated with administration of aspirin in viral fever. Aspirin triggers an underlying metabolic condition, masked by viral infection. It is an efficient antipyretic agent as it causes irreversible COX inhibition but contraindicated in children with viral fever as it triggers Reye's syndrome.

Drug of Choice: Acetaminophen (Paracetamol)

RATIONALE

Acetaminophen (Paracetamol) is preferred to aspirin as an anti-pyretic in children with viral infection as it is **rapidly acting, very effective, safe**, usually **well tolerated** with minimal GIT side effects. **Aspirin** is an **irreversible** COX inhibitor, more efficient as antipyretic compared to other NSAIDs but **contraindicated** in children with fever of viral origin as it can **trigger** Reye's syndrome.

10. *Acetaminophen (paracetamol)/Diclofenac in osteoarthritis.*

BACKGROUND

Osteoarthritis, a disease of aging occurs more commonly in women. It causes degeneration of cartilage and hypertrophy of articular bone margins. Inflammation is minimal but pain and restriction of joint movements is troublesome, joint effusion and inflammation of synovial fluid is absent. In view of the above, the need for anti-inflammatory drug does not arise.

ACETAMINOPHEN (PARACETAMOL)

Acetaminophen (Paracetamol) has minimal anti-inflammatory but a very potent analgesic action. Frequent administration does not result in cardiovascular and GIT toxicity. It is also devoid of uricosuric effects. Since long-term therapy is required in osteoarthritis acetaminophen (paracetamol) is preferred as it is less toxic.

DICLOFENAC

Diclofenac is a much more potent analgesic and anti-inflammatory agent but its toxicity profile outweighs its therapeutic benefits in osteoarthritis because prolonged therapy is required. Increase in serum transaminases level and renal toxicity occur on prolonged use.

Drug of Choice: Acetaminophen (Paracetamol)

RATIONALE

Management of pain in osteoarthritis is a continuous process where an analgesic has to be given on a daily basis for a long period of time. Since the predominant feature is **pain** and **not inflammation**, a drug with excellent analgesic action is usually better tolerated than an analgesic, anti-inflammatory drug for long-term therapy. NSAIDs with anti-inflammatory property have higher toxicity profile and are unsuitable for continuous, daily administration. Therefore, **acetaminophen (paracetamol)** is preferred as the **first line analgesic** in osteoarthritis.

12

Pharmacotherapy of Gout

1. *Nonsteroidal anti-inflammatory drugs/Colchicine in acute gout.*

BACKGROUND

Gout is a familial metabolic disease due to abnormal uric acid level. Hyperuricemia is either due to over production of uric acid or due to its reduced excretion. Inflammation and gouty pain are caused by precipitation of monosodium urate crystals. Acute gouty arthritis has a sudden onset and occurs most frequently during night.

NONSTEROIDAL ANTI-INFLAMMATORY DRUGS

Nonsteroidal anti-inflammatory drugs (NSAIDs) are analgesic and anti-inflammatory agents so are preferred. They are very effective in acute gout if given within first 24 hours. At higher doses, they cause substantial reduction of pain and inflammation. Such high doses are nephrotoxic and induce severe gastritis. They are therefore contraindicated in peptic ulcer and renal dysfunction.

COLCHICINE

Colchicine has good therapeutic efficacy and causes excellent pain relief in gout. Symptoms like pain and swelling disappear within 12 hours in 70% of patients but colchicine is highly toxic and has a narrow therapeutic index. Therefore, colchicine is considered only as second line drug in acute gout.

Drug of Choice: Nonsteroidal Anti-inflammatory Drugs

RATIONALE

The onset of acute gout is **nocturnal** and often **sudden**. The symptoms are usually very severe. Pain and inflammation respond very well to both NSAIDs and colchicine if given immediately after the onset of symptoms. Although the therapeutic efficacy of **colchicine** is superior to NASIDs, the **therapeutic window is narrow**. NSAIDs are better tolerated. Hence, NSAIDs are preferred to colchicine in acute gout.

2. *Naproxen/Aspirin in the treatment of acute gouty arthritis.*

BACKGROUND

Acute gout resolves on its own even if left untreated but therapy with anti-inflammatory agents promotes faster recovery. NSAIDs effectively control pain and inflammation of acute gouty arthritis. They act by inhibiting the synthesis of prostaglandins. NSAIDs indicated in the treatment of acute gout are naproxen, indomethacin and sulindac.

NAPROXEN

Naproxen is more commonly used NSAID. It is a reversible COX inhibitor and has long duration of action. It is a very effective analgesic and as an anti-inflammatory agent. Uric acid anionic transporter (URAT) is responsible for reabsorption of urate and uric acid is transported through this transporter in bidirectional manner. Naproxen does not interfere with uric acid transport. Naproxen at the dose of 500 mg twice daily is very effective.

ASPIRIN

The action of aspirin is influenced by its dose. Lower dose of aspirin inhibits, while higher dose stimulates URAT. Aspirin at 1 to 2 g/day, leads to retention of uric acid by inhibiting its excretion. If given between 2 to 3 g/day, it does not interfere with urate excretion. It displays uricosuric action only at a high dose of more than 5 g/day but such a high dose can result in renal damage and can also potentiate the risk of nephrolithiasis. Since the anti-inflammatory dose of aspirin causes uric acid retention it should be avoided in the treatment of acute gout.

Drug of Choice: Naproxen

RATIONALE

NSAIDs are generally indicated in the treatment of gouty arthritis for immediate control of inflammation and pain. The NSAID **aspirin** should **not** be used due to its **variable action** in plasma level of uric acid. At **anti-inflammatory dose**, it inhibits uric acid excretion **increasing serum uric acid level** and worsening the clinical picture of gout. Very high dose is required for uricosuric action of aspirin and such a high dose can cause renal calculi and analgesic nephropathy. Hence, naproxen is preferred to aspirin in the treatment of acute gout.

3. *NSAIDs/Allopurinol in acute gout.*

BACKGROUND

Acute gout is characterized by onset of severe nocturnal pain. Urate crystals provoke the inflammatory process and an anti-inflammatory agent is more effective in terminating acute attacks.

NSAIDs

Naproxen, indomethacin, sulindac, celecoxib and etoricoxib are effective. Aspirin should be avoided as its toxicity outweighs its usefulness. NSAIDs inhibit synthesis of prostaglandins, reduce pain and swelling.

ALLOPURINOL

Allopurinol inhibits action of enzyme xanthine oxidase. Allopurinol is an analog of hypoxanthine, the precursor of uric acid. Xanthine oxidase mediates synthesis of uric acid from hypoxanthine and inhibits oxidation of hypoxanthine and xanthine. During initial administration, allopurinol increases plasma uric acid level by mobilizing tissue stores of uric acid to plasma but this pharmacological effect worsens the clinical picture of acute gout. Allopurinol actually increases the incidence of acute attacks of gout. Hence, allopurinol should be avoided during acute gouty arthritis.

Drug of Choice: NSAIDs

RATIONALE

NSAIDs like **naproxen** are **preferred** in the management of acute attacks of gouty arthritis. As analgesic and anti-inflammatory agents, they inhibit prostaglandin synthesis thereby reducing pain and inflammation. During early months of treatment, instead of reducing uric acid level, **allopurinol** actually increases its plasma concentration **potentiating** the risk of **acute gouty attacks**. Hence, allopurinol should be avoided during acute gout.

4. *Allopurinol/Colchicine in the treatment of chronic gout.*

BACKGROUND

Chronic gout is associated with repeated episodes of acute attack. It is characterized by precipitation of uric acid crystals in joints. The main aim of treatment is to lower uric acid level to prevent recurrent attacks.

ALLOPURINOL

Allopurinol is an inhibitor of xanthine oxidase enzyme, inhibiting the enzyme competitively at low doses and noncompetitively at higher doses. Its metabolite oxypurinol also suppresses xanthine oxidase. Inhibition of xanthine oxidase prevents the conversion of hypoxanthine to uric acid. Low uric acid level prevents the precipitation of monosodium urate crystals reducing inflammatory pain induced by urate crystals. Allopurinol inhibits the progression of chronic gout by reducing plasma urate level. It also facilitates the dissolution of gouty tophi.

COLCHICINE

Colchicine is antimitotic and inhibits neutrophil motility. It inhibits release of neutrophil chemotactic factors induced by urate crystals. It is more effective in controlling the acute episodes rather than chronic gout. Hence, allopurinol is the most widely used medication in chronic gout.

Drug of Choice: Allopurinol

RATIONALE

Chronic gout is characterized by frequent acute attacks of gouty arthritis. **Allopurinol** is traditionally the most widely used drug as it inhibits the synthesis of uric acid. It **inhibits progression** of chronic gout and **facilitates dissolution** of tophi. **Colchicine does not inhibit** synthesis of **uric acid** but inhibits inflammatory reactions during acute gout. It has a minimal safety profile. Hence, colchicine is more suited for acute therapy while **allopurinol** is **effective** in **chronic therapy**.

5. *Allopurinol/Febuxostat in chronic gout.*

BACKGROUND

The therapeutic target in chronic gout is reduction of uric acid level. Xanthine oxidase inhibitors cause significant reduction of uric acid. Allopurinol and febuxostat are xanthine oxidase inhibitors and they dissolve uric acid crystals in tophi.

ALLOPURINOL

The clinical efficacy of allopurinol is similar to febuxostat but is less potent. It is well tolerated but may cause Stevens-Johnson syndrome and this risk is expected only in the initial period of two months. Hence, it has a better safety profile than febuxostat.

FEBUXOSTAT

Febuxostat is a non-purine inhibitor of enzyme xanthine oxidase inhibiting the catalytic function of xanthine oxidase. It lowers reduced and oxidized form of this enzyme by forming a stable complex. Febuxostat causes prompt and prominent reduction of uric acid concentration. Febuxostat is more potent and has clinical supremacy over allopurinol in achieving target urate level but has questionable safety profile. It results in higher incidence of myocardial infarction and stroke.

Drug of Choice: Allopurinol

RATIONALE

The clinical efficacy of **allopurinol** in achieving target serum uric acid concentration is lower than febuxostat but has a **better safety profile**. **Febuxostat** is a **novel xanthine oxidase inhibitor** that competitively inhibits the function of xanthine oxidase. It is more potent and has greater clinical supremacy over allopurinol but has **higher toxicity profile** as it increases the risk of **myocardial infarction** and **stroke**.[24] Hence, it is not preferred in chronic gout.

6. *Probenecid/Benzbromarone as an alternative agent to allopurinol.*

BACKGROUND

Probenecid and benzbromarone are uricosuric agents and increase the rate of excretion of uric acid. They are used as alternative uricosuric agents to allopurinol.

PROBENECID

Probenecid inhibits reabsorption of uric acid mediated through URAT-1. It competes with uric acid for this transporter and reduces the uric acid level. Since increased excretion of uric acid may cause nephrolithiasis, the patient should be advised to take adequate fluid therapy. Probenecid is the uricosuric agent of choice in patients intolerant to allopurinol.

BENZBROMARONE

Benzbromarone is a reversible inhibitor of urate anionic transporter. Its metabolites also have uricosuric action but can result in hepatotoxicity so are not preferred.

Drug of Choice: Probenecid

RATIONALE

Probenecid and benzbromarone are uricosuric agents. Uric acid is freely filtered at the glomerulus. These drugs inhibit the reabsorption of uric acid. **Benzbromarone** is a potent uricosuric agent but may cause **hepatotoxicity**. **Probenecid** is preferable and is very **effective** in reducing the plasma urate concentration. Since it causes nephrolithiasis, the patient should be advised to take plenty of fluids.

Rheumatoid Arthritis

1. *NSAIDs/DMARDs in rheumatoid arthritis.*

BACKGROUND

Rheumatoid arthritis is a chronic inflammatory disease involving multiple joints. It is an autoimmune condition, three times more prevalent in women than men. The risk factor is HLA DRB1 allele encoding a 5 amino acid sequence or 'shared epitope'. Treatment aims at reduction of pain and inflammation, with preservation of function.

DMARDs

Disease modifying antirheumatoid drugs are known as DMARDs. They include both biological and nonbiological or synthetic agents. They reduce the severity of the disease and retard the progression of arthritis thereby improving the quality of life.

NSAIDs

NSAIDs are analgesic, anti-inflammatory agents and reduce pain and inflammation. Their clinical action is mediated through inhibition of prostaglandin synthesis. They provide only symptomatic relief but do not inhibit the progression of disease.

Drug of Choice: DMARDs

RATIONALE

Being a chronic inflammatory autoimmune condition, rheumatoid arthritis affects multiple joints and requires prolonged therapy.

Although **NSAIDs** offer **symptomatic** relief, they do not affect the course of disease. **DMARDs** act after a **lag period** but they are effective in **arresting** the **progression** of disease. In view of the above, DMARDs are preferred to NSAIDs for long-term management.

2. *Synthetic DMARDs/Biologic DMARDs in rheumatoid arthritis.*

BACKGROUND

DMARDs should be started soon after confirmation of the diagnosis. Only then they are effective in retarding the tissue destruction.

SYNTHETIC DMARDs

Methotrexate, sulfasalazine and leflunomide are few of the synthetic DMARDs. Nonbiological DMARDs are effective for mild to moderate disease. They are given either as monotherapy or in combination with other DMARDs.

BIOLOGIC DMARDs

Tumor necrosis factor inhibitors (TNF) are biologic DMARDs. They are very effective in arresting the progression of disease. They inhibit TNF, main mediators of rheumatoid arthritis but have a very severe toxicity profile and need to be used cautiously. They increase the risk of serious infections, lymphomas and other malignancies. Therefore, their clinical use should be weighed against their potential toxic profile. They are preferred only in patients with extra-articular involvement and bony erosions and can be combined with either NSAIDs or with nonbiologic DMARDs.

Drug of Choice: Synthetic DMARDs

RATIONALE

Nonbiologic DMARDs are effective mainly in **mild** to **moderate** rheumatoid arthritis but **biologic DMARDs** are effective even in **severe** form of rheumatoid arthritis as they inhibit TNF, main mediator of the disease. **Biologic DMARDs** have a **higher**

toxicity profile. Hence, they are not preferred for monotherapy in the treatment of rheumatoid arthritis.

3. *Methotrexate/Sulfasalazine as a DMARD in rheumatoid arthritis.*

BACKGROUND

Both methotrexate and sulfasalazine are anti-inflammatory agents. They are synthetic DMARDs and they retard the course of disease. As anti-inflammatory agents, they reduce pain and swelling of joints.

METHOTREXATE

Rheumatoid arthritis is an autoimmune condition, causing immune reactions. Methotrexate is more effective as it is an immunosuppressant agent. It is a folate antagonist and an anticancer drug. If given in the dose of 7.5 to 15 mg/week it causes relief from symptoms within 2 to 6 weeks but can cause gastric irritation, stomatitis and bone marrow depression. Usually well tolerated even by children, yet should be avoided in pregnancy as it is a teratogenic agent.

SULFASALAZINE

Sulfasalazine, an anti-inflammatory agent, is a second line drug in this condition. Its active ingredient is 5-aminosalicylic acid that inhibits TNF-α and PAF. It has only modest efficacy but results in rashes, hemolysis and blood dyscrasias. Twenty five percent of patients do not tolerate this drug and suffer from neutropenia and thrombocytopenia so monitoring of blood count is essential for all patients treated with sulfasalazine.

Drug of Choice: Methotrexate

RATIONALE

Synthetic DMARDs are started as initial treatment in rheumatoid arthritis as they **retard** the course of disease. Since rheumatoid arthritis is an **autoimmune** condition, the immunosuppressant **methotrexate** is preferred as **first line** drug. It is effective in reducing the symptoms, well tolerated for long-term treatment, can safely be combined with other nonbiological DMARDs but it should not be used in hepatitis and pregnancy. **Sulfasalazine** is **not an immunosuppressant**. It has only modest efficacy as an **anti-inflammatory** agent but can result in severe toxicity. In view of the above, sulfasalazine is not preferred.

4. *Etanercept/Abatacept in refractory rheumatoid arthritis.*

BACKGROUND

Tumor necrosis factor (TNF) is a proinflammatory cytokine and is one of the main mediators in pathogenesis of this condition. Etanercept and abatacept are TNF inhibitors effective in refractory rheumatoid arthritis.

ABATACEPT

Abatacept is a T cell modulator and inhibits T cell activation. Patients refractory to methotrexate or biologic DMARDs respond well to abatacept. It is better tolerated but can increase risk for upper respiratory tract infection. Very rarely, it causes infusion related hypersensitivity reactions and lymphomas. When compared to etanercept, the toxicity profile of abatacept is limited. It is suitable as monotherapy and preferred due to its clinical superiority.

ETANERCEPT

Etanercept binds to TNF-α and prevents its interaction with its receptors. It is effective in patients who do not respond to methotrexate monotherapy. It is more effective when combined with methotrexate than when given alone. It causes injection site reactions such as erythema and swelling in one third of the patients and also increases risk of serious bacterial and granulomatous infections.

Drug of Choice: Abatacept

RATIONALE

Etanercept and abatacept are effective in patients with rheumatoid arthritis who do not respond to methotrexate or combination of methotrexate and other drugs. **Etanercept** is **more effective** only when combined with methotrexate **potentiating** the chances for **serious side effects** in one third of patients. **Abatacept** is a T cell modulator, has **clinical superiority** with **better safety profile** and can be used as monotherapy in refractory rheumatoid arthritis.

Opioid Analgesics

1. *Morphine/Pentazocine as analgesic in acute myocardial infarction.*

BACKGROUND

Pain in acute myocardial infarction is of severe intensity and builds up rapidly. Patients suffering from acute MI are usually apprehensive and anxious. The heart rate may range from bradycardia in inferior wall infarction or tachycardia. Similarly, blood pressure may be high in hypertensive patients or low in shock. If pain is not relieved by nitroglycerin or mild analgesics only then opioids are helpful.

MORPHINE

Morphine is preferred because it is a potent analgesic. It allays apprehension and causes euphoria. It also results in a favorable hemodynamic effect in MI patients. It releases histamine from mast cells resulting in peripheral vasodilatation. It decreases heart rate and cardiac contractility by reducing the cardiac work load and reduces myocardial oxygen consumption. Morphine shunts blood from pulmonary to systemic circulation thereby alleviating dyspnea and preventing pulmonary edema. Morphine sulfate 8 mg IV is given initially, repeated if necessary.

PENTAZOCINE

Pentazocine is a weak antagonist and partial agonist at μ receptor and an agonist at κ receptor. Analgesia induced by pentazocine is comparable to morphine and mediated through both μ and κ receptors. It results in unfavorable hemodynamic actions in patients with MI. Unlike other opioid analgesics, pentazocine increases heart rate and blood pressure so it is contraindicated in patients with coronary artery disease.

Drug of Choice: Morphine

RATIONALE

In patients with acute MI, if pain is not relieved after sublingual nitroglycerin, opioids are indicated. Even though **pentazocine** is an opioid analgesic it is **contraindicated** as it **increases** the **heart rate, blood pressure and cardiac work load. Morphine** is **preferred** not only because it is a potent analgesic when compared to pentazocine but also because it **reduces the cardiac workload, myocardial oxygen consumption** and prevents the development of pulmonary edema.

2. *Meperidine (Pethidine)/Fentanyl as obstetric analgesic during labor.*

BACKGROUND

Opioids are used as obstetric analgesics due to their analgesic and euphoric actions but they can cause maternal hypoxemia, postural hypotension, nausea, vomiting, sedation, drowsiness and fetal respiratory depression. Meperidine (pethidine) and fentanyl are commonly used in obstetric analgesia.

FENTANYL

Fentanyl is 1000 times more potent when compared to meperidine (pethidine). If administered intravenously it results in peak analgesic action within 5 minutes. Epidural administration of fentanyl offers a similar degree of analgesia and reduces its plasma concentration thereby reducing the placental transfer. Therefore, it reduces the potential for fetal respiratory depression. Low dose fentanyl is frequently co-administered with a local anesthetic which minimizes the side effects of both agents.

MEPERIDINE (PETHIDINE)

Intravenous meperidine (pethidine) reaches peak plasma concentration within 15 minutes. It neither delays labor nor interferes with uterine contraction during delivery and does not affect involution of uterus. It does not cause postpartum hemorrhage but may delay fetal respiration and decrease oxygen saturation. The concentration of free form of meperidine (pethidine) compared to bound form is high in fetus. Besides nor-meperidine (nor-pethidine), the toxic metabolite of meperidine (pethidine) has higher half-life in fetus, accumulates in fetal blood inducing CNS toxicity.

Drug of Choice: Fentanyl

RATIONALE

Although **meperidine (pethidine)** and fentanyl offer **similar degree** of analgesia and do not prolong labor, **fentanyl** is **preferred** to meperidine (pethidine) as it is **more potent**. Epidural administration offers greater advantage by reducing the placental transfer and neonatal respiratory depression. The dose of fentanyl can be further reduced by combining it with a local anesthetic, a **synergistic combination** minimizing its side effects while retaining the therapeutic benefit.

3. *Meperidine (Pethidine)/Fentanyl for chronic pain management.*

BACKGROUND

Chronic pain can occur in malignant or non-malignant conditions. Repeated daily administration of opioids results in tolerance and physical dependence. Opioids should be the last line drugs in non-malignant chronic pain. They can be tried only after failure of NSAIDs, antidepressants and antiepileptics. Opioids are indicated in chronic cancer pain due to analgesic and euphoric action in spite of their tendency to develop physical dependence.

FENTANYL

Fentanyl has quick onset of action and rapid termination of effect. It is also available as transdermal patches that release the drug for

72 hours and can be given as lollypop lozenges as well as buccal tablets for break through cancer pain. Hence, fentanyl is preferred for chronic pain management.

MEPERIDINE (PETHIDINE)

Meperidine (Pethidine) is metabolized to nor-meperidine (nor-pethidine) which crosses the blood brain barrier. Nor-meperidine (Nor-pethidine) has a longer half-life compared to short half-life of meperidine (pethidine). Frequent administration of meperidine (pethidine) results in accumulation of nor-meperidine (nor-pethidine) in CNS causing hyper excitability and seizures that cannot be reversed even by naloxone, its complete antagonist. Therefore, even though it is a potent analgesic, meperidine (pethidine) is not recommended.

Drug of Choice: Fentanyl

RATIONALE

Meperidine (Pethidine) is **not suitable** for chronic pain management due to accumulation of its **toxic metabolite nor-meperidine (nor-pethidine)** that crosses BBB. If meperidine (pethidine) is given at repeated, short intervals it causes **hyper-excitability** and seizures. Unlike meperidine (pethidine) **fentanyl does not produce a toxic metabolite**. It has quick **onset** and **rapid termination** of effect. Hence, transdermal or buccal fentanyl is preferred to meperidine (pethidine) as analgesic in chronic pain.

4. *Morphine/Meperidine (Pethidine) in postanesthetic shivering.*

BACKGROUND

Shivering occurs frequently during surgery and in postoperative period as the core temperature set point is lowered by volatile general anesthetics. It is an important complication of hypothermia an involuntary oscillatory muscle activity, increasing the metabolic heat production. It stimulates carbon dioxide production and increases cardiac work load. Maintenance of body temperature is vital and hypothermia during surgery may augment perioperative morbidity. It may also interfere with and delay the postoperative wound healing.

MEPERIDINE (PETHIDINE)

Opioids lower the equilibrium point of hypothalamic temperature regulating center causing fall in body temperature. Meperidine (Pethidine) slightly increases threshold for sweating when compared to other opioids but decreases the threshold for vasoconstriction thereby decreasing the threshold for shivering. Small single dose of meperidine (pethidine) is effective in arresting postanesthetic shivering.

MORPHINE

Morphine is less effective than meperidine (pethidine) in controlling postoperative shivering. Besides, it causes release of histamine and stimulates bronchoconstriction. Other opioids useful in this condition are tramadol and alfentanil.

Drug of Choice: Meperidine (Pethidine)

RATIONALE

Shivering, the important complication of hypothermia, where the core temperature set point is lowered increases metabolic heat production through involuntary oscillatory muscle activity. Opioids lower equilibrium point of hypothalamic temperature regulating center. Shivering is managed by a **single small dose of meperidine (pethidine)** as it decreases the threshold for vasoconstriction and shivering. Although **morphine** is indicated in this condition, it is **less effective**, and causes **release of histamine** so, no longer used.

5. *Morphine/Fentanyl as anesthetic adjuvant.*

BACKGROUND

Anesthetic adjuvant helps in reducing the dose of coadministered anesthetics and augments anesthetic parameters specifically.

Given with anesthetics, opioids cause analgesia in perioperative period reducing the hemodynamic changes provoked by pain. Synthetic phenylpiperidine opioids are preferred for this purpose as they have quick onset and shorter duration of action.

FENTANYL

Being more potent and highly lipid soluble than morphine, fentanyl crosses blood brain barrier better than morphine. It has a rapid onset of action, attains peak concentration quickly, has a short duration of action and rapid termination of action. It has relative hemodynamic stability and does not result in histamine release. It has very minimal myocardial depressant action, so can be safely used as primary anesthetic for cardiovascular surgery. Fentanyl is also preferred as an anesthetic adjuvant and can be given through epidural, intrathecal or intravenous routes.

MORPHINE

Morphine causes histamine release resulting in peripheral vasodilatation. It inhibits baroreceptor reflexes, leads to orthostatic hypotension and fainting attacks. It crosses blood brain barrier at a slower rate than fentanyl.

Drug of Choice: Fentanyl

RATIONALE

Being less lipophilic **morphine** crosses blood brain barrier slowly when compared to fentanyl. It degranulates mast cells, causes **histamine release**, vasodilatation, **hypotension** and fainting attacks making it **unsuitable** as an anesthetic. **Fentanyl** is **highly lipid soluble**, attains good CSF concentration quickly and it has **rapid onset**, does not cause histamine release and has relative **cardiovascular stability**. Hence, it is preferred to morphine as anesthetic adjuvant.

6. *Fentanyl/Remifentanil as neuroanesthetic in neurosurgical procedures.*

BACKGROUND

The opioids fentanyl, sufentanil and remifentanil have more hemodynamic stability. They do not increase intracranial pressure and maintain cerebral perfusion pressure and are used as anesthetic adjuncts for neurosurgical procedures. Prolonged anesthetic effect delays postoperative assessment in neurosurgery. Therefore, rapid emergence from anesthesia is an important factor in neurosurgery. Remifentanil and fentanyl are both equipotent and are given as intravenous infusion.

REMIFENTANIL

Remifentanil has more rapid onset of action compared to fentanyl. Peak analgesic action occurs within 1 to 1.5 minutes. Similarly, recovery is also very quick compared to fentanyl. Remifentanil results in rapid emergence from anesthesia hence it is a more suitable adjuvant in neurosurgery and helps for early neurologic evaluation. It is formulated with glycine, an inhibitory neurotransmitter and should never be given through intrathecal administration.

FENTANYL

Fentanyl is a commonly used potent opioid anesthetic adjuvant. Its onset and duration are short and quick but the recovery rate of fentanyl is a little slow.

Drug of Choice: Remifentanil

RATIONALE

Remifentanil has **faster onset** of action and **rapid termination** of effect when compared to fentanyl. It has **rapid emergence rate** from anesthesia, an important factor contributing to **success rate** in neurosurgical procedures. Hence, it is preferred as neuroanesthetic to fentanyl but it should **never** be **administered** through **intrathecal** route.

7. *Loperamide/Diphenoxylate in acute nonspecific diarrhea.*

BACKGROUND

As early as 3rd century BC, opium was used by Arabians for traveler's diarrhea. Opioids should not be used as primary treatment in infective diarrhea. They are also used in diarrhea due to ulcerative colitis.

LOPERAMIDE

Loperamide is 40 to 50 times more potent than morphine as antidiarrheal agent. It acts locally on the GIT as it is poorly absorbed after oral administration. It interacts with opioid receptors in intestine and reduces intestinal secretions. Unlike other opioids it inhibits both circular and longitudinal muscles of intestine and therefore increases anal sphincter tone prolonging the intestinal transit time. It does not cross BBB as CNS entry is prevented by the efflux pump, P-glycoprotein does not result in euphoria or dependence or addiction. Overdose can cause CNS effects and paralytic ileus. Loperamide has higher efficacy and safety when compared to diphenoxylate. Hence, loperamide is preferred as antidiarrheal agent.

DIPHENOXYLATE

Diphenoxylate is a meperidine (pethidine) congener and difenoxin is its active metabolite and approved for treatment of diarrhea as it causes constipation. It is more potent than morphine as an antidiarrheal agent. It has very good bioavailability, extensively absorbed, deesterified to its metabolite difenoxin which has a half-life of 12 hours. It causes nonpropulsive high amplitude contractions of circular muscles of intestine. Such an action adds to its therapeutic benefit resulting in constipation. Although small dose produce little CNS action, higher doses can result in euphoria and chronic therapy results in physical dependence, drug abuse and toxic mega colon.

Drug of Choice: Loperamide

RATIONALE

Opioids are given only in noninfective and nonspecific diarrhea. **Loperamide** is more **potent** than morphine as an antidiarrheal agent, acts on both **longitudinal** and **circular** muscles of intestine. It prolongs intestinal transit time and increases anal sphincter tone. It **does not** cause **euphoria, dependence** and **addiction** as it does not cross BBB. But injudicious use can cause paralytic ileus and unwanted CNS side effects. **Diphenoxylate**, although potent antidiarrheal, acts **only** on **circular** muscles thereby increasing intestinal spasm and can also cause **drug addiction**. Hence, loperamide is preferred to diphenoxylate as an antidiarrheal agent.

8. *Morphine/Diclofenac in biliary colic.*

BACKGROUND

Classic biliary pain is severe, constant and acute in nature. Pain is mainly due to obstruction of common bile duct by gallstones.

DICLOFENAC

Intramuscular diclofenac 50 to 75 mg relieves biliary colic pain effectively. Ketorolac, the NSAID can also be used in this condition. Diclofenac does not potentiate biliary spasm or increase the intrabiliary pressure. NSAIDs relieve pain and reduce progression of biliary colic to cholecystitis. Hence, diclofenac is preferred to morphine in biliary colic.

MORPHINE

Morphine is a potent narcotic analgesic used commonly in acute pain conditions but contraindicated in biliary colic as it aggravates the condition. It contracts circular muscles causing spasm of bile duct and sphincter of oddi thereby increasing intrabiliary pressure up to 10 times. Further it increases fluid pressure of gallbladder and worsens the biliary colic. Morphine also stimulates CTZ and results in nausea and vomiting. Similarly, if opioids are used in this condition it will also increase the biliary spasm. Hence, all opioids should be avoided in biliary colic.

Drug of Choice: Diclofenac

RATIONALE

Morphine is **contraindicated** in **acute abdomen**. Even though it is a potent analgesic it should not be given in biliary colic as it causes spastic contraction of circular muscles, **augmenting intrabiliary pressure, worsening** the **biliary colic. Diclofenac relieves** pain and **does not interfere** with **intrabiliary pressure**.

9. *Nalorphine/Naloxone in the treatment of acute morphine poisoning.*

BACKGROUND

Pinpoint pupils, respiratory depression and coma are triad of symptoms occurring in morphine poisoning. By inhibiting the respiratory centers, morphine causes respiratory depression. It reduces respiratory rate, minute volume and tidal exchange and suppresses the response of respiratory center to hypercapnic drive. Its effects on respiration are mainly mediated through μ and δ receptors. Nalorphine is an agonist antagonist whereas naloxone is a complete antagonist.

NALOXONE

Naloxone blocks all three types of opioid receptors. It antagonizes the action of morphine at μ, κ and δ receptors. Naloxone not only blocks the respiratory depression caused by morphine but in addition it reverses morphine action on respiration causing stimulation. The capacity of naloxone to stimulate respiration in morphine poisoning is known as "overshoot phenomenon". Hence, naloxone is given in morphine poisoning. Naloxone when given IV in the dose of 0.4 to 0.8 mg completely reverses the action of morphine. It increases the respiratory rate within 1 to 2 minutes.

NALORPHINE

Nalorphine is a competitive antagonist at µ receptor and an agonist at κ receptor. It is highly lipid soluble and crosses BBB freely. Nalorphine has agonist action and fails to block all symptoms of morphine poisoning.

Drug of Choice: Naloxone

RATIONALE

Death occurs due to respiratory failure in acute morphine poisoning. **Nalorphine** is only an **agonist antagonist** whereas **naloxone** is a **complete antagonist** of morphine. **Naloxone** blocks all three opioid receptors and also **reverses** the **respiratory depression** induced by over dose of morphine. It results in **'overshoot phenomenon'** stimulating the respiration. Hence, naloxone is preferred to nalorphine in acute morphine poisoning.

15

Antiepileptic Drugs

1. *Carbamazepine/Sodium valproate as first line drug in complex partial seizures.*

BACKGROUND

Complex partial seizure is characterized by loss of consciousness and unwanted movements. Since epilepsy requires long-term therapy, efficacy, adverse effects as well as cost play a major role in the selection of a drug. When compared to newer antiepileptic drugs older drugs are preferred as their efficacy and long-term toxicities are well documented. Carbamazepine and sodium valproate are both effective in complex partial seizures and they delay the rate of recovery of inactivated voltage activated sodium channels.

CARBAMAZEPINE

Carbamazepine is more effective than sodium valproate in complex partial seizures.[25] Modulation of sodium channels stabilizes neuronal membranes inhibiting the spread of seizure to other areas. Skin rash is the most common adverse effect of carbamazepine. Diplopia, blurred vision, ataxia and vertigo are neurotoxic side effects but tolerance can develop to these effects on long-term administration.

SODIUM VALPROATE

Sodium valproate, in addition to sodium channel modulation inhibits voltage activated T type calcium channels. The choice between both drugs is determined by their safety profile as they should be given for a long period. Sodium valproate causes tremor, weight gain and 40% increase in hepatic transaminases. Tolerance does not develop to its neurotoxic side effects.

Drug of Choice: Carbamazepine

RATIONALE

Carbamazepine and sodium valproate are both used in complex partial seizures. They act by **slowing down** the **rate of recovery** of inactivated voltage gated sodium channels stabilizing neuronal membrane thereby preventing the spread of seizures. Although **sodium valproate** has an **additional** inhibitory **action** on T type calcium channels, it results in **higher incidence** of **side effects**. **Carbamazepine** is **better tolerated** by patients but **tolerance** can develop to its **neurotoxic side effects** but not to sodium valproate. Carbamazepine is preferred due to its efficacy and safety.

2. *Carbamazepine/Oxcarbazepine in simple partial seizures.*

BACKGROUND

The clinical manifestations of simple partial seizures depend upon the area of cortex stimulated. While muscular movements occur due to stimulation of motor cortex, paresthesia occurs as a result of stimulation of the sensory cortex. Consciousness is always preserved and duration of seizures extends from 20 to 60 seconds. They are both sodium channel modulators, and they prolong the recovery rate of inactivated channels.

CARBAMAZEPINE

Carbamazepine is absorbed slowly and its peak plasma concentration is delayed up to 24 hours. It is an enzyme inducer and has a variable half-life ranging from 20 to 40 hours. It is also available as extended release formulation. The incidence of hepatotoxicity is high but it causes minimal nausea and vomiting. Besides, it is more potent and cost effective than oxca bazepine.

OXCARBAZEPINE

Oxcarbazepine is a prodrug but is converted immediately to its active metabolite carbamazepine. It has a different pharmacokinetic profile and its capacity to induce microsomal enzymes is minimal. Therefore, it does not result in many drug interactions. Half-life of oxcarbazepine is only 1 to 2 hours and it is less potent than carbamazepine and produces equivalent therapeutic benefit at a higher dose only. It increases the occurrence of hyponatremia.

Drug of Choice: Carbamazepine

RATIONALE

Carbamazepine and oxcarbazepine have **similar pharmacodynamic** but **different pharmacokinetic** profiles. **Carbamazepine** is **preferred** to oxcarbazepine in simple partial seizures[26] as it is **more potent and available as extended release formulation**. **Oxcarbazepine** is absorbed quickly, **better tolerated** and leads to **minimal enzyme induction** but it is **twenty times costlier**, has a short half-life and has to be given at a **higher dose** more frequently hence increasing the incidence of adverse effects. Therefore, carbamazepine is the drug of choice in simple partial seizures.

3. *Carbamazepine/Lamotrigine in trigeminal neuralgia and glossopharyngeal neuralgia.*

BACKGROUND

Trigeminal neuralgia occurs due to persistent compression of trigeminal nerve and characterized by paroxysmal, intense pain along the branches of trigeminal nerve. The pain is sharp and stabbing in nature and triggered by activities such as talking, chewing or brushing. Although glossopharyngeal neuralgia is uncommon, it causes similar intense pain. Pain in glossopharyngeal neuralgia occurs over tonsillar area and may radiate towards ear.

CARBAMAZEPINE

Carbamazepine is preferred as it is cost effective and reduces intensity of pain substantially. It stabilizes neuronal membranes and blocks the propagation of action potential. It results in neurotoxicity, hypersensitivity and multiple drug interactions.

LAMOTRIGINE

Lamotrigine is at least eight times costlier than carbamazepine. The adverse effect ranges from diplopia to Stevens-Johnson syndrome. Its efficacy and superiority to carbamazepine is not well established. Therefore, it is a second line drug in patients who do not tolerate carbamazepine.

Drug of Choice: Carbamazepine

RATIONALE

Neuralgias are painful conditions where analgesics do not offer complete relief. In case of trigeminal and glossopharyngeal neuralgias, a drug is required to provide complete pain relief as the degree of pain is very severe. These drugs **act** by **inhibiting** the **transmission of nerve impulses**, but **carbamazepine** is preferred as it is **more effective, cheaper** and provides **significant relief** of pain when compared to lamotrigine.[27] Lamotrigine is reserved as a second line drug in the treatment of trigeminal and glossopharyngeal neuralgias.

4. *Felbamate/Rufinamide in Lennox-Gastaut syndrome.*

BACKGROUND

Lennox-Gastaut syndrome is an epileptogenic encephalopathy occurring in either sex in the age group of 1 to 7 years. It is characterized by either tonic or atonic type of seizures (drop attacks) and causes cognitive and behavioral impairments. They are both indicated in this condition and clobazam can be an adjunctive because it can reduces the rate of drop attacks.

RUFINAMIDE

Rufinamide potentiates slow inactivation of voltage sensitive sodium channels. It is approved for treatment of seizures associated with

Lennox-Gastaut syndrome. It has better tolerability and minimal side effects, so preferred for long-term therapy.

FELBAMATE

Felbamate has dual action. It inhibits NMDA mediated excitatory neurotransmission and also potentiates GABA mediated inhibitory neurotransmission.[28] It decreases the frequency as well as total number of tonic seizures and drop attacks and improves the quality of life of patients but can cause aplastic anemia and hepatotoxicity. So it cannot be used, as long-term therapy is required for this condition.

Drug of Choice: Rufinamide

RATIONALE

The seizures associated with Lennox-Gastaut syndrome are of either tonic or atonic type. Although **felbamate** has **dual action** and controls the frequency and total number of seizures in this condition, it has **higher toxicity profile** that makes it unsuitable for use since prolonged drug administration is required for effective control of seizures. **Rufinamide** potentiates the slow inactivation of sodium channels and is much **safer for long-term administration**.[29]

5. *Gabapentin/Topiramate for prophylaxis of migraine.*

BACKGROUND

Family history is common among patients suffering from migraine. It is due to dysfunctioning of monoaminergic system in brainstem and thalamus. Pulsatile headache occurs due to dilatation of blood vessels around trigeminal nerve. Prophylaxis is indicated in patients experiencing five or more attacks per month. Antiepileptic drugs are proved to be effective in prophylaxis of migraine. Drugs commonly used are topiramate, sodium valproate and, gabapentin.[30]

TOPIRAMATE

Topiramate has at least three different mechanisms of action. It is a sodium channel modulator and also potentiates GABA mediated inhibition. It antagonizes AMPA/kainite subtype of glutamate receptor as an additional mechanism. It is also a weak inhibitor of enzyme carbonic anhydrase. If given at a dose of 100 to 200 mg per day, for a period of two months it reduces the mean monthly frequency and severity of migraine. It has been proved to be highly effective in prophylaxis of migraine. Sodium valproate is also found to be equally effective but is more toxic. Topiramate is better tolerated but results in weight loss and nephrolithiasis.

GABAPENTIN

Gabapentin is a GABA agonist but does not have GABA mimetic action. It acts by binding to $\alpha 2\delta$-1 subunit modulating voltage sensitive calcium channels. There is conflicting and inadequate evidence to prove its usefulness in migraine.[31]

Drug of Choice: Topiramate

RATIONALE

Antiepileptic drugs are indicated for prophylaxis of migraine. **Topiramate** has **multiple mechanisms** of action and is found to be safer. It is **well-tolerated** when compared to equieffective dose of sodium valproate. Topiramate **reduces** the **frequency** of attacks. Gabapentin is less effective when compared to topiramate. Hence, the antiepileptic drug topiramate is preferred in prophylaxis of migraine.

6. *Sodium valproate/Tiagabine in absence seizures.*

BACKGROUND

Absence seizure presents as abrupt loss of consciousness for about 30 seconds. The patient appears stunned, unaware of the ongoing activities and continues to stare vacantly. It is due to stimulation of thalamus and cerebral cortex. EEG shows bilateral spike and wave discharges at a frequency of three per second.

SODIUM VALPROATE

Sodium valproate, a broad spectrum antiepileptic, is the drug of choice. It stabilizes neuronal membranes by modulating the sodium channel. It also inhibits T type voltage gated calcium channel and alters GABA metabolism by inhibiting GABA degrading enzymes and stimulating GABA synthetic enzyme. Sodium valproate is rapidly and completely absorbed and its CSF concentration equilibrates its plasma concentration. Transient GIT symptoms and alopecia, weight gain and hepatotoxicity are common side effects.

TIAGABINE

Tiagabine reduces reuptake of GABA by inhibiting its transporter GAT-1. In absence seizure, it facilitates spike and wave discharge, worsening the condition resulting in generalized absence seizures.[32] Hence, tiagabine is contraindicated in absence seizures.

Drug of Choice: Sodium Valproate

RATIONALE

In absence seizures EEG shows bilateral spike and wave discharges at a frequency of 3 per second. **Sodium valproate modulates** the **sodium channel, inhibits T type calcium channel**, and **prolongs GABA** action in the synaptic terminal. Its multiple actions make it the drug of choice in absence seizures. On the other hand, **Tiagabine** potentiates firing rate and the condition deteriorates to generalized absence seizures, so it is **contraindicated**.

7. *Topiramate/Zonisamide in refractory partial seizures.*

BACKGROUND

Carbamazepine and phenytoin are preferred in simple partial seizures. Carbamazepine is superior to sodium valproate in complex partial seizures. If seizures become unresponsive to these drugs, the necessity for another drug arises. Topiramate and zonisamide are effective in refractory partial seizures. They effectively control simple and complex partial seizures.

TOPIRAMATE

Topiramate is effective as initial monotherapy and abolishes the need for another drug. It prolongs the inactivation of sodium channels and modulates GABA receptor. Further it blocks the activity of glutamate and inhibits carbonic anhydrase.[33] It can cause cognitive impairment, dysgeusia, renal calculi and weight loss.

ZONISAMIDE

Zonisamide as monotherapy in refractory partial seizures is not well proven. It inhibits T type calcium channels and prolongs inactivation of sodium channels. Ataxia, renal calculi and metabolic acidosis are common side effects. It can be used only as an adjuvant or as add on therapy with other drugs.

Drug of Choice: Topiramate

RATIONALE

Zonisamide is well-tolerated, acts by inhibiting calcium channels and by prolonging the rate of recovery of inactivated sodium channels but it is effective **only as an adjuvant** in **refractory** partial seizure and has **inadequate efficacy** when given as **monotherapy**. **Topiramate** acts through **multiple mechanisms** and is effective as monotherapy during initial stages, a **definite therapeutic advantage** as it avoids the need for an additional drug and improves patient's compliance.

8. *Carbamazepine/Lamotrigine in prophylaxis of SUNCT (Short term unilateral neuralgiform unilateral attacks with conjunctival injection and tearing).*

BACKGROUND

It is a rare primary headache syndrome characterized by unilateral headache. The three basic patterns are single stab, group of stabs or saw tooth phenomenon. In trigeminal neuralgia a clear refractory period is usually present. Unlike trigeminal neuralgia, refractory period is absent between attacks. Usually it does not respond to analgesics like indomethacin. Attacks last for only a short period and prophylaxis is more helpful.

LAMOTRIGINE

Lamotrigine is the drug of choice and very effective at 200 to 400 mg. Topiramate and gabapentin are also equally effective. Lamotrigine and carbamazepine stabilize neuronal membranes due to prolonged inactivation of sodium channels. The T type or transient type calcium channels are present in neurons of thalamus and are activated at negative membrane potential (–55 mv). Stimulation of such channels results in repetitive firing of action potential in thalamus[34] and lamotrigine causes blockade of T type calcium channels. This additional mechanism of lamotrigine differentiates it from carbamazepine and therefore it is thus very effective in prophylaxis of SUNCT.

CARBAMAZEPINE

Carbamazepine 400 to 500 mg per day has only a moderate activity in SUNCT. It stabilizes neuronal membrane but has no additional mechanism like lamotrigine. Hence, it is not preferred in prophylaxis of SUNCT.

Drug of Choice: Lamotrigine

RATIONALE

Severe continuous stabbing pain without any interval due to repetitive firing of neurons is the characteristic feature of SUNCT. Carbamazepine and lamotrigine prolong the recovery of inactivated sodium channels thereby making them very effective in this condition. **Lamotrigine** is **more effective** as it **additionally blocks** the T or **transient type calcium channel**, a mechanism by which calcium channel blockers are found to be useful in prophylaxis of migraine. Hence, lamotrigine shows more efficacy than carbamazepine as a prophylactic in SUNCT.

9. *Phenytoin/Sodium valproate in juvenile myoclonic seizure.*

BACKGROUND

Juvenile myoclonic seizure is bilateral myoclonus without loss of consciousness and characterized by irregular shock like movements. Contraction of muscles occurs for a very short period of time. Myoclonus may be restricted to few muscles or may be generalized. Most often, seizure occurs early in the morning. Cluster jerks occur frequently before generalized tonic clonic seizures. It is more common in mid to late childhood, in children between 10 to 16 years of age.

SODIUM VALPROATE

Sodium valproate is the drug of choice and levetiracetam is a second line drug. Sodium valproate prolongs the duration of sodium channel inactivation and also inhibits transient T type calcium channels. Alopecia, anorexia, ataxia and hepatotoxicity are a few side effects.

PHENYTOIN

Phenytoin is effective in tonic clonic seizures but not in juvenile myoclonic seizures. Besides it facilitates the progression of seizure to more severe cluster jerks.[35] Since it aggravates juvenile myoclonic seizure, it is contraindicated.

Drug of Choice: Sodium Valproate

RATIONALE

In juvenile myoclonic seizure, myoclonic jerks occur for a very short period of time. Sodium valproate is found to be effective in the treatment of juvenile myoclonic seizure. **Phenytoin** on the other hand **worsens** the **seizure** and **facilitates** its **progression** to more severe cluster jerks and so is absolutely contraindicated in this condition.

10. *Lorazepam/Diazepam in management of status epilepticus.*

BACKGROUND

Status epilepticus is a medical emergency requiring immediate treatment. Benzodiazepines are used initially to control prolonged, repeated seizures. They prevent systemic and neurological sequelae if given early. Lorazepam and diazepam are both used as they have broad spectrum effect.

LORAZEPAM

Lorazepam has greater tolerance[36] and addiction liability, but still preferred. It has lower lipid solubility and has a distribution half-life of 2 to 3 hours but binds with GABA receptors much more tightly than diazepam. Thus, it has longer duration of action with a greater clinical advantage. The anticonvulsant effect of lorazepam persists for 6 to 12 hours and the required dose is only 4 mg. Hence, lorazepam is preferred in acute management of status epilepticus.

DIAZEPAM

Diazepam is highly lipid soluble and crosses blood brain barrier rapidly but gets quickly redistributed to other tissues within 10 to 15 minutes. Hence, it has a shorter duration of action, reducing its clinical benefit. Despite such faster distribution half-life, its elimination half-life is 24 hours aggravating its sedative effect following repeated administration. The dose requirement of diazepam is around 10 to 20 mg. Common adverse effects of both drugs are vertigo and sedation.

Drug of Choice: Lorazepam

RATIONALE

In any medical emergency, the drug should have immediate but sustained action. **Diazepam acts quickly** but the effect is **short lived** due to its high lipid solubility and quick **redistribution**. **Lorazepam** has lower lipid solubility, **binds** more **tightly** with GABA receptors and has a **longer duration** of action. The dose requirement is also less compared to diazepam. Hence, lorazepam is preferred to diazepam[37] in acute management of status epilepticus although it results in greater tolerance and addiction liability.

16

General Anesthetics

1. *Propofol/Nitrous oxide as inducing agent with minimal post-operative nausea and vomiting.*

BACKGROUND

The incidence of postoperative nausea and vomiting is around 25 to 30%. Aspiration of GIT contents into lung is the common complication of vomiting. The vomiting center is situated in brainstem and chemoreceptor trigger zone (CTZ) is located in the area postrema. Anesthetics stimulate these centres through activation of vestibular system but suppress afferent stimulation from pharynx. The neurotransmitters dopamine, acetylcholine, histamine and 5HT mediate nausea and vomiting through CTZ.

PROPOFOL

Propofol is an antiemetic with the least incidence of nausea and vomiting, which is probably due to modulation of subcortical pathways. It inhibits spontaneous movements induced by dopaminergic activity and also causes occulogyric crisis indicating antidopaminergic activity. Dopamine antagonism may be the principal reason for antiemetic action of propofol as it has no known anticholinergic and antiserotonergic action. It reduces the incidence of postoperative nausea and vomiting.

NITROUS OXIDE

Nitrous oxide is a potent emetic and induces intense postoperative nausea and vomiting through three different mechanisms.

It stimulates opioid receptors in CTZ, stimulates intestines directly and diffuses into middle ear stimulating the vestibular system.

Drug of Choice: Propofol

RATIONALE

Nitrous oxide is a potent **emetogenic** drug[38] resulting in higher incidence of postoperative nausea and vomiting mediated through stimulation of opioid receptors. **Propofol,** on the other hand has **antiemetic action**[39] through its **antidopaminergic activity** and causes minimal postoperative nausea and vomiting.

2. *Ketamine/Propofol for patients with high risk of developing hypotension and shock.*

BACKGROUND

Anesthetics can induce the risk of postoperative hypotension and shock. Ketamine and propofol are both intravenous anesthetics used for induction as well as maintenance of anesthesia. Their pharmacokinetic property is based on their hydrophobicity (lipophilicity) hence they accumulate in brain, resulting in anesthesia quickly within a single circulation time.

KETAMINE

Ketamine acts through inhibition of (N Methyl D Aspartate) NMDA receptors. It is a potent analgesic and produces dissociative anesthesia. Dissociation is a state of hypnosis associated with amnesia, analgesia and catatonia. As a cardiostimulatory drug, it increases blood pressure, heart rate and cardiac output. Cardiac effects are either through direct CNS stimulatory action or indirect inhibitory action mediated by decreased norepinephrine reuptake mechanism. Therefore, it is preferred in patients with high risk of cardiogenic or septic shock.

PROPOFOL

Propofol is a GABA mimetic and potentiates the action of GABA. It is a vasodilator and inhibits myocardial contractility. Therefore, it produces a dose dependent fall in blood pressure. Besides, it blunts baroreceptor reflex and inhibits sympathetic activity. On account of these reasons propofol should be avoided in patients with risk for hypotension.

Drug of Choice: Ketamine

RATIONALE

Ketamine, a dissociative anesthetic blocks NMDA receptors. It has cardiostimulatory actions and **increases blood pressure**. It is often preferred in patients who are at high risk for developing hypotension and shock. **Propofol** has GABA mimetic action. It reduces blood pressure and **worsens shock** and should be **avoided** in high risk patients prone for developing hypotension and shock.

3. *Ketamine/Propofol for short term surgical procedures in outpatient unit.*

BACKGROUND

Anesthetics with short duration of action are preferred for short surgical procedures but the anesthetic used should have relative hemodynamic stability. It should not cause undesirable side effects that limit patient's mobility.

PROPOFOL

Propofol is a GABA mimetic and has unique pharmacokinetic feature and both onset of action as well as reversal are rapid following administration. Rapid emergence is due to short elimination half-life and rapid clearance rate. Postoperative nausea and vomiting are minimal due to its antiemetic action. A dose of 1 to 2.5 mg/kg will act for 4 to 8 minutes. The patient becomes ambulant immediately after reversal. This advantage makes it more suitable for short-term OP procedures. It is also used an inducing and maintenance agent. It is useful in long-term anesthetic maintenance.

KETAMINE

The duration of action of ketamine at a dose of 0.5 to 1.5 mg/kg is around 10 to 15 minutes. It is associated with 'emergence delirium' during reversal, most often during the first hour. Since it causes delusions and hallucinations patient cannot be discharged immediately. Hence, ketamine is unsuitable for short-term surgical procedures in OP unit.

Drug of Choice: Propofol

RATIONALE

Propofol is **preferred** for short-term OP procedures as it has **rapid onset** of action with **rapid reversal** and the patient is ambulant immediately after reversal. **Ketamine** is associated with postoperative **'emergence delirium'** and the patient needs to be **monitored closely** for at least 12 hours, so, it is not suitable for OP procedures.

4. *Clonidine/Dexmedetomidine as an anesthetic adjuvant.*

BACKGROUND

Clonidine and dexmedetomidine are both α_2 agonists and are being used as anesthetic adjuncts. Stimulation of α_{2A} receptors decreases nociceptive transmission in spinal cord.

DEXMEDETOMIDINE

Dexmedetomidine, a selective α_{2A} agonist is approved for short-term sedation. It causes sedation and analgesia through stimulation of α_{2A} receptors but does not result in amnesia and patients can be easily aroused. The degree of hypotension induced by dexmedetomidine is relatively minimal and it causes lower incidence of rebound hypotension. Nausea and bradycardia are other common side effects. When compared to clonidine it has eight times higher affinity to α_2 receptors which results in prolonged sensory and motor blockade. Since it exerts its action and has relative hemodynamic stability, it is preferred to clonidine as an anesthetic adjuvant.

CLONIDINE

Clonidine is a less selective α_{2A} agonist when compared to dexmedetomidine. The incidence of 'rebound hypertension' is high with clonidine. It is not approved by FDA for this purpose and anesthetic adjuvant is 'off-label' use of clonidine.

Drug of Choice: Dexmedetomidine

RATIONALE

Although clonidine and dexmedetomidine are both used as anesthetic adjuncts, only **dexmedetomidine** is **approved by FDA** and preferred to clonidine as it is more selective and results in **prolonged** sensory and motor blockade.[40,41] The **degree of hypotension** due to dexmedetomidine is **relatively minimal** and it can be used safely.

5. *Ketamine/Propofol as inducing agent in patients with bronchial asthma.*

BACKGROUND

Since the airway resistance is high in patients with bronchial asthma, anesthetics causing bronchoconstriction should not be used. Bronchodilator anesthetics are preferred in such patients. Some anesthetics cause histamine release and potentiate bronchoconstriction.

KETAMINE

Ketamine has a direct bronchodilating activity and also causes bronchodilatation indirectly through sympathomimetic action. It maintains muscle tone of upper airway and preserves airway reflexes. It is a very potent bronchodilator, well suited for patients prone to bronchospasm.

PROPOFOL

The degree of respiratory depression produced by propofol is high. Conflicting reports are available about its safety in bronchial asthma as it causes histamine release but does not induce bronchospasm in all patients. Therefore, propofol is better avoided in patients with bronchial asthma.

Drug of Choice: Ketamine

RATIONALE

The sympathomimetic action and direct bronchodilating action of ketamine causes bronchodilatation so, it is safe in asthmatics. Although propofol is being used in patients with bronchial asthma it can release histamine and can aggravate bronchospasm[42] in sensitive individuals.[43] Hence, it is better avoided in patients with bronchial asthma.

6. *Ketamine/Etomidate in patients with CAD and cerebrovascular disease.*

BACKGROUND

The drug used to induce anesthesia should be safe and should not interfere with cardiac functions. It should not alter cardiac, pulmonary or systemic circulation. It is wiser to use an anesthetic that does not increase either intracranial pressure or intraocular pressure.

ETOMIDATE

Etomidate decreases intraocular pressure moderately and is used in ocular lesions. It decreases cerebral blood flow and cerebral oxygen utilization. It can be safely used even in the presence of space occupying lesions. Cardiac output, peripheral or pulmonary circulation are unaffected by etomidate. Therefore, it poses no threat if used in patients with cardiomyopathy or CAD.

KETAMINE

Ketamine increases heart rate, blood pressure and cardiac output. It inhibits norepinephrine reuptake both centrally and peripherally.

It also increases myocardial oxygen consumption. In view of the above, it should not be used in patients with myocardial ischemia. It increases blood flow to anterior cingulate gyrus, thalamus and frontal cortex. While its S-enantiomer increases cerebral blood flow and metabolic rate, its R-enantiomer decreases both metabolic rate and cerebral blood flow. Ketamine is the racemic mixture of both enantiomers and increases blood flow and metabolic rate. It has a unique property of increasing both intraocular pressure (IOP) and intracranial pressure (ICP). It increases intracranial pressure secondary to cerebral vasodilatation hence should not be used in patients with cerebrovascular disease. Moderate and transient increase in intraocular pressure by ketamine is reported. It is contraindicated in ocular laceration as it increases the intraocular pressure. It should also be avoided in CAD, cardiomyopathy and open eye wounds.

Drug of Choice: Etomidate

RATIONALE

Ketamine is an efficient **anesthetic** and a good **analgesic but increases** blood pressure, **intraocular pressure**[44] and **intracranial pressure**. So, it is not suited in patients with open eye wounds, CAD, cardiomyopathy and cerebrovascular disease. **Etomidate** is not an **analgesic** but has **additional advantage** as it moderately **reduces IOP**[45] **and ICP**.[46] It has no effect on cardiac output and peripheral circulation and so preferred to ketamine in these conditions.

7. *Halothane/Sevoflurane as inducing agent.*

BACKGROUND

Some anesthetics have poor solubility in blood and other tissues. Such anesthetics achieve good equilibrium very quickly. Since equilibrium determines the speed of induction of anesthesia, drugs with poor solubility are preferred as inducing agents. The rate of increase of alveolar partial pressure is high for drugs with lower solubility and so such drugs result in effective 'minimum alveolar concentration' or MAC. MAC determines the potency of an anesthetic to induce surgical anesthesia.

SEVOFLURANE

The solubility of sevoflurane is very low in blood and tissues hence it provides very rapid induction at 2 to 4% concentration. Its poor solubility also causes rapid changes in depth of anesthesia leading to rapid reversal after discontinuation. Further, it does not irritate the airway and produces bronchodilatation. Among inhalational anesthetics, it is the most potent bronchodilator. Due to rapid induction and recovery it is most suitable as inducing agent.

HALOTHANE

Halothane is highly soluble in blood, fat and other body tissues and accumulates in these places. Higher solubility causes slower induction of anesthesia and prolongs the recovery. Therefore, it is not suitable for induction.

Drug of Choice: Sevoflurane

RATIONALE

Sevoflurane has **lower solubility** and has the capacity for **rapid induction** and **recovery**. It is also a **potent bronchodilator** and it is widely used as an **inducing agent** among inhalational anesthetics. **Halothane** is highly **soluble**, accumulates in both fat and tissues and has **slow induction and recovery** hence not preferred.

8. *Sevoflurane/Desflurane as an inducing agent.*

BACKGROUND

Solubility of an inhalational anesthetic determines the equilibrium which occurs when partial pressure of inspired gas equals that of alveolar gas. Sevoflurane and desflurane have lower blood-gas partition coefficient and do not accumulate in fat and other tissues. Their low solubility helps in achieving higher rates of equilibrium. They have rapid onset of action and cause rapid changes in depth of anesthesia resulting in quick reversal hence these drugs can be used as anesthetics in outpatient surgery.

SEVOFLURANE

Similar to other fluorinated anesthetics, sevoflurane is a broncho-dilator but it is not an irritant to respiratory tract. It increases respiratory rate and reduces tidal volume. It increases partial pressure of carbon dioxide and is a potent bronchodilator. Hence, sevoflurane is preferred to desflurane as an inducing agent especially in children.

DESFLURANE

Desflurane on the other hand, is an irritant to airway provoking cough and excessive respiratory secretions. Not only does it augment cough but it also potentiates laryngospasm. Therefore, desflurane is more suitable for maintenance of anesthesia and not for induction.

Drug of Choice: Sevoflurane

RATIONALE

Sevoflurane and desflurane are anesthetic agents with lower solubility. They result in rapid onset and recovery enabling them to be preferentially used for induction during minor surgical procedures in out patients. While sevoflurane is a bronchodilator and preferred for induction, desflurane is an irritant to airway and should be avoided as an inducing agent.

9. *Sevoflurane/Isoflurane in closed system technique.*

BACKGROUND

Closed system technique is used for expensive anesthetics because re-breathing of exhaled air reduces the quantity of anesthetic required. This technique uses soda lime to absorb carbon dioxide present in exhaled air. Soda lime contains calcium hydroxide that helps in absorption of carbon dioxide. The exhaled air goes through a canister containing soda lime which removes carbon dioxide allowing for recirculation of anesthetic. As this chemical reaction proceeds, the pH drops and becomes more acidic changing the color of soda lime from white to blue indicating the need for replacement. Absorption of carbon dioxide results in exothermic reaction.

ISOFLURANE

Isoflurane is volatile but noninflammable anesthetic can be safely used through closed technique because it does not undergo exothermic reaction. Ninety-nine percent of isoflurane is not metabolized and is exhaled unchanged. 0.2% is metabolized and the metabolites do not produce renal or hepatotoxicity.

SEVOFLURANE

Sevoflurane is a noninflammable and nonexplosive liquid but undergoes exothermic reaction with desiccated soda lime leading to spontaneous ignition, fire and explosion, causing airway burns. Interaction of sevoflurane with soda lime can also generate carbon monoxide harming patients during the rebreathing process. Compound A is a decomposition product produced due to interaction of sevoflurane with soda lime. It is highly nephrotoxic if inhaled by patients in the closed circuit technique. Hence, sevoflurane should be avoided in closed system technique.

Drug of Choice: Isoflurane

RATIONALE

Sevoflurane when used in closed circuit, results in **exothermic reaction** with desiccated soda lime, generating heat. This can lead to explosion and fire causing damage to patient's airway. Besides, rebreathing of exhaled air increases possibility of breathing carbon monoxide and a nephrotoxic compound A. Hence, sevoflurane should not be used in closed system. **Isoflurane** is **not exothermic**, does not produce significant quantities of toxic metabolites and can be safely used in closed system technique.

10. *Desflurane/Sevoflurane in patients prone to myocardial infarction.*

BACKGROUND

During cardiac surgeries desflurane and sevoflurane are both reported to be safe. Yet, in patients with myocardial infarction, sevoflurane is the drug of choice.

SEVOFLURANE

Sevoflurane causes concentration dependent fall in blood pressure. Unlike desflurane, it does not cause transient increase in blood pressure during induction and does not result in reflex tachycardia. It reduces tidal volume, increases respiratory rate and causes bronchodilatation. Hence, it is an agent of choice in patients prone to myocardial infarction.

DESFLURANE

Desflurane decreases blood pressure mainly by reducing peripheral resistance but results in transient increase in heart rate during induction. Tachycardia occurs due to stimulation of adrenergic system when given through a closed system, toxic carbon monoxide is produced by desflurane. It is an irritant causing laryngospasm and copious respiratory secretions.

Drug of Choice: Sevoflurane

RATIONALE

Even transient increase in blood pressure increases the risk in patients prone to myocardial infarction. Desflurane and sevoflurane can both be safely used as anesthetics during cardiac surgeries but **desflurane** cannot be used in patients with underlying cardiac problem and in those prone for **myocardial infarction** as it causes transient increase in blood pressure, during induction of anesthesia.[47] Since sevoflurane does not alter the blood pressure, it is **preferred** in patients prone for **cardiac problem**. Besides, sevoflurane is not an irritant to respiratory tract and does not cause laryngo-spasm like desflurane.

11. *Halothane/Nitrous oxide as anesthetic for labor and vaginal delivery.*

BACKGROUND

Anesthetics used in obstetrics should not interfere with the progress of labor and should be safe to mother, fetus and neonates. A good analgesic rather than a good anesthetic is preferred during delivery. Halothane and other fluorinated anesthetics have lower safety margin.

NITROUS OXIDE

Nitrous oxide causes rapid induction and rapid reversal. It is a very good analgesic even at lower concentrations. It neither interferes with uterine contractions nor with progress of labor. It does not interfere with the physiological role of oxytocin. It is simpler to administer and does not require sophisticated equipment. It crosses placenta but does not result in undesirable effects in both mother and fetus.[48] Ninety-nine percent of nitrous oxide is eliminated through lungs without any metabolic alteration. Short comings of nitrous oxide are nausea and vomiting.

HALOTHANE

Halothane causes relaxation of uterine smooth muscle and it delays labor by inhibiting uterine contractions. As a smooth muscle relaxant it causes vasodilatation increasing blood loss during delivery. It is not a good analgesic and results in slow induction, qualities unfavorable in labor. Hence, it is not a preferred anesthetic for labor.

Drug of Choice: Nitrous Oxide

RATIONALE

Halothane is **not** a **good analgesic**. It relaxes uterine smooth muscle, delays labor and **increases blood loss** during delivery.

Nitrous oxide is a potent analgesic, causes rapid induction and recovery and **does not interfere with uterine contractions**. It is safe for mother, fetus and neonates. It does not interfere with the function of oxytocin and is easy to administer. Hence, it is preferred to halothane as anesthetic in labor and for vaginal delivery.

12. *Administration of 100% oxygen/Plain air during discontinuation of nitrous oxide.*

BACKGROUND

Nitrous oxide is highly insoluble hence has rapid induction and quick reversal. It helps in rapid uptake of halogenated anesthetics administered along with it. This mechanism is called as 'second gas effect'. The advantage of this phenomenon is to quicken the induction of anesthesia.

100% OXYGEN

On discontinuation of nitrous oxide, it quickly diffuses from blood to alveoli. This process dilutes the oxygen present in lung causing hypoxia and this effect is termed as 'diffusional hypoxia'. 100% oxygen administered during discontinuation of nitrous oxide helps in the reversal of diffusional hypoxia.

PLAIN AIR

Air alone is inadequate to reverse the diffusional hypoxia. Hence, plain air does not prevent nitrous oxide induced dilution of oxygen.

Drug of Choice: 100% Oxygen

RATIONALE

Nitrous oxide causes **diffusional hypoxia** during discontinuation as it quickly diffuses from blood to alveoli. To **overcome** this problem **100% oxygen** should be administered during its discontinuation as **plain air** is **insufficient** to prevent diffusional hypoxia.

13. *Midazolam/Lorazepam as an adjuvant with anesthetics.*

BACKGROUND

Anesthetic adjuncts are given to potentiate a particular component of anesthesia and reduce the required dose of anesthetics. Benzodiazepines can also be used either alone to induce sedation or as adjuvants to induce amnesia, sedation and to reduce anxiety. Midazolam and lorazepam are both used as adjuvants with anesthetics.

MIDAZOLAM

Midazolam is water soluble and can be given intravenously. It has rapid onset of action with shorter duration of action. Sedative effect of IV midazolam starts within 2 minutes and lasts for 30 minutes. Its elimination is seven times quicker than lorazepam. Minimal venous irritation is reported for midazolam when compared to lorazepam.

LORAZEPAM

Lorazepam is very potent and causes profound amnesia but it has delayed onset and its duration of action is longer. Due to these reasons, lorazepam is highly unsuitable as adjunct.

Drug of Choice: Midazolam

RATIONALE

Midazolam and lorazepam are both used as anesthetic adjuncts to produce amnesia, sedation and to reduce anxiety prior to surgical procedures. **Midazolam** has **quick onset**, **rapid elimination** and **shorter duration** of action when compared to lorazepam hence, it is preferred to lorazepam.

Therapeutic Gases

1. *Nitric oxide/100% Oxygen for pulmonary hypertension in newborn.*

BACKGROUND

Incidence of pulmonary hypertension in newborn is around 2% and responsible for one-third of neonatal mortality. COX_1 is upregulated during late gestation increasing prostacyclin levels. Nitric oxide, prostacyclin and endothelin pathway are involved in stimulating vasodilatation. In affected neonates these normal pathways are disrupted causing pulmonary hypertension.

NITRIC OXIDE

Nitric oxide synthases produce nitric oxide from L-arginine stimulating cyclic GMP mediated vasodilatation. It has selective action on pulmonary vasculature and dilates the pulmonary vessels. It does not modify the tone of systemic vessels but decreases pulmonary vascular resistance and arterial pressure thereby improving pulmonary oxygenation. It is useful in pulmonary hypertension, right heart failure and pulmonary embolism. FDA has approved the use of nitric oxide in pulmonary hypertension of newborn.

100% OXYGEN

Hypoxia due to pulmonary conditions can be partially relieved by oxygen. However, oxygen cannot be used safely in a newborn. 100% oxygen can change lung function within 12 hours of administration but it damages pulmonary endothelium and increases the capillary permeability thereby increasing the incidence of pulmonary interstitial edema. In premature infants and newborn it can lead to abnormal neovascularization. Fibrovascular proliferation of retina causes blindness. Hence, 100% oxygen should not be used for pulmonary hypertension in newborn.

Drug of Choice: Nitric Oxide

RATIONALE

Hundred percent oxygen causes **damage** to the **pulmonary epithelium** increasing capillary permeability and interstitial edema. It also results in fibrovascular proliferation of retina in newborn leading to **blindness**. **Nitric oxide improves pulmonary oxygenation** by selectively dilating the pulmonary vessels. Hence, nitric oxide is preferred to 100% oxygen for the treatment of pulmonary hypertension.

CHAPTER
18

Alcohol, Sedatives and Hypnotics

1. *Zolpidem/Benzodiazepines (BDZ) as a sedative hypnotic.*

BACKGROUND

Sleep pattern is characterized by stages 0, 1, 2, 3 and 4. Stages 0 to 3 are wakefulness, sleepiness, arousable and not easily arousable sleep. Stage 4 is deep, rapid eye movement (REM) sleep or stage of dreams and nightmares.

ZOLPIDEM

Zolpidem is a gamma-aminobutyric acid (GABA) agonist approved by Food and Drug Administration (FDA) for sleep onset insomnia. Zolpidem shortens sleep latency and prolongs total sleep time. Compared to benzodiazepine (BDZ), suppression of REM sleep by zolpidem is relatively minimal. It does not produce residual day time sedation, dizziness or amnesia. Hence, it is far superior to benzodiazepines as a sedative and hypnotic.

BENZODIAZEPINES

Benzodiazepines exert GABA mimetic action by binding with GABA-A receptor. They cause sedation, hypnosis and anterograde amnesia and reduce the time taken for onset of sleep and also reduce the number of nocturnal awakenings. Benzodiazepines improve the quality of sleep. The duration of stage 0, 1, 3 and 4 are reduced by benzodiazepines but stage 2 is prolonged, so it is unsuitable for those having difficulty in falling asleep. The time taken from stage 3 to REM sleep is increased by benzodiazepines and it shortens REM sleep, increasing number of REM cycles and total sleep time. BDZ decrease upper airway muscle tone causing sleep apnea. They also suppress arousal response to hypoxia resulting in residual hangover, light headedness and motor in coordination.

Drug of Choice: Zolpidem

RATIONALE

Benzodiazepines increase total sleep time but **prolong** the time spent in stage of **descending wakefulness**. They also result in **residual hangover** and light headedness. BDZ worsen sleep apnea. **Zolpidem** on the other hand, **shortens sleep latency**, prolongs total sleep time with **minimal suppression of REM sleep** and does not produce any residual **effects, the next morning. Hence, zolpidem is preferred to benzodiazepines as an ideal** sedative and hypnotic.

2. *Eszopiclone/Ramelteon as an ideal agent for both transient and chronic insomnia.*

BACKGROUND

The hypnotic used should not disturb the normal pattern of sleep. It should not cause hangover or day time sedation or rebound insomnia on discontinuation.

RAMELTEON

Higher concentrations of melatonin can cause good sleep. Ramelteon is a melatonin congener and binds to melatonin receptors to induce sleep. It shortens sleep latency for onset of sleep and prolongs total duration of sleep. It does not result in impairment of cognitive function the following morning. Tolerance is not reported even after six months of continuous administration. It does not result in rebound insomnia or withdrawal effects.

ESZOPICLONE

Eszopiclone is an active S- enantiomer of zopiclone. Patients who have difficulty in falling asleep or in staying asleep are benefited by eszopiclone. It is approved by FDA for both transient and chronic insomnia. It decreases time taken to fall asleep and improves the quality of sleep. Eszopiclone reduces the number of awakenings during sleep and tolerance does not develop even after 12 months of therapy. It does not result in rebound insomnia on discontinuation but has a bitter taste and can result in abnormal dreams and anxiety.

Drug of Choice: Ramelteon

RATIONALE

Eszopiclone and ramelteon shorten sleep onset latency and improve the quality of sleep. They do not develop tolerance to their hypnotic action. Rebound insomnia does not occur on discontinuation of either drug. **Ramelteon** is **devoid** of **withdrawal symptoms** but **eszopiclone** results in **abnormal dreams** and **anxiety**. Hence, ramelteon is the drug of choice for transient and chronic insomnia.

3. *Triazolam/Flurazepam for prevention of early morning insomnia.*

BACKGROUND

For prevention of early morning insomnia, the drug should have a sustained action. Benzodiazepines have high lipid solubility and their CSF level equilibrates with their plasma levels.

FLURAZEPAM

Flurazepam has short half-life of about 2 hours but its metabolite, N-des-alkyl-flurazepam has prolonged half-life of 40 to 100 hours due to high plasma protein binding and enterohepatic circulation. So, flurazepam is preferred for prevention of early morning insomnia.

TRIAZOLAM

Triazolam is a short acting benzodiazepine with a short half-life of 6 hours. It results in early morning insomnia as the effect of drug wanes off quickly. Besides, triazolam results in serious paradoxical disinhibition reactions such as cognitive impairment, paranoia, depression and suicidal tendencies. Triazolam has been banned in UK for these disinhibition reactions. Further it results in greater degree of anterograde amnesia.

Drug of Choice: Flurazepam

RATIONALE

Sedative hypnotic with rapid onset and sustained action is preferred for preventing early morning insomnia. **Flurazepam** is **preferentially chosen** for this purpose as its metabolite has **longer duration** of action besides, **paradoxical psychological** effects occur occasionally. **Triazolam** is better **avoided** as it has a short duration of action making it **unsuitable** for **preventing early morning insomnia** moreover it can cause serious **paradoxical disinhibition reactions** such as paranoia and suicidal tendencies as well as cognitive impairment.

4. *Diazepam/Eszopiclone in anxiety related gastrointestinal disorders.*

BACKGROUND

Hypothalamus and locus coeruleus are associated with stress and anxiety and amygdala and hippocampus activates hypothalamus at times of stress. Corticotropin releasing factor secreted from hypothalamus is the key mediator of stress. Anxiety related gastrointestinal tract (GIT) disorders vary from stress ulcers to functional dyspepsia, irritable bowel syndrome, inflammatory bowel disease and gastroesophageal reflux disease (GERD).[49]

DIAZEPAM

In addition to being an anxiolytic, diazepam also reduces nocturnal gastric secretion. Hence, it is very effective as an adjuvant in acid peptic disease and GERD. It is also a centrally acting skeletal muscle relaxant. Since stress and related conditions result in insomnia, an anxiolytic is effective in GIT related stress disorders.

ESZOPICLONE

It is an S-enantiomer of zopiclone and acts on α-1 subunit of GABA-A receptor. Eszopiclone is a sedative hypnotic, has a calming effect on patients. It is a better hypnotic but an inferior anxiolytic when compared to benzodiazepines so it does not provide any additional benefit in anxiety related GIT conditions. Besides, it can cause nausea and vomiting due to its bitter taste.

Drug of Choice: Diazepam

RATIONALE

Diazepam has both **direct** and **indirect** effect in anxiety related disorder. It has direct effect in acid peptic disease and in GERD as it **reduces** nocturnal gastric **acid secretion**. It also acts indirectly through its anxiolytic action. **Eszopiclone**, being a sedative hypnotic calms the patient but is not effective in anxiety related GIT disorders. Although it is an anxiolytic, it is **inferior** to diazepam. Besides, it results in minor GIT side effects.

5. *Zolpidem/Zaleplon as hypnotic for inducing sleep of short duration.*

BACKGROUND

Short-term insomnia extends from three days to three weeks. Intermittent use of hypnotics for short term insomnia is indicated. Zaleplon and zolpidem are both effective in treating sleep–onset insomnia. They are given initially for a period of one week to ten days to relieve insomnia. These drugs act selectively on α-1 subunit of GABA-A receptor. They decrease sleep latency without causing rebound insomnia on discontinuation.

ZALEPLON

Zaleplon has a very short half-life, reaches peak concentration within one hour. Therefore, zaleplon results in a short sleep for four hours. It has only 30% bioavailability due to high first pass metabolism and can be administered safely, four hours before the anticipated waking time. So, it is preferred for those having difficulty in falling asleep past bed time.

ZOLPIDEM

Half-life of zolpidem is about 2 hours and it produces 8 hours sleep. Zolpidem, if administered late at night, past bed time causes residual hangover. Sedation, motor incoordination and anterograde amnesia occur if administered late. Zaleplon is the drug of choice for inducing sleep of short duration.

Drug of Choice: Zaleplon

RATIONALE

Zolpidem and zaleplon reduce the time taken for onset of sleep and are devoid of rebound insomnia on discontinuation. **Zolpidem** produces **eight hours of sleep** whereas **zaleplon** produces only **four hours** of sleep. So, if patient needs a **hypnotic past bed time, zaleplon** is the drug of choice because it induces **short sleep without** morning **hangover** whereas zolpidem, if given late at night can cause unpleasant hangover the next morning.

6. *Benzodiazepines/Barbiturates overdose is treated by flumazenil.*

BACKGROUND

Benzodiazepines and barbiturates are both GABA agonists and act at GABA-A receptor subtype increasing chloride conductance. Benzodiazepines increase the frequency of chloride channel opening. Barbiturates prolong the duration of interaction at GABA-A receptor site. It allows more time for regular chloride channel bursts without increasing the frequency of chloride channel opening. Barbiturates act only at α and β subunits of GABA-A. Benzodiazepines act at α, β and γ subunits of GABA receptors.

FLUMAZENIL IN BENZODIAZEPINE OVERDOSE

Flumazenil is an imidazobenzodiazepine and a benzodiazepine antagonist. It is an inverse agonist and competitive antagonist of

GABA-A receptor. It is effective only in the treatment of benzodiazepine overdose. It is usually given as multiple small dose injections and not as a bolus injection. A dose of 1 to 5 mg is given for a period of 2 to 10 minutes. Lack of response indicates that overdose may be due to other drugs and not due to benzodiazepines.

FLUMAZENIL IN BARBITURATE OVERDOSE

Flumazenil is ineffective when given in overdose of barbiturates. Flumazenil is reported to cause seizures if given in overdose of barbiturates. Therefore, flumazenil is contraindicated in barbiturates poisoning.

Drug of Choice: Benzodiazepines

RATIONALE

Benzodiazepines and barbiturates act on **GABA-A** receptor. Benzodiazepines act on α, β and γ subunits of GABA-A while barbiturates act only on α and β subunits of GABA. Barbiturates prolong the duration of interaction at GABA-A while benzodiazepines increase the frequency of chloride channel opening at GABA-A. **Flumazenil** is a **competitive antagonist** of **benzodiazepines** and is effective in management of benzodiazepines overdose. It is **contraindicated** for **overdose** of **barbiturates** as it causes seizures if given in this condition.

7. *Acamprosate/Naltrexone as adjunct for de-addiction in those abstained from alcohol.*

BACKGROUND

Acamprosate and naltrexone are both approved as adjuncts in alcohol de-addiction.[50] Acamprosate is a GABA agonist and a weak NMDA antagonist. Naltrexone is a complete opioid antagonist. They block alcohol activated dopaminergic reward pathways.

NALTREXONE

Naltrexone effectively reduces craving for alcohol, prolongs the abstinence period. Further it improves patient's compliance and reduces relapse rate. Even short term administration of naltrexone can prevent the relapse rate. It is well tolerated, given at a daily dose of 50 mg and causes nausea, headache, sedation and anxiety in only 10% of individuals. Dose related hepatotoxicity is its severe adverse effect.

ACAMPROSATE

The efficacy of acamprosate is lower in prolonging the abstinence period. Its capacity in reducing relapse rate is much lower compared to naltrexone. Acamprosate does not reduce the craving for alcohol and has poor compliance rate as it needs to be given thrice a day. It is contraindicated in severe renal impairment and can cause nausea, vomiting, diarrhea, dyspepsia, flatulence and headache.

Drug of Choice: Naltrexone

RATIONALE

Acamprosate and naltrexone are both used as adjuncts in alcohol de-addiction. They are approved for patients abstained from alcohol to prevent further relapse. Naltrexone is a complete opioid antagonist and acamprosate is a GABA agonist with weak NMDA antagonistic action. Naltrexone is given once daily and **improves** the **compliance rate** while treating alcoholism. Acamprosate is given thrice daily, so has poor compliance. Naltrexone **reduces craving, prolongs abstinence** and **reduces relapse rate** but acamprosate is less effective. Besides, naltrexone is better tolerated. Hence, naltrexone is the drug of choice[51,52] in alcohol de-addiction.

8. *Ethyl alcohol/Fomepizole in methyl alcohol poisoning.*

BACKGROUND

Methanol causes GIT distress, pancreatitis, blindness and metabolic acidosis. Hemodialysis should be the first step in methyl alcohol poisoning before initiating pharmacotherapy. Formaldehyde and formic acid, the metabolites of methanol are responsible for these toxicities.

FOMEPIZOLE

Fomepizole is an inhibitor of alcohol dehydrogenase and suppresses conversion of methanol to formaldehyde. Fomepizole has predictable pharmacokinetics hence, given on a fixed dose regimen based on body weight. Therefore, it does not need frequent serum monitoring. Fomepizole causes headache, nausea, metallic taste, drowsiness and dizziness. Although ethanol is still being given as standard therapy as it is cost effective fomepizole is preferred due to the above said advantages.[53]

ETHYL ALCOHOL

Ethanol is a competitive substrate for alcohol dehydrogenase responsible for conversion of methanol to formaldehyde. It competes with methanol for alcohol dehydrogenase and gets converted to acetaldehyde thereby preventing the conversion of methanol to formaldehyde. Ethanol has unpredictable pharmacokinetics needs serum level monitoring and causes hypoglycemia, pancreatitis, agitation or loss of consciousness.

Drug of Choice: Fomepizole

RATIONALE

Ethanol is only a competitive substrate of alcohol dehydrogenase. Even though ethanol is still the standard therapy in methanol poisoning it has the disadvantage of causing unpredictable serum levels and serious side effects. **Fomepizole** is an inhibitor of alcohol dehydrogenase and prevents conversion of methanol to its toxic metabolites. It has **better safety profile** and has **predictable serum levels**. Hence, **if available**, fomepizole should be preferred to ethanol in the treatment of methanol poisoning.[54]

CHAPTER
19
Cerebrodegenerative Disorders

1. *Apomorphine/Ropinirole in Parkinson's disease as an alternative to levodopa.*

BACKGROUND

Apomorphine and ropinirole are direct dopamine agonists in neostriatum. They are effective alternatives and have longer duration of action. They are used in patients suffering from dyskinesia or "on/off" phenomenon as they reduce the need for endogenous as well as exogenous dopamine.

ROPINIROLE

Ropinirole has selective action on D_2 receptors and has good oral bioavailability. It has long half-life, so it is given once daily, improving patient compliance and reduces side effects. Nausea, hypotension and hallucination are minimized by starting at a small dose. The required dose is gradually increased. Although uncommon, somnolence could be quite severe. Patients treated by ropinirole should be warned about this side effect.

APOMORPHINE

Apomorphine has high affinity for D_4 receptors and has moderate affinity for D_2, D_3, D_5 and α adrenergic receptors. It is highly emetic and has to be given as subcutaneous injection. Main disadvantage of apomorphine is its ability to prolong QT interval. It causes profound hypotension when combined with ondansetron hence it is preferred for acute intermittent treatment for "wearing off" phenomenon only. Apomorphine is given as a 'rescue therapy' for this condition.

Drug of Choice: Ropinirole

RATIONALE

Apomorphine and ropinirole are both dopamine agonists and reduce the need for exogenous and endogenous dopamine. **Ropinirole** is **superior** because of its **selective** activity at D_2 receptors, good oral bioavailability, **longer duration** of action and tolerable side effects. Apomorphine is indicated only for intermittent management of "wearing off" phenomenon as it is a strong emetic, has a nonselective action on dopamine receptors, prolongs QT interval and results in other severe side effects.

2. *Entacapone/Tolcapone in the treatment of Parkinsonism as an adjuvant to levodopa.*

BACKGROUND

Entacapone and tolcapone are catechol-O-methyltransferase (COMT) inhibitors and prevent peripheral conversion of levodopa. These drugs facilitate the entry of dopamine into central nervous system (CNS) and are given with levodopa/carbidopa to reduce the "wearing off" phenomenon.

ENTACAPONE

Entacapone has short half-life and has to be administered frequently. It is usually administered with every dose of levodopa-carbidopa. Common adverse effects are nausea, orthostatic hypotension and bizarre dreams. Entacapone does not result in hepatotoxicity unlike tolcapone so it is preferred.

TOLCAPONE

Tolcapone has long half-life and inhibits COMT both centrally and peripherally. Tolcapone induces hepatotoxicity and increases serum aspartate aminotransferase (AST) and alanine aminotransferase (ALT). Adverse effects of tolcapone make it unsuitable as drug of choice.

Drug of Choice: Entacapone

RATIONALE

Catechol-o-methyltransferase (COMT) inhibitors prevent the peripheral metabolism of levodopa and facilitate its entry into CNS. Tolcapone and entacapone share the same mechanism of action and have some common side effects but **tolcapone** causes **hepatotoxicity** with a **black box warning** to its label. Entacapone does not increase serum AST and ALT and **does not need monitoring**. On account of its short half-life it can be administered conveniently with each dose of levodopa-carbidopa. Hence entacapone is preferred to tolcapone as an adjunct to levodopa in the treatment of Parkinsonism.

3. *Clozapine/Quetiapine for management of hallucination induced by levodopa.*

BACKGROUND

Progression of Parkinson's disease often results in deterioration of motor functions progressing to psychological and cognitive symptoms. Hallucination and paranoid delusion are common in due course of disease and can be are overcome by atypical antipsychotic drugs such as clozapine and quetiapine.

QUETIAPINE

Quetiapine is a weak D_2 blocker also blocks $5HT_{2A}$, H_1, M_1, M_3 and α_1 receptors. It also reduces the frequency of paranoid delusion and hallucination and improves psychotic symptoms without worsening motor functions.[55] It is more tolerable and causes mainly sedation as its side effect. It has short half-life and has to be given twice daily. Quetiapine is usually well tolerated and does not result in agranulocytosis and seizures so it is preferred.

CLOZAPINE

Clozapine blocks D_2, D_4, $5HT_{2A}$ and α_1 receptors but has only weak D_2 blockade. It improves symptoms of psychosis without deteriorating motor functions. Clozapine reduces frequency of hallucination and paranoid delusion but causes neutropenia, leukopenia, agranulocytosis, sleepiness, fatigue and weight gain. It also reduces seizure threshold.

Drug of Choice: Quetiapine

RATIONALE

Atypical antipsychotic drugs clozapine and quetiapine are both weak D_2 blockers and are found to be equally effective in reducing the frequency of hallucination and paranoid delusion but **clozapine** causes **agranulocytosis** necessitating frequent **blood picture** monitoring. It also causes seizures, sedation and weight gain. Quetiapine is well tolerated, results mainly in sedation and preferred to clozapine in treating hallucination induced by levodopa.[56]

4. *Phenelzine/Selegiline in Parkinson's disease as adjuncts with levodopa.*

BACKGROUND

For any given dose of levodopa the clinical response declines in due course of time, becoming less predictable due to progression of disease. The reason is mainly due to increased catabolism of dopamine by striatal monoamine oxidase (MAO) enzyme. It can be overcome by coadministration of monoamine oxidase inhibitors (MAOI).

SELEGILINE

Selegiline is an irreversible, selective MAO-B inhibitor. Selegiline selectively inhibits MAO-B in striatum resulting in beneficial effects. Besides it does not inhibit catecholamine metabolism peripherally therefore it can be coadministered with food containing tyramine. It can also be taken safely with levodopa.

PHENELZINE

Phenelzine is a nonselective, irreversible MAO inhibitor acting on both MAO-A and MAO-B. It inhibits metabolism of serotonin, norepinephrine, epinephrine and dopamine potentiating the action of levodopa causing life-threatening hypertensive crisis. Hence, it should not be used along with levodopa in Parkinsonism. Coadministration of food rich in tyramine causes dangerous hypertensive crisis.

Drug of Choice: Selegiline

RATIONALE

Monoamine oxidase inhibitors are given along with levodopa to promote its pharmacological action and to augment its benefit. **Phenelzine** is a **nonselective** MAO inhibitor and inhibits both MAO-A and MAO-B irreversibly. If given with levodopa, it **causes life-threatening hypertensive crisis**. **Selegiline** is a **selective**, **irreversible** inhibitor of MAO-B and acts specifically in neostriatum, does not inhibit metabolism of catecholamine peripherally, can **safely** be **administered** with levodopa and so is preferred to phenelzine.

5. *Selegiline/Rasagiline in treatment of Parkinsonism.*

BACKGROUND

Selective, irreversible MAO-B inhibitors inhibit MAO-B in striatum. Therefore, these drugs inhibit dopamine metabolism and prolong its action. Selegiline and rasagiline are both given as monotherapy in early Parkinson's disease. They can also be combined with levodopa in advanced Parkinson's disease. These drugs have neuroprotective effect as they reduce catabolism of dopamine and they prevent the formation of free radicals. They should not be coadministered with selective serotonin reuptake inhibitor (SSRI), and tricyclic antidepressants (TCA).

RASAGILINE

Rasagiline is an irreversible inhibitor of MAO-B enzyme and has greater degree of neuroprotective action than selegiline. The metabolite of rasagiline does not have amphetamine like action. Rasagiline results in dry mouth, loss of appetite, weight loss, orthostatic hypotension and joint pain.

SELEGILINE

Selegiline should not be given for those with pre-existing cognitive impairment because it exaggerates motor and cognitive symptoms in such patients. Its metabolites amphetamine and methamphetamine cause anxiety and insomnia. Selegiline has low oral bioavailability and available as transdermal patch. Adverse effects are severe headache, intense nausea, vomiting, weight loss, photophobia and orthostatic hypotension.

Drug of Choice: Rasagiline

RATIONALE

Selegiline and rasagiline have neuroprotective action and can delay the progression of Parkinson's disease. **Selegiline** can **potentiate** the **motor** and **cognitive impairment** caused by levodopa. If given orally, it causes unwanted side effects such as anxiety and insomnia due to its metabolites and transdermal administration can reduce these unwanted side effects. **Rasagiline** is preferred to selegiline as it has a greater degree of neuroprotective action. It is not metabolised into amphetamine and has a **better safety profile**.

6. *Amantadine/Trihexyphenidyl for drug induced Parkinsonism in elderly patients.*

BACKGROUND

Antipsychotics chlorpromazine and haloperidol cause drug-induced Parkinsonism due to their capacity to block D_2 receptors. They result in bradykinesia, rigidity, tremor and shuffling gait and these symptoms usually occur within the first month of therapy. Drug-induced Parkinsonism is more common in elderly individuals.

AMANTADINE

Amantadine blocks presynaptic dopamine reuptake and facilitates dopamine release potentiating dopamine action on its receptors. It is well tolerated by elderly individuals without any alteration to cognition and memory. It causes very minimal and reversible anticholinergic side effects.

TRIHEXYPHENIDYL

Trihexyphenidyl is a centrally acting anticholinergic drug. It freely crosses blood brain barrier and blocks muscarinic cholinergic receptors in neostriatum modulating dopamine release. It primarily inhibits dopamine reuptake transporter thereby increasing dopamine availability in synaptic clefts. It is very effective in treating drug induced Parkinsonism but not advisable for elders. It causes cognitive impairment, loss of memory and urinary retention, dry mouth and cycloplegia. It can aggravate pre-existing glaucoma and prostatic hypertrophy in elderly.

Drug of Choice: Amantadine

RATIONALE

Trihexyphenidyl is a centrally acting anticholinergic drug and increases the synaptic availability of dopamine. But, in elders, it can result in **impaired cognition, memory** and other unwanted **peripheral anticholinergic side effects**. Hence, it should be avoided in drug induced Parkinsonism in elders. **Amantadine facilitates dopamine release** and action, is **well tolerated** by elders causing only minimal anticholinergic side effects. It **does not result** in **loss of memory** and **exaggeration** of pre-existing **glaucoma** and **prostatic hypertrophy**.[57]

7. *Amantadine/Memantine in Alzheimer's disease as adjunct to anticholinesterases.*

BACKGROUND

Alzheimer's disease is a chronic neurodegenerative disease. It is characterized by cognitive impairment and dementia. Amantadine and memantine are both N-methyl-D-aspartate (NMDA) antagonists.

MEMANTINE

Memantine causes non-competitive blockade of NMDA-glutamate receptor reducing the excitotoxicity induced by glutamate. It inhibits clinical progression of Alzheimer's disease. It causes mild reversible side effects such as headache or dizziness. Memantine has a higher degree of neuroprotective action and unlike amantadine it does not have antidyskinetic property. Abnormal phosphorylation of Tau proteins is responsible for neuronal death and memantine inhibits and reverses such abnormal phosphorylation. It exhibits a disease modifying role in Alzheimer's disease so it is preferred.

AMANTADINE

Amantadine is useful in Parkinson's disease but not effective in Alzheimer's disease. It is an NMDA antagonist and exerts a neuroprotective action. It modulates dopamine release and facilitates dopamine action. It has antidyskinetic property. Hence, amantadine is more effective in Parkinsonism.

Drug of Choice: Memantine

RATIONALE

Although **amantadine** blocks NMDA receptors, it is **more effective** in controlling symptoms of Parkinsonism as it is also a **dopamine facilitator**. Memantine is a **better neuroprotective**, inhibits excitotoxicity of glutamate, reverses abnormal phosphorylation of Tau proteins and delays the clinical progression of Alzheimer's disease, causing only mild reversible side effects so, it is preferred to amantadine.

8. *Donepezil/Rivastigmine in Alzheimer's disease.*

BACKGROUND

Deficiency of acetylcholine is the principal pathophysiology of Alzheimer's disease so facilitation of cholinergic neuronal transmission is the main line of treatment. Anticholinesterases control mild cognitive impairment that occurs in early stage and prevent progression of mild cognitive impairment to full fledged disease. Donepezil and rivastigmine are both reversible cholinesterase inhibitors.

RIVASTIGMINE

Rivastigmine inhibits both acetylcholinesterase and butyrylcholinesterase. Butyrylcholinesterase is present in serum and liver and upregulated in the brain of patients suffering from Alzheimer's disease. By inhibiting butyrylcholinesterase rivastigmine is more effective than donepezil. It is also effective in dementia associated with Parkinson's disease. Rivastigmine is metabolized only by plasma esterases. Therefore, it causes minimal drug interactions and offers greater benefit and improvement in cognition and behavior.

DONEPEZIL

Acetylcholinesterase is the major cholinesterase in brain. Donepezil selectively inhibits acetylcholinesterase but it does not reverse Parkinson's disease induced dementia. Donepezil is metabolized by CYP_2D_6 and CYP_3A_4 hence, it is prone for drug interactions as most drugs are metabolized by these enzymes.

Drug of Choice: Rivastigmine

RATIONALE

Cholinesterase inhibitors prevent progression of Alzheimer's disease. **Rivastigmine** inhibits both acetyl as well as butyrylcholinesterases offers significant **improvement in cognition** and **behavior** and causes minimal drug interactions. **Donepezil** inhibits only acetylcholinesterase and **does not offer** any significant **advantage over rivastigmine.**[58] Donepezil is prone for many drug interactions so it is not preferred in Alzheimer's disease.

9. *Memantine/Riluzole in amyotrophic lateral sclerosis.*

BACKGROUND

Amyotrophic lateral sclerosis (ALS) is a progressive condition affecting both lower and upper motor neurons. Due to abnormal excitatory neurotransmitter glutamate reuptake, it causes accumulation of glutamate increasing excitotoxicity.

RILUZOLE

Riluzole blocks NMDA receptors and inhibits sodium channels. It also blocks glutamate action, inhibiting its release and antagonizing its receptors. It prolongs the survival period of patients affected by ALS by 2 to 3 months. Food interferes with absorption of riluzole and has to be given on empty stomach. It has a good safety profile resulting in mild nausea and diarrhea.

MEMANTINE

Memantine is an NMDA type glutamate receptor blocker more effective in Alzheimer's disease. It is an antagonist of the excitatory amino acid glutamate. Riluzole and memantine are both neuroprotective in nature. Memantine is not effective if given alone in ALS. It improves the clinical picture of ALS only if combined with riluzole.

Drug of Choice: Riluzole

RATIONALE

Riluzole and memantine are both NMDA receptor blockers. They inhibit glutamate action, prevent its excitotoxicity and are neuroprotective in nature. **Memantine** is **more specific** to Alzheimer's disease as it **inhibits** and reverses **phosphorylation of Tau proteins. Riluzole** has **additional inhibitory action** on voltage dependent sodium channels. It is reported to **prolong the survival rate** of patients affected by ALS by two months.[59] Hence, riluzole is preferred in ALS.

CHAPTER
20
Antipsychotics and Drugs in Bipolar Disorder

1. *Clozapine/Aripiprazole as monotherapy in treatment-resistant schizophrenia.*

BACKGROUND

Treatment-resistance indicates lack of improvement of symptoms. If administration of antipsychotic drugs over a period of time does not improve positive and negative symptoms, it indicates that it is a case of resistant schizophrenia.

CLOZAPINE

Clozapine is gold standard for management of treatment-resistant schizophrenia effective in almost 30% of individuals. It is a weak antagonist at D_2, D_4, $5HT_2$ receptors and a potent blocker of H_1 and α adrenergic receptors. Even after chronic therapy, the D_2 receptor occupancy rate of clozapine is only 47%. Therefore, it does not cause extrapyramidal side effects. About 60% of patients benefit after six months of clozapine therapy. It reduces polydipsia and hyponatremia in many patients but causes leucopenia, weight gain, sedation and orthostatic hypotension. It lowers seizure threshold and should be avoided in epileptics.

ARIPIPRAZOLE

Aripiprazole is a partial agonist at D_2, D_3 and $5HT_{1A}$ receptors, but aripiprazole antagonizes the $5HT_2$ receptors. It is less effective when given as monotherapy. It reduces the occurrence of weight gain, hyperprolactinemia and sedation, tremor and extrapyramidal symptoms. It improves symptoms of obsessive-compulsive neurosis better than clozapine[60] but causes insomnia, agitation, akathisia and rhabdomyolysis. It is preferred mainly for augmentation therapy with clozapine.

Drug of Choice: Clopazine

RATIONALE

Antipsychotics are used for augmentation therapy and are rarely effective as monotherapy in treatment-resistant schizophrenia. **Clozapine** is the **gold standard** for the management of this condition in spite of its adverse effects, offering 60% benefit. **Aripiprazole** is **not effective** as **monotherapy** but ideal only for augmentation therapy with clozapine.

2. *Clozapine/Olanzapine in schizophrenic patients with suicidal behavior.*

BACKGROUND

Patients with chronic schizophrenia suffer from affective symptoms such as depression and that low self-esteem contributes to suicidal tendencies. Schizophrenic patients have eight-fold risks for suicidal tendencies. About 5–10% of patients with schizophrenia commit suicide. The incidence of patients who attempt suicide is around 20–50%. Antipsychotic drugs form the main approach of therapy in reducing suicidal tendencies.

CLOZAPINE

Clozapine is an atypical antipsychotic drug used to prevent suicidal tendencies and has the strongest evidence for being an anti suicidal drug. It blocks D_2, D_4, $5HT_{2A}$ receptors, does not result in extrapyramidal side effects and suppresses suicidal thoughts. Clozapine is cost effective but can cause leucopenia necessitating weekly white cell counts. It also causes weight gain, elevated blood sugar levels and can provoke seizures. Clozapine lowers the seizure threshold.

OLANZAPINE

Olanzapine is an alternative to clozapine in reducing the negative symptoms. Olanzapine blocks muscarinic, $5HT_2$, D_1, D_2 and D_4 receptors. It too does not result in extrapyramidal side effects. Although it controls negative symptoms of schizophrenia, it is not as effective as clozapine. Headache, somnolence, weight gain and increase in blood sugar levels occur.

Drug of Choice: Clozapine

RATIONALE

Clozapine has a **superior** efficacy in **reducing suicidal behavior**, so is considered to be the first treatment option in a patient prone for suicidal tendencies.[61] It is **cost effective**, **devoid of extrapyramidal side effects** and has **proven efficacy** in suppressing suicidal thoughts. It results in **blood dyscrasias** necessitating weekly blood counts. **Olanzapine controls negative symptoms** in schizophrenia but is **not** as **effective** in **reducing suicidal thoughts** and is only considered to be a second line drug. Both drugs cause weight gain, type-2 diabetes and can provoke seizures. Hence, olanzapine is only an alternative to clozapine in schizophrenic patients with suicidal behavior.

3. *Paliperidone/Olanzapine for maintenance in patients, nonadherent to oral therapy*

BACKGROUND

Although long-acting antipsychotic is preferred in those who tend to miss regular medication, their nonadherence to therapy is due to severe adverse effects of the drug being used. Therefore, a better drug should be tried before long-acting formulation is initiated.

OLANZAPINE

Olanzapine pamoate is available as depot preparation, given once in 2–4 weeks. Elimination half-life is 30 days and it reaches steady state concentration in approximately 12 weeks.[62] Oral supplementation of olanzapine is not necessary. The efficacy and safety of parenteral formulations are similar to oral olanzapine. Side effects are weight gain, elevated blood sugar and increased incidence of seizures. Post-injection delirium sedation syndrome (PDSS) is reported in a few patients. Olanzapine results in significant antipsychotic effect and it delays exacerbation of symptoms[63] so, it is preferred.

PALIPERIDONE

Paliperidone is a primary active metabolite of risperidone. Paliperidone palmitate injection is given once monthly. It has the advantage of lower incidence of weight gain, diabetes mellitus and hyperlipidemia. It can easily be converted from oral to parenteral formulation during therapy and does not need an overlap with oral drug during such conversion but it is very expensive and increases the risk of QT prolongation in high-risk patients.

Drug of Choice: Olanzapine

RATIONALE

Long-acting injectable preparations are used in patients whose compliance in taking oral medication is very poor. Paliperidone, an active metabolite of risperidone has many advantages such as low incidence of metabolic disorder and it does not require overlap with oral formulation but it is very expensive and has the potential to prolong QT interval in high-risk patients. Hence, it is not preferred. Olanzapine has good efficacy, cost effective, needs no oral supplementation, devoid of extrapyramidal side effects. Therefore, it is preferred.

4. *Trihexyphenidyl/Clonazepam in acute akathisia due to antipsychotic drugs.*

BACKGROUND

Twenty percent of patients suffer from akathisia during early days of therapy with antipsychotic drugs. High doses of high potency antipsychotics result in akathisia. Even second generation drugs such as aripiprazole and quetiapine with weak D_2 blockade can result in mild akathisia. It is characterized by constant movement, inability to sit or stand and restlessness. Akathisia is of extrastriatal origin and is very often accompanied by dysphoria but nigrostriatal pathway responsible for extrapyramidal symptoms is not involved.

CLONAZEPAM

First line treatment is clonazepam at the dose of 0.5–1 mg thrice a day. It is gamma-aminobutyric acid (GABA) mimetic and has significant cortical activity so it is effective in controlling acute akathisia induced by antipsychotic drugs. Therefore, coadministration of anticholinergic drugs during clonazepam therapy is not required. Another alternative is non-selective beta blocker propranolol with good central nervous system (CNS) penetration.

TRIHEXYPHENIDYL

Anticholinergics are useful only in Parkinsonism induced by antipsychotics and in dystonia and their clinical utility in akathisia remains unclear. Trihexyphenidyl is a centrally acting anticholinergic drug. A dose of 2–5 mg three times daily is helpful but therapy is limited by its side effects.

Drug of Choice: Clonazepam

RATIONALE

Akathisia is characterized by restless movements with an inability to stand or sit. It occurs mainly due to high doses of first generation antipsychotics. **Clonazepam** is centrally acting **GABA mimetic** drug with **significant cortical activity** and effectively controls acute akathisia induced by antipsychotic drugs. Therefore, it is the drug of choice for this condition. Trihexyphenidyl is effective only in Parkinsonism induced by antipsychotic drugs. In akathisia, its use is limited and not preferred.

5. *Ziprasidone/Clozapine as antipsychotic in obese patients.*

BACKGROUND

Cardiac problems and type 2 diabetes mellitus occur frequently in schizophrenia and their prevalence is two-fold high in such patients. Baseline blood glucose, serum lipids and cardiac assessment have to be done in schizophrenia. These assessments are necessary and required as per guidelines. Antipsychotic drugs usually result in metabolic side effects such as dyslipidemia, hypertriglyceridemia and impaired glycemic control. Antipsychotic induced hypertriglyceridemia is independent of weight gain. It is temporary and resolves if the drug is discontinued. Hyperglycemia and alteration of glucose-insulin homeostasis can occur and the risk of diabetes mellitus is also independent of weight gain.

ZIPRASIDONE

Among atypical antipsychotics, ziprasidone has high efficacy. It causes the least weight gain compared to clozapine. It controls both positive and negative symptoms of schizophrenia due to blockade of both dopamine and serotonin receptors. It does not cause significant weight gain, diabetes mellitus or hypertriglyceridemia. It causes torsades de pointes or prolongation of QT interval. So, patients on ziprasidone should be screened for cardiac risk factors. Pretreatment cardiac assessment is necessary for high-risk individuals. Hence, ziprasidone and not clozapine is preferred in obese patients but ziprasidone necessitates constant cardiac monitoring.

CLOZAPINE

Clozapine causes severe hyperglycemia and hypertriglyceridemia promoting weight gain and increasing the risk of diabetes mellitus. Hence, clozapine should be avoided in obese patients.

Drug of Choice: Ziprasidone

RATIONALE

Clozapine should be **avoided** in **obese** patients as it causes weight gain, hyperglycemia and hypertriglyceridemia. It also increases the risk of diabetes mellitus. **Ziprasidone** is effective in **controlling** both **positive** and **negative** symptoms of schizophrenia. Among the atypical antipsychotic drugs ziprasidone **causes** least **weight gain**, does not result in hypertriglyceridemia or diabetes mellitus so it is preferred in obese patients. Since it has a **higher tendency** to cause **QT prolongation**, the patient should be **monitored** continuously to avoid the risk of **ventricular arrhythmia**.

6. *First generation/Second generation antipsychotics as first line drug in schizophrenia.*

BACKGROUND

Antipsychotic therapy is aimed at reducing symptoms of schizophrenia such as agitation, hostile behavior, hallucinations and social withdrawal. First generation (typical) and second generation (atypical) drugs are used in therapy. They are equally effective in controlling positive symptoms like agitation.

SECOND GENERATION ANTIPSYCHOTICS

Atypical or second generation antipsychotic (SGA) agents are devoid of extrapyramidal and anticholinergic side effects. Atypical antipsychotics are more effective in controlling the negative symptoms such as social withdrawal. Besides, the side effect profile and the dose required for therapy of atypical drugs (SGA) are lower than typical drugs. Lower dose reduces the incidence of orthostatic hypotension due to atypical drugs. Therefore, they have better efficacy with minimal extrapyramidal symptoms and anticholinergic side effects. So, they are preferred to typical antipsychotic drugs.

FIRST GENERATION ANTIPSYCHOTICS

First generation antipsychotics (FGA) such as haloperidol are highly potent. They antagonize D_2 receptors. Since they result in severe D_2 blockade, the incidence of extrapyramidal symptoms is high. They cause muscular rigidity, tremor and bradykinesia. Chlorpromazine is a low potent typical drug. It causes sedation, orthostatic hypotension, blurring of vision and dryness of mouth. This is due to blockade of histamine, α_1 and muscarinic receptors. Typical drugs such as thioridazine, mesoridazine, pimozide inhibit cardiac K channels. Since they prolong QT interval, they are highly cardiotoxic.

Drug of Choice: Second Generation Antipsychotics

RATIONALE

The main goal of treatment in schizophrenia is to control both positive and negative symptoms as well as to improve cognition. Although **typical agents (FGA) control positive symptoms** as effectively as atypical agents (SGA), they have **minimal efficacy** in **controlling negative symptoms** and do not improve cognition. Besides, the dose requirement is high and such high doses given for prolonged periods result in undesired side effects like extra-pyramidal side effects, orthostatic hypotension and anticholinergic side effects. Since **atypical** antipsychotics (SGA) **control both positive and negative symptoms even at low doses, improve cognition**, have better safety profile they are preferred to typical antipsychotics (FGA).

7. *Lithium/Divalproex during first week of acute episodes of mania.*

BACKGROUND

Symptoms of acute mania begin abruptly and are progressive over many days. Patients suffer from lack of sleep, increased activity and faulty judgment. Atypical antipsychotics can be given for initial management of acute mania.

DIVALPROEX

Divalproex has a better gastrointestinal tract (GIT) tolerability and is more effective than lithium during the initial period and it acts immediately. It offers good therapeutic benefit within 3–5 days. Immediate release preparations of divalproex control symptoms quickly. While sustained release preparations are effective for about

24 hours. Divalproex is usually combined with either antiepileptic drugs or antipsychotics or both.

LITHIUM

Lithium is the main line of treatment in acute episodes of mania but it is not effective in the initial stages of acute mania. Its action starts only after a lag period because it requires 5–7 days to achieve a steady state concentration. It is initially distributed widely in extracellular fluid and therefore, accumulates in various tissues and achieves steady state concentration slowly. So, it is unsuitable as monotherapy for immediate control of symptoms in acute mania.

Drug of Choice: Divalproex

RATIONALE

Symptoms of acute mania start abruptly and should be controlled immediately. Although **lithium** is the main line drug in treatment of acute mania, it is **not effective immediately** as its **onset** of action is **delayed** for a period of 5–7 days. **Divalproex acts immediately** and controls symptoms quickly. Hence, it is preferred to lithium for acute mania. However, lithium is combined with divalproex as soon as symptoms start. The initial control is by divalproex and lithium acts after one week.

8. *Olanzapine/Quetiapine as monotherapy for bipolar depression.*

BACKGROUND

The period of depression exceeds that of mania in bipolar depression. The depressive phase is more frequent and continues for a longer duration than manic phase. Greater risk of suicidal thoughts and behaviors occur during this phase. Antidepressants are effective only in unipolar depression and are not effective in bipolar depression. Lithium has only modest efficacy in controlling bipolar depression.

QUETIAPINE

Quetiapine is very effective in controlling symptoms of both mania and depression. It acts by moderate blockade of D_2 and $5HT_2$ receptors. It is the first antipsychotic approved as monotherapy for the treatment of depression.[64] It is effective at a dose of 300 to 600 mg per day. It does not increase the risk of patients switching over to mania from depressive phase. It can result in akathisia and it causes very minimal weight gain.

OLANZAPINE

Olanzapine is not approved for monotherapy but approved for combination therapy with fluoxetine for bipolar depression. It acts by blocking dopamine and $5HT_2$ receptors. It results in weight gain and increases the risk of diabetes mellitus but does not result in extrapyramidal symptoms. It shows only moderate efficacy in controlling depression of bipolar disorder. Hence, it has to be combined with the selective serotonin reuptake inhibitor (SSRI) fluoxetine.[65]

Drug of Choice: Quetiapine

RATIONALE

The depressive phase in bipolar disorder continues for a longer period and occurs more frequently. **Quetiapine** is approved for **monotherapy** in the management of depressive phase as it is very effective at a daily dose of 300 to 600 mg but can **cause akathisia**. **Olanzapine** is effective **only** when **combined** with SSRI, **fluoxetine**. Quetiapine is the drug of choice.[66]

CHAPTER
21   Antidepressants and Antianxiety Drugs

1. *Selective serotonin reuptake inhibitors (SSRI)/Tricyclic antidepressants (TCA) as antidepressants.*

BACKGROUND

The incidence of major or unipolar depression in women is twice that of men. It is characterized by pessimism, mental slowing, altered activity, poor concentration and frequently a feeling of sadness.

SELECTIVE SEROTONIN REUPTAKE INHIBITORS

The SSRIs are fluvoxamine, fluoxetine, sertraline, citalopram and escitalopram. They inhibit neuronal reuptake of serotonin. Since they inhibit reuptake of serotonin, they enhance serotonin transmission. They are well tolerated, have good efficacy with immediate onset without a lag period and do not affect cognition. SSRIs do not cause sedation, agitation, weight gain, postural hypotension and cardiac problems. They do not lower seizure threshold. They can cause insomnia, anxiety, irritability, vomiting and diarrhea. They decrease libido due to stimulation of $5HT_2$ receptors. Hence, SSRIs are preferred to TCAs as first line drugs in major depression.

TRICYCLIC ANTIDEPRESSANTS

Imipramine, amitriptyline and doxepin inhibit reuptake of norepinephrine and 5HT. Tricyclic antidepressants (TCAs) antagonize norepinephrine and serotonin transporters and also block muscarinic, α adrenergic and histaminergic receptors. Therefore, they enhance serotonergic and noradrenergic transmission but due to poor safety profile, they are not preferred as first line drugs in depression. They cause sedation due to blockade of H_1 receptors, postural hypotension through α_1 blockade and anti-cholinergic side effects such as blurred vision, dry mouth, constipation and impaired cognition. TCAs also lower seizure threshold and cause weight gain. They cause inversion of T-wave and inhibit cardiac conduction leading to arrhythmias. Several days to weeks are required to achieve steady state plasma concentration. Therefore, antidepressant action of TCAs starts only after a lag period of 2–4 weeks.

Drug of Choice: Selective Serotonin Reuptake Inhibitors (SSRIs)

RATIONALE

The TCAs result in sedation, postural hypotension, weight gain, impairment of cognition, cardiac and anticholinergic side effects. SSRIs cause insomnia, anxiety, GIT-related side effects and decreased libido due to serotonin over activity. **SSRIs** are preferred to TCAs for the treatment of unipolar depression as they are **more effective, well tolerated with quick onset** of action and a **better safety profile**.

2. *Sertraline/Paroxetine in post-traumatic stress disorder (PTSD).*

BACKGROUND

Post-traumatic stress disorder (PTSD) is a psychosomatic disorder characterized by improper concentration, fatigue and sleep disturbance with night sweats. PTSD can either be acute or chronic and is a highly difficult condition to treat. Sertraline and paroxetine are the only approved SSRIs for treatment of PTSD.[67] Neuronal reuptake through 5HT transporters terminates 5HT neurotransmission and SSRIs block such reuptake enhancing serotonin transmission at neuronal terminals. They are more selective to serotonin transporters (SERT) than norepinephrine transporters (NET). Increased availability of serotonin stimulates postsynaptic serotonin receptors as well as presynaptic autoreceptors but, prolonged treatment causes desensitization of autoreceptors. Hence, efficacy of these drugs is not reduced during long-term therapy.

SERTRALINE

Sertraline is more effective than paroxetine, well tolerated and is devoid of severe side effects. Although sertraline and paroxetine can potentiate the risk of seizures, sertraline is preferred in PTSD on account of its efficacy.

PAROXETINE

Vomiting, diarrhea, sedation, anorgasmia, erectile dysfunction and congenital malformations are few side effects of paroxetine. Intense withdrawal syndrome occurs if the drug is discontinued or due to intentional or unintentional failure of drug intake.

Drug of Choice: Sertraline

RATIONALE

Acute or chronic PTSD is very difficult to treat. Sertraline and paroxetine are both approved for treatment of PTSD. They are more selective to SERT (neuronal serotonin transporters) than to NET (neuronal norepinephrine transporters), and enhance serotonin transmission at neuronal terminals. **Paroxetine** causes sedation, erectile dysfunction, congenital malformations and an **intense withdrawal syndrome. Sertraline** is **more effective, well tolerated and devoid of severe side effects** so preferred to paroxetine for treatment of PTSD.

3. *Sertraline/Clomipramine in obsessive-compulsive disorder (OBD).*

BACKGROUND

Obsessive compulsive disorder (OCD) is characterized by repetitive behavior of obsessions and compulsions. It is a chronic disorder and early treatment will reduce the symptoms.

CLOMIPRAMINE

Clomipramine is a tricyclic antidepressant (TCA). It inhibits the norepinephrine transporters (NET) so, it prevents the reuptake of norepinephrine at neuronal terminals. It antagonizes muscarinic, α adrenergic and histaminergic receptors. It causes dry mouth, blurring of vision, tachycardia and urinary retention due to muscarinic blockade. It also results in orthostatic hypotension due to adrenergic blockade and sedation due to histaminergic blockade. Further, it potentiates conduction abnormalities and seizures.

SERTRALINE

Sertraline, the SSRI, is more specific to SERT and enhances the action of serotonin. The patient responds within a week after starting sertraline and it inhibits relapse. It leads to early improvement and causes remissions[68] hence, it is preferred.

Drug of Choice: Sertraline

RATIONALE

Repetitive obsessive thoughts and compulsive behavior are the symptoms of OCD. Clomipramine and sertraline are both indicated in this condition but **sertraline** is **preferred** as it is more **effective, well tolerated and devoid of sedation, anticholinergic** and **anti-adrenergic** side effects. It also **inhibits relapse. Clomipramine** is not preferred due to its side effects and requires a **lag period** for its therapeutic action.

4. *Fluvoxamine/Fluoxetine in binge eating disorder.*

BACKGROUND

Binge eating disorder is due to lack of control in eating food. It occurs at least twice a week followed by a feeling of guilt after eating. It may or may not be associated with obesity and is more common in women. Cognitive behavioral therapy is the main line of treatment but SSRIs are also helpful in reducing the symptoms. Fluvoxamine and fluoxetine are both SSRIs and are effective in this condition.

FLUVOXAMINE

The elimination half-life of fluvoxamine is only 18 hours and it is given once daily. When given at the dose of 300 mg per day, it does not induce seizures. It does not cause agitation, sedation, cardiac effects but causes GIT and sexual side effects. Fluvoxamine enhances the efficacy of cognitive behavioral therapy.[69]

FLUOXETINE

Fluoxetine is long acting because of its active metabolite and has a long elimination half-life of 53 hours. Its active metabolite, norfluoxetine has a longer elimination half-life of 240 hours. Hence, it can be administered once in a week but there is time delay in the onset of its therapeutic action. It results in agitation, sedation, cardiac effects, vomiting and diarrhea, and sexual side effects such as erectile dysfunction. It does not promote cognitive behavioral therapy.

Drug of Choice: Fluvoxamine

RATIONALE

Cognitive behavioral therapy is the main line of treatment in binge eating disorder. The SSRIs useful in this condition are fluvoxamine and fluoxetine. **Fluoxetine** is **not preferred** as it does not result in immediate action, **induces seizures** and has **no effect on cognitive behavioral therapy**. **Fluvoxamine** is preferred as it **acts quickly**, does **not cause seizures**, agitation and more importantly, **enhances the efficacy of cognitive behavioral therapy**.

5. *Venlafaxine/Escitalopram in preventing vasovagal symptoms in menopausal women.*

BACKGROUND

Vasovagal symptoms occur frequently in menopausal women. Venlafaxine is a serotonin/norepinephrine reuptake inhibitor (SNRI). Escitalopram is a selective serotonin reuptake inhibitor (SSRI).

ESCITALOPRAM

Escitalopram is an SSRI, and an active S-enantiomer of citalopram. It is effective at 10 mg/day at just half the dose of citalopram. Escitalopram has an elimination half-life of 30 hours. It is cost effective, given once daily thereby improving the patient compliance. It is the safest SSRI but causes erectile dysfunction, vomiting and diarrhea. It is devoid of sedation and anticholinergic side effects. It is more effective than venlafaxine in preventing vasovagal symptoms. It does not cause agitation, weight gain, seizures and hypotension like other SSRI. Hence, escitalopram, the safest SSRI, is preferred to SNRI, venlafaxine.[70]

VENLAFAXINE

Venlafaxine prevents the reuptake of both serotonin and norepinephrine. It is administered at 75 mg in three divided doses leading to poor patient compliance. The overall cost of therapy is higher than escitalopram. It is very effective in controlling vasovagal symptoms in postmenopausal women and does not cause sedation, seizures or anticholinergic side effects. It can cause agitation, cardiotoxicity, sexual disturbances and gastrointestinal tract (GIT) side effects.

Drug of Choice: Escitalopram

RATIONALE

Venlafaxine is an SNRI, effective in controlling the vasovagal symptoms in postmenopausal women and does not cause sedation, seizures, anticholinergic side effects but can cause **agitation** and **cardiotoxicity**. **Escitalopram**, an S-enantiomer of citalopram is the safest SSRI available, **more potent, effective** in preventing symptoms, **does not cause agitation and cardiotoxicity** hence it is preferred.

6. *Pregabalin/Duloxetine in fibromyalgia pain.*

BACKGROUND

Fibromyalgia is persistent and widespread musculoskeletal pain with tenderness. Middle-aged women are more frequently affected than men. Pain stimulus can originate from deep muscle, fascia or tissue. It is very severe and often disturbs sleep and causes fatigue. Increased corticotropin releasing factor (CRF), stimulation of N-methyl-D-aspartate (NMDA) and neurokinin receptors are reasons for pain. Corticosteroids and nonsteroidal anti-inflammatory drugs (NSAIDs) are usually ineffective and do not alleviate pain.

DULOXETINE

Duloxetine is an SNRI and is effective in controlling the pain. It inhibits the reuptake of serotonin and norepinephrine at the level of dorsal horn in descending pain pathway. As an antidepressant, it reduces depression associated with chronic and severe pain.[71] It causes anticholinergic, antihistaminergic and antiadrenergic side effects.

PREGABALIN

Pregabalin is an antiepileptic and regulates neuronal excitability. It binds to $\alpha2\delta$-1 subunit of voltage-gated calcium channel. It is particularly useful in neuropathic pain as it has analgesic property. The therapeutic efficacy of duloxetine is superior to pregabalin.

Drug of Choice: Duloxetine

RATIONALE

Pain due to fibromyalgia is often, severe and widespread. **Pregabalin** is an **antiepileptic** and by **modulating** the **neuronal excitability** of calcium channel, it is effective in neuropathic pain. **Duloxetine**, the **SNRI**, inhibits reuptake of serotonin and norepinephrine, **relieves depression associated with pain**, results in **better therapeutic benefit** and therefore is preferred to control pain in fibromyalgia despite adverse effects.

7. *Gabapentin/Duloxetine in diabetic neuropathy.*

BACKGROUND

Gabapentin, an analog of gamma-aminobutyric acid (GABA) is an antiepileptic. Duloxetine is an SNRI, inhibits reuptake of 5HT and norepinephrine.

DULOXETINE

Duloxetine prevents the reuptake of 5HT and norepinephrine in neuronal terminals. It is cost effective, is administered once daily improving patient compliance. Since chronic pain conditions are associated with depression, the antidepressant duloxetine is more effective than gabapentin. It modulates ascending corticospinal monoamine pain pathway resulting in superior therapeutic benefit. Hence, duloxetine is preferred in the treatment of diabetic neuropathy.

GABAPENTIN

Gabapentin does not mimic the action of GABA. It binds to $\alpha2\delta$-1 subunit of voltage-gated calcium channel. It regulates neuronal excitability and its analgesic action is mediated through modulation of calcium channel excitability. It is well absorbed orally, not bound to plasma proteins and excreted unchanged as it is not metabolized. It has to be given thrice daily resulting in poor compliance. It can result in somnolence (irresistible sleep), dizziness and fatigue hence, not preferred.

Drug of Choice: Duloxetine

RATIONALE

Gabapentin, an antiepileptic agent modulates calcium channel excitability and useful as an analgesic in diabetic neuropathy. It is **expensive**, has to be given thrice daily causing inconvenience to patients interfering with compliance.[72] **Duloxetine** modulates monoaminergic ascending corticospinal pathways, relieves depression associated with chronic pain, **cost effective** and can be administered once daily, resulting in better patient compliance. Hence, duloxetine is preferred to gabapentin in diabetic neuropathy.

8. *Escitalopram/Alprazolam in generalized anxiety disorder (GAD).*

BACKGROUND

Generalized anxiety disorder (GAD) is characterized by enormous anxiety or apprehension in daily activities. It decreases the concentrating ability causing excessive worries and poor ability to cope up with skills. Patient is tired, restless and irritable due to sleep disturbance. Symptoms persisting for more than 6 months is the criteria for diagnosis. There is impairment of cognition and social interaction. Cognitive behavioral therapy is more effective in bringing down the symptoms. It deals with relaxation techniques, coping skills and cognitive enhancement.

ESCITALOPRAM

The SSRIs are the drugs of choice in both acute and chronic GAD but they should be avoided in children or adolescents because they can cause suicidal tendencies in this age group. The SSRI, escitalopram, at 10 mg is very effective, well tolerated and has minimal relapse rate. It does not result in addiction and drug dependence but costlier than alprazolam. It causes side effects such as vomiting, decreased libido and insomnia.

ALPRAZOLAM

Benzodiazepines are more commonly used as they are anxiolytic. Alprazolam, a benzodiazepine, is well tolerated and relieves anxiety as it reaches steady state plasma concentrations quickly. Alprazolam is an intermediate-acting drug and results in moderate response especially in the initial few weeks of therapy. It relieves somatic symptoms but does not improve cognitive or psychic symptoms. It has a higher relapse rate than SSRIs and results in greater degree of anterograde amnesia. Tolerance develops to sedation, drowsiness and psychomotor slowing. Alprazolam causes dependence and withdrawal symptoms on discontinuation.

Drug of Choice: Escitalopram

RATIONALE

Cognitive behavioral therapy is more effective in the management of GAD. SSRIs are more effective in controlling both cognitive and somatic symptoms of GAD but they should be avoided in children and adolescents as they induce suicidal tendencies.

Escitalopram, an SSRI, is **well tolerated**, causes **minimal relapse** and results in tolerable side effects. **Alprazolam**, a benzodiazepine is prescribed more commonly for GAD. It is cheaper, **not very effective** therapeutically, leads to **more relapse**, does not improve cognitive symptoms and may result in dependence, tolerance and withdrawal symptoms on discontinuation. Hence, escitalopram is preferred to alprazolam.

9. *Sertraline/Alprazolam for long-term treatment in panic disorder.*

BACKGROUND

Panic disorder is characterized by spontaneous episodes of panic attacks with intense fear followed by anxiety of a possible new attack. Patients suffer from both psychological and physical symptoms. About 70% of patients with panic disorder develop 'agoraphobia'. They confine themselves in familiar environment. About 30% suffer from recurrent panic attacks during sleep. Benzodiazepines (BDZ) are more commonly used to control initial agitation but SSRIs are preferred for sustained treatment. Since SSRIs act after a lag period, BDZ can be added to initial therapy to achieve immediate therapeutic benefit.

SERTRALINE

Panic disorder is a chronic problem and SSRIs are first line agents for long-term treatment. They are very effective and are usually well tolerated. Sertraline is started at a low dose of 25 mg per day as it can cause initial agitation. After one week, it is gradually increased to 50 mg per day. It does not result in dependence and causes only tolerable side effects.

ALPRAZOLAM

Alprazolam offers equal therapeutic benefit as sertraline but effective only at very high dosages. It is highly potent, usually started at 0.5 mg per day and increased up to 6 mg per day. Such high doses given for long period often causes dependence and withdrawal symptoms on sudden discontinuation. As patients suffer from depression, alprazolam monotherapy is not effective.

Drug of Choice: Sertraline

RATIONALE

Short-term administration of high-potency BDZ, alprazolam for 4–6 weeks with sertraline may result in rapid therapeutic response but **alprazolam** is **not preferred** for long-term treatment as the dose required to control panic symptoms is high and such high dose if continued for a long period may produce **dependence and discontinuation leads to withdrawal symptoms.**[73] **Sertraline** is preferred for **long-term treatment** as it is an antidepressant with **tolerable side effects ahead of equally effective alprazolam.**

10. *Venlafaxine ER/Paroxetine in social anxiety disorder (SAD).*

BACKGROUND

Social anxiety disorder (SAD) is characterized by persistent fear and avoidance of social situations. Psychosocial functioning is impaired significantly in this condition. It follows a long unremitting course and resolves only with treatment. Venlafaxine is an SNRI and paroxetine is an SSRI.

VENLAFAXINE ER

Venlafaxine inhibits reuptake of both serotonin and nor-epinephrine. It is not safe and contraindicated during pregnancy. Venlafaxine extended release (ER) is more effective than paroxetine. Unlike paroxetine, it does not result in agitation in early phase of treatment. It is cost effective and does not result in hypotension, sedation or seizures. Venlafaxine ER has greater efficacy and tolerability than paroxetine. Venlafaxine induces agitation and abdominal pain. It also lowers libido and causes conduction abnormalities.

PAROXETINE

As an SSRI, paroxetine inhibits reuptake of serotonin. It causes agitation during early phases of treatment and contraindicated during pregnancy. It causes agitation, sedation, vomiting, diarrhea and anticholinergic side effects. It also decreases libido.

Drug of Choice: Venlafaxine ER

RATIONALE

Social anxiety disorder (SAD) follows a long unremitting course and resolves only with treatment. **Paroxetine**, an SSRI, **causes agitation in early phase of treatment** while **venlafaxine ER does not result in agitation**. Venlafaxine ER has greater efficacy, is well tolerated, cost effective[74,75] but cardiac monitoring is essential in patients taking venlafaxine.

CHAPTER
22

Drug Addiction

1. *Rimonabant/Bupropion for nicotine de-addiction.*

BACKGROUND

Nicotine stimulates CNS, releases endogenous opioids and gluco-corticoids. It increases dopamine level and activates nucleus accumbens reward system in brain. Nicotine is highly addictive, leads to withdrawal symptoms if stopped suddenly.

BUPROPION

Bupropion is an aminoketone antidepressant. Its hydroxyl meta-bolite is responsible for its therapeutic benefits. It prevents reuptake of norepinephrine and dopamine. Bupropion inhibits nicotine craving and also reduces withdrawal symptoms. It resists the urge to smoke by inhibiting activation of limbic and prefrontal areas. Bupropion SR given for 7 to 12 weeks improves the abstinence rates. It causes dizziness, agitation, seizures, insomnia, headache and dry mouth.

RIMONABANT

Cannabinoid receptors are highly concentrated in mesolimbic pathway. These receptors modulate excitatory and inhibitory inputs of dopaminergic neurons. Endocannabinoids are released from dopaminergic neurons. These substances activate nucleus accumbens reward system. Rimonabant is a cannabinoid receptor inverse agonist. As CB_1 receptor agonist, rimonabant improves abstinence rates but results frequently in depression and neurologic symptoms.

Varenicline is a partial agonist of nicotinic cholinergic receptors and prolongs abstinence but has black box warning for suicidal tendencies.

Drug of Choice: Bupropion

RATIONALE

Bupropion is an antidepressant **inhibits nicotine craving** and **improves abstinence rates**. **Rimonabant** is a cannabinoid receptor inverse agonist and inhibits dopamine mediated reward system. It **improves abstinence period** in nicotine addiction. Although drugs such as rimonabant and varenicline have novel, superior mechanisms of action compared to bupropion, they are not preferred in nicotine de-addiction as they **cause depression and suicidal tendencies**. Even though, not many long term reports are available for bupropion in nicotine de-addiction, it is still preferred, as it improves abstinence rates and has a better safety profile but it is contraindicated in epileptic patients.

2. *Methadone/Clonidine in opioid de-addiction.*

BACKGROUND

Opioids cause severe physical and psychological dependence and it is unwise to stop the drug suddenly as it can result in severe withdrawal symptoms. Drug craving, irritability, insomnia, dysphoria, algesia and restlessness can occur due to sudden discontinuation.

METHADONE

Methadone causes milder but similar pharmacological effects like morphine. It is a μ agonist, effective orally with long duration of action. It binds to plasma proteins firmly and accumulates in various tissues including brain. It is slowly released from tissues after discontinuation. Hence, it results in mild, tolerable withdrawal syndrome. Methadone withdrawal is slower in onset but it lasts longer and so drug craving is minimal. Hence, it is the drug of choice in opioid de-addiction. Although protracted withdrawal syndrome occurs up to 6 months after tapering methadone it is usually very mild and most tolerable. 1 mg of methadone is substituted for 4 mg of morphine and 2 mg of heroin. It is administered at higher dose for longer period in methadone maintenance therapy. It causes tolerance so euphoric effects of opioids may not be experienced by patients. Daily dose of 10 to 40 mg of methadone is given and it has cumulative effect.

CLONIDINE

Clonidine, the α_2 agonist inhibits adrenergic neurotransmission from locus coeruleus. Opioids suppress locus coeruleus and their discontinuation releases the inhibition precipitating withdrawal symptoms. Nausea, hypertension, sweating and tachycardia are mediated through autonomic system. Clonidine inhibits the autonomic symptoms due to opioid withdrawal. It does not inhibit the psychological symptoms that occur mainly due to stimulation of locus coeruleus. Besides, it does not inhibit drug craving and does not prolong the abstinence.

Drug of Choice: Methadone

RATIONALE

The severe symptoms of opioid withdrawal are due to physical and psychological dependence. Hence, it is unwise to discontinue opioids abruptly. **Methadone** acts as a **substitute** for opioids as it is a µ agonist and it results in similar but **mild** pharmacological **actions** and **prevents drug craving**. It binds to plasma proteins and accumulates in tissues. So, the **effects** of methadone **persist even after its discontinuation** as it is slowly released from these storage sites. **Clonidine inhibits only** the **autonomic symptoms** and has **no effect** on psychological symptoms of **drug craving**. It does not effectively prolong abstinence period so it is not preferred.

Cardiovascular System

Antianginal Drugs and Drugs in Peripheral Vascular Disease

1. *Beta blockers/Calcium channel blockers in prophylaxis of exertional angina.*

BACKGROUND

Exertional angina occurs due to unaccustomed physical activity and terminates if patient takes rest but worsens when the patient resumes physical activity. The pain is severe, distressing and is rarely localized. If treated promptly, it usually subsides without any residual discomfort. Prophylaxis is required for prevention of further attacks and to improve cardiac performance during exertion.

BETA BLOCKERS

Beta blockers reduce the severity and frequency of anginal attacks. They prolong life expectancy in patients with coronary artery disease (CAD) and in post myocardial infarction (MI) patients. Drugs used are timolol, atenolol, metoprolol and propranolol. The beta blockers atenolol and metoprolol are cardioselective but timolol and propranolol are nonselective. Timolol, propranolol and metoprolol are highly lipid soluble. Since these drugs are devoid of intrinsic sympathomimetic activity, they are suitable for prophylaxis. Metoprolol and propranolol have an additional membrane stabilizing property. Beta blockers reduce heart rate, contractility and ventricular wall stress. This reduces myocardial oxygen demand not only at rest but also during exercise improving the cardiac performance during exertion thereby reducing mortality and sudden cardiac death. Nonselective beta blockers are contraindicated in patients with bronchial asthma and heart failure.

CALCIUM CHANNEL BLOCKERS

The calcium channel blockers do not reduce number of anginal attacks as they do not improve the performance of heart during exertion. They have not been reported to reduce mortality rate or to prolong the survival period. They reduce myocardial oxygen demand secondary to reduction in double product. Heart rate and blood pressure are two components that determine the double product. Nifedipine, the dihydropyridine causes reflex tachycardia. Calcium channel blockers such as verapamil and diltiazem result in AV block. In view of the above, calcium channel blockers are not preferred for prophylaxis of exertional angina.

Drug of Choice: Beta Blockers

RATIONALE

Calcium channel blockers reduce oxygen demand by dilating coronary vessels and by decreasing double product but they can result in reflex tachycardia and AV nodal block. **Beta blockers reduce heart rate**, **cardiac contractility** and are specifically **effective** in exercise induced angina. They **reduce** number of anginal attacks as well as **mortality rate** and **sudden cardiac death**. Hence, they are preferred to calcium channel blockers for prophylaxis of exertional angina.

2. *Amlodipine/Nicardipine to prevent cerebral vasospasm associated with stroke.*

BACKGROUND

Autoregulation of cerebral blood flow is difficult in patients with cerebral ischemia. Amlodipine and nicardipine are dihydropyridine calcium channel blockers. They have similar mechanism of action and block L type calcium channels by binding to domains III and IV of its α subunit. They dilate both coronary as well as peripheral arterioles. The arterioles are more sensitive than veins, to the action of nicardipine and amlodipine.

NICARDIPINE

Nimodipine and nicardipine have peculiar cerebrovascular profile. They have high affinity to cerebral vessels and prevent cerebral vasospasm in stroke. Although nimodipine has been withdrawn recently, nicardipine is still available and safe. It is effective in preventing cerebral vasospasm in stroke. Prolonged release formulation of nicardipine administered intraarterially, reduces the incidence of vasospasm. Nicardipine also delays ischemic deficits due to cerebral vasospasm and improves cognition and does not cause coronary steal syndrome[76] but still should be used with caution in coronary ischemia.

AMLODIPINE

Amlodipine reduces peripheral resistance and decreases blood pressure. It also dilates coronary arterioles improving blood supply to heart. It has long half-life and causes minimal reflex tachycardia and given once a day. Amlodipine does not have action on cerebral blood vessels. Peripheral edema, fatigue and headache are some frequent side effects of amlodipine.

Drug of Choice: Nicardipine

RATIONALE

Amlodipine is more suitable for peripheral conditions as it **does not act** on **cerebral vessels**. It is effective in reducing systemic blood pressure, improves coronary blood flow but **not useful in cerebral ischemia**. **Nicardipine** has **high affinity** to **cerebral vessels** and is recommended for prevention of cerebral vasospasm associated with stroke. It also improves cognition and delays ischemic deficits. It is administered intra-arterially or as sustained release implants to improve its cerebral action.

3. *Beta blockers/Calcium channel blockers for prophylaxis in variant angina.*

BACKGROUND

Variant angina or Prinz-metal angina occurs due to coronary vasospasm in normal as well as in stenosed coronary arteries. Focal vasospasm results in severe myocardial ischemia leading to symptoms of angina. It is associated with transient ST segment elevation with pain at rest. Calcium channel blockers with nitrates are very effective in acute attacks but nitrates are not preferred for long-term prophylaxis as they result in tolerance.

CALCIUM CHANNEL BLOCKERS

Calcium channel blockers cause vasodilatation of coronary arteries relieving vasospasm and improving blood flow. Therefore, they reduce the myocardial oxygen demand and increase exercise tolerance. Amlodipine and long acting nifedipine preparations are preferred and are highly effective in prophylaxis of variant angina. Nifedipine should be used with caution in patients with left ventricular dysfunction.

BETA BLOCKERS

By antagonizing beta receptors, beta blockers can lead to unopposed alpha action causing vasoconstriction and worsening vasospastic angina. Hence, beta blockers are not preferred in variant angina and are more effective for the prophylaxis of exertional angina.

Drug of Choice: Calcium Channel Blockers

RATIONALE

Pain in Prinz-metal angina or variant angina is of severe intensity and occurs not only during exertion but also at rest. Coronary vasospasm causes severe myocardial ischemia. Coadministration of nitrates with calcium channel blockers is effective in relieving acute attacks. **Calcium channel blockers** are preferred instead of beta blockers for prophylaxis as they cause **coronary vasodilatation**

without much **systemic action**. Beta blockers, on the other hand, worsen the condition by causing vasoconstriction due to unopposed alpha action.

4. *Nitrates/Calcium channel blockers in classic acute angina.*

BACKGROUND

Acute angina can be triggered by exertion, exercise, stress and emotion. Nocturnal angina occurs as a result of improper oxygenation due to changes in respiratory pattern during sleep. Recumbent position during sleep increases blood volume leading to higher end diastolic volume and greater wall tension resulting in greater myocardial oxygen demand. The primary cause in acute angina is the imbalance between oxygen demand and supply.

NITRATES

Organic nitrates dilate veins and cause peripheral pooling of blood. They reduce venous return and decrease the preload. Nitrates reduce the workload of heart, left ventricular end diastolic pressure and cardiac output. Nitrates reduce peripheral resistance decreasing the afterload, through systemic arteriolar dilatation. They also decrease the left ventricular wall tension thereby decreasing the myocardial oxygen demand. They dilate coronary arteries and improve blood flow to subendocardial regions. Hence, they relieve 'subendocardial crunch'. Initial pain responds well to sublingual nitrates or repeated buccal spray at interval of five minutes. Sublingual nitroglycerin is the main drug of choice for immediate relief in angina and preferred due to its rapid action. The cost of nitrates is low and they have good efficacy. IV nitroglycerin is indicated only if pain persists after three doses of sublingual nitrates.

CALCIUM CHANNEL BLOCKERS

Calcium channel blockers are useful only as prophylactic agents in variant angina but not useful in acute pain. They reduce myocardial contractility and decrease left ventricular wall stress. This ensures reduction of myocardial oxygen demand. Their efficacy in relieving pain in acute angina is not superior to organic nitrates.

Drug of Choice: Nitrates

RATIONALE

The pain is very severe in classic acute angina and requires immediate management. **Sublingual glyceryl trinitrate** reduces **both preload** and **afterload**, dilates coronary arteries, reduces myocardial oxygen requirement and is **most preferred** due to its **quick onset** of action and **good efficacy**. Although **calcium channel blockers** increase myocardial oxygen supply through coronary vasodilatation, they **reduce only** the **afterload** and do not reduce workload of heart as effectively as nitrates and so are not preferred.

5. *Ranolazine/Beta blockers in chronic angina coexisting with heart failure.*

BACKGROUND

During ischemia, metabolism of myocardium shifts to fatty acid oxidation increasing oxygen requirement needed for the production of ATP. The energy expenditure of heart is increased causing overload to heart worsening the performance of already failing heart.

RANOLAZINE

Ranolazine reduces cardiac contractility by inhibiting calcium entry. This action is mainly mediated by blockade of late sodium channel. It is also a pFox inhibitor and suppresses the fatty acid oxidative pathway. It chiefly inhibits the fatty acid oxidative pathway in myocardium. In addition, it also acts as a metabolic modulator and it inhibits 3-ketoacyl thiolase, the enzyme required for fatty acid oxidation. Therefore, myocardial energy is obtained from glucose oxidation instead of fatty acid oxidation. Extended release (ER) preparation does not affect heart rate or blood pressure and prolongs exercise duration. It can be safely used in asthmatic patients with coexisting angina. Erectile dysfunction is commonly seen in patients suffering from angina. Ranolazine ER can be safely coadministered with drugs used in erectile dysfunction because it does not affect heart rate or blood pressure. Since it can cause QT prolongation, it should not be used in acute angina.

BETA BLOCKERS

Beta blockers reduce heart rate and cardiac contractility thereby reducing myocardial oxygen requirement. They are contraindicated in heart block, heart failure and hypotension. They worsen heart failure by inhibiting cardiac contractility. Peripheral vasoconstriction occurs due to unopposed alpha receptor mediated action. Hence, they cannot be used in chronic angina coexisting with heart failure.

Drug of Choice: Ranolazine

RATIONALE

Ranolazine is a **pFox inhibitor, reduces cardiac contractility** by blocking sodium current and inhibiting calcium entry. It also inhibits the fatty acid oxidative pathway in myocardium. Ranolazine ER does not affect heart rate or blood pressure and can be **safely** used in patients with heart failure. **Beta blockers** are given as prophylaxis for chronic angina but **contraindicated** in patients with **heart failure** as they worsen the condition by inhibiting cardiac contractility and through alpha receptor mediated peripheral vasoconstriction.

6. *Cilostazol/Pentoxyfylline in lower extremity claudication in absence of heart failure.*

BACKGROUND

Claudication of lower extremities is common in patients with peripheral vascular disease. Obstruction of blood flow to lower extremities causes ischemia of peripheral muscles. Impaired blood flow is unable to compensate the oxygen requirement during exertion. Intermittent pain or intermittent claudication occurs during exercise but disappears when these blood vessels dilate at rest. If this condition progresses, it leads to pain at rest and formation of ulcers due to ischemia.

PENTOXYFYLLINE

Pentoxyfylline is a rheologic modifier and increases RBCs deformability permitting easy flow of blood through partially obstructed arteries. Although it facilitates blood flow and improves the exercise tolerance, it does not effectively relieve lower extremity claudication.

CILOSTAZOL

Cilostazol increases cyclic AMP of blood platelets by inhibiting of phosphodiesterase-3 enzyme preventing platelet aggregation and promotes vasodilatation. It is very effective in intermittent claudication affecting lower extremities but contraindicated in heart failure as it can cause ventricular tachycardia. Due to its vasodilatory action, cilostazol increases the incidence of headache.

Drug of Choice: Cilostazol

RATIONALE

Vasodilators are effective in treating intermittent claudication due to impaired blood flow to lower extremities. Pentoxyfylline and cilostazol are vasodilators and are used in treating peripheral vascular disease. **Pentoxyfylline** is a **rheologic modifier** and causes **RBC deformity** but **not effective** in **lower extremity claudication**. **Cilostazol** increases cyclic AMP in platelets, **prevents platelet aggregation**, promotes **vasodilatation** and is more effective in lower extremity claudication but it should not be used in patients with heart failure.

CHAPTER
24
Pharmacotherapy of Hypertension

1. *Long acting/Short acting dihydropyridine calcium channel blockers for therapy of hypertension.*

BACKGROUND

Dihydropyridine calcium channel blockers increase myocardial blood flow through coronary vasodilatation. They are used as antihypertensive drugs as they reduce blood pressure through peripheral vasodilatation but cause baroreceptor mediated reflex tachycardia as a compensatory mechanism.

LONG ACTING CALCIUM CHANNEL BLOCKERS

Long acting calcium channel blockers have a gradual onset of action and reduce BP gradually resulting in minimal feedback stimulation of sympathetic system. Amlodipine and extended release nifedipine are preferred. Slow and sustained absorption of amlodipine prolongs the duration of action. Besides, amlodipine has a long half-life of 35 to 50 hours and cumulative plasma level due to daily administration adds to its clinical efficacy. Long acting calcium channel blockers result in minimal tachycardia and are not associated with adverse cardiac events like myocardial infarction (MI).

SHORT ACTING CALCIUM CHANNEL BLOCKERS

Short acting preparations lead to rapid fall in blood pressure and such a quick response is secondary to the reduction in total peripheral vascular resistance but reflex tachycardia occurs as a compensatory mechanism due to stimulation of sympathetic system.

Regular nifedipine has short half-life and potentiates reflex tachycardia which is prominent during its peak plasma concentration. Immediate release nifedipine preparations mediate catecholamine release. In hypertension coexisting with angina, short acting drugs cause intense tachycardia potentiating adverse cardiac events. Therefore, drugs acting for short duration should be avoided in post-MI patients. Hence, these preparations are not preferred for long term treatment.

Drug of Choice: Long Acting Calcium Channel Blockers

RATIONALE

Long acting calcium channel blockers are used in the treatment of hypertension. **Amlodipine** and **extended release nifedipine** are preferred as they have **gradual** onset of action, **do not result in reflex tachycardia** and are not associated with adverse cardiac events.[77] Short acting preparations are not preferred as they cause severe reflex tachycardia, a compensatory measure for sudden fall in blood pressure that potentiates adverse cardiac events like MI.

2. *Angiotensin-converting enzyme (ACE) inhibitors/Amlodipine for hypertension in patients with diabetes mellitus.*

BACKGROUND

Progression of diabetes mellitus often results in diabetic nephropathy. Prolonged hyperglycemia causes accumulation of proteinaceous substances stimulating mesangial proliferation leading to thickening of basement membrane. Matrix deposition further narrows down the arterial lumen. These factors compromise renal function and reduce glomerular filtration rate.

ANGIOTENSIN-CONVERTING ENZYME (ACE) INHIBITORS

ACE inhibitors offer renoprotection in patients with diabetes mellitus by reducing albuminuria and preventing the progression of nephropathy and retinopathy. They reduce blood pressure, dilate renal efferent arterioles and increase the glomerular filtration rate. They prevent mesangial proliferation induced by proteinaceous substances, inhibits matrix production and thickening of basement membrane. Since they inhibit the synthesis of angiotensin II they reduce the mesangial proliferation and prevent glomerular injury secondary to increased glomerular capillary pressure.[78]

AMLODIPINE

Amlodipine, a calcium channel blocker, reduces albuminuria[79] but does not inhibit mesangial cellular proliferation or matrix deposition. Amlodipine does not arrest the progression of nephropathy in diabetes mellitus. So, it is used only as second line drug for management of hypertension in diabetes mellitus.

Drug of Choice: Angiotensin-Converting Enzyme (ACE) Inhibitors

RATIONALE

ACE inhibitors offer **renoprotection** and **prevent** the **progression** of nephropathy by inhibiting mesangial cellular proliferation and matrix production. These actions are secondary to their antihypertensive action. Hence, they are the drugs of choice in the management of hypertension in patients with diabetes mellitus. Among the ACE inhibitors, ramipril reduces cardiovascular events in high risk patients and excretion of fosinopril is not altered in renal impairment as it is eliminated by both liver and kidney. Amlodipine, the calcium channel blocker reduces albuminuria but does not offer other beneficial effects of ACE inhibitors.

3. *Nicardipine/Sodium nitroprusside in hypertensive emergency following ischemic stroke.*

BACKGROUND

Diastolic blood pressure shoots beyond 130 mg of Hg in hypertensive emergency. BP needs to be reduced quickly to prevent death. Myocardial infarction, encephalopathy, intracranial hemorrhage and preeclampsia are a few conditions predisposing to hypertensive emergency. Irritability and confusion occur due to cerebral ischemia in encephalopathy. Choice of drug is based on etiology of hypertensive emergency. Parenteral therapy is absolutely essential to bring down the blood pressure quickly. Initial fall in BP should be rapid within few minutes but total percentage of fall should not exceed 25% in the first two hours. After two hours, BP should be reduced gradually over a period of 2 to 6 hours. Drastic reduction in BP can cause coronary, cerebral or renal ischemia. Ideally, a drug should result in dose dependent, transient and predictable action.

NICARDIPINE

Intravenous nicardipine has quick onset resulting in rapid fall in BP. The duration of action of nicardipine is about 6 hours. It causes predictable, transient action that does not necessitate dose monitoring. Nicardipine has more selective action on coronary and cerebral vessels. It is a non-sedative drug. It does not increase intracranial pressure although it improves cerebral circulation through dilatation of cerebral vessels. Hence, it is the drug of choice in hypertensive encephalopathy.

SODIUM NITROPRUSSIDE

Sodium nitroprusside is a nonselective vasodilator dilating both arterioles and venules. Its dose has to be titrated otherwise, it can cause excessive vasodilatation. Such excessive vasodilatation results in rapid fall in BP and severe reflex tachycardia. It increases intracranial pressure, reduces cerebral blood flow and is not preferred.

Drug of Choice: Nicardipine

RATIONALE

Hypertensive emergency due to ischemic stroke is a crisis situation where high BP has to be reduced quickly. Since the symptoms are mainly due to cerebral ischemia, a drug that improves cerebral circulation is preferred. **Nicardipine**, a calcium channel blocker, has

immediate onset of action and acts within 1 to 5 minutes. It results in **quick fall** in BP and dilates cerebral and coronary vessels but does not increase intracranial pressure. Hence, nicardipine is the drug of choice. **Sodium nitroprusside** is a nonselective vasodilator dilating both arteries as well as veins but can cause **severe reflex tachycardia** and potentiate cerebral ischemia.[80]

4. *Enalapril/Amlodipine as antihypertensive in patients with bronchial asthma or COPD.*

BACKGROUND

Bronchial hyper-responsive patients are sensitive to bronchoconstrictors. The antihypertensive drug used should not cause bronchoconstriction. ACE inhibitors, the first line antihypertensive agents are not indicated in asthma.

AMLODIPINE

Calcium channel blocker amlodipine is preferred in these patients. Amlodipine abolishes hyper-responsiveness of airway to such stimulants.[81] It also relaxes the bronchial smooth muscles. In view of this, it is preferred as an antihypertensive drug in patients prone for airway resistance.

ENALAPRIL

Enalapril acts by preventing the synthesis of angiotensin II from angiotensin I. It inhibits angiotensin converting enzyme and suppresses bradykinin metabolism increasing the plasma level of bradykinin. It also stimulates prostaglandin biosynthesis. Enalapril is a cardio-protective agent as it increases natural stem cell regulator. Excess angiotensin-I is converted to angiotensin peptide 1-7 a potent vasodilator. The pharmacological effect of enalapril is mediated through bradykinin which accumulates in lungs causing intractable dry cough. Enalapril also results in accumulation of substance P and prostaglandins (PGs) that potentiate the hyper-responsiveness of airway. Cough is very troublesome and necessitates immediate withdrawal of the drug and disappears following its discontinuation. Enalapril is not preferred in patients with bronchial asthma[82] or COPD. The angiotensin receptor blockers are more tolerable and do not result in cough.[83]

Drug of Choice: Amlodipine

RATIONALE

Being an ACE inhibitor, **enalapril** increases **bradykinin** level, **substance P** and **prostaglandins** aggravating the hyper-responsiveness of airway, worsening the already compromised function of airway in patients with bronchial asthma and COPD. The **angiotensin receptor blockers** are **more tolerable** than ACE inhibitors and do not result in cough. Amlodipine, a calcium channel blocker, relaxes bronchial musculature, prevents airway resistance and preferred in such patients.

5. *Oral clonidine/Immediate release nifedipine capsules in hypertensive urgency.*

BACKGROUND

In hypertensive urgency the diastolic blood pressure is around 120 mm of Hg. Hypertensive urgency does not result in acute end organ damage. Perioperative hypertension and pre-eclampsia are few such conditions. It occurs in those who are nonadherent to their routine antihypertensive therapy. The blood pressure has to be reduced gradually over a period of a few hours. The drug should cause rapid, smooth and predictable reduction of blood pressure. Patient comfort, cost, efficacy and safety are other factors determining the selection of drug. Oral drug having quick onset of action is the first line therapy. Parenteral administration is not required in hypertensive urgency.

ORAL CLONIDINE

Clonidine satisfies most of the above said criteria. Hence, it is the drug of choice for hypertensive urgency.[84] Clonidine is an α_2 agonist and acts centrally to reduce blood pressure. 0.1 to 0.2 mg every hour is given initially and followed by half the dose every hour. A maximum dose of 0.8 mg effectively reduces blood pressure. Sedation is the frequent side effect of clonidine. Risk of rebound hypertension is high in those who stop the drug abruptly. Immediate outpatient follow-up for 24 hours is mandatory in patients treated with clonidine.

NIFEDIPINE

Nifedipine is a calcium channel blocker, has potent peripheral than cardiac action. Immediate release nifedipine has quick onset but has unpredictable action. It causes hypotension due to intense fall in blood pressure and reflex tachycardia. Since it potentiates the risk of myocardial infarction, it is not preferred and should be avoided.

Drug of Choice: Oral Clonidine

RATIONALE

The need to reduce blood pressure drastically does not arise in hypertensive urgency. Hence, orally acting drugs that reduce blood pressure over a period of a few hours are indicated as first line therapy. **Clonidine**, the α_2 agonist and **centrally acting** antihypertensive agent is the drug of choice as it leads to predictable fall in blood pressure over a period of time. It **does not result** in intense **hypotension** but can cause sedation and rebound hypertension if stopped suddenly. Immediate release nifedipine acts in an unpredictable manner causing intense hypotension, reflex tachycardia and should be avoided.

6. *Labetalol/Hydralazine in hypertensive emergency associated with pregnancy.*

BACKGROUND

Eclampsia and pre-eclampsia are the major causes of hypertensive emergency associated with pregnancy.

LABETALOL

Labetalol exists in four different forms of stereo-isomers. Each displays different pharmacodynamic and pharmacokinetic properties. The commercially available labetalol is a selective mixture of these stereo-isomers. It is a selective α_1 and nonselective β blocker with partial agonistic action on β_2 receptors. The selective α_1 blockade reduces the vasoconstriction mediated through α_1 receptors causing rapid fall in BP. Its action on β_2 receptors mediates vasodilatation, further reducing the blood pressure. Since it blocks β_1 receptors of heart, the risk of reflex tachycardia is negligible. The dosage is 20 to 40 mg every 10 minutes and the maximum dose is 300 mg. The onset of action starts within 5 to 10 minutes when given as intravenous infusion. The total duration of action persists for 6 hours. It has poor lipid solubility and minimal placental transfer. It is safe in pregnancy and is the first line therapy in hypertensive emergency.

HYDRALAZINE

Hydralazine relaxes arteriolar smooth muscles. It also reduces peripheral vascular resistance. Only arterioles and not veins are dilated hence it results in postural hypotension. It can cause headache, hypotension, palpitations, tachycardia, dizziness and SLE. It induces reflex tachycardia and increases myocardial oxygen demand causing ischemia. Hydralazine increases fetal heart rate and reduces Apgar score in neonates.[85]

Drug of Choice: Labetalol

RATIONALE

Hypertensive emergency during pregnancy occurs in patients with eclampsia and pre-eclampsia. **Labetalol**, the selective α_1 and nonselective beta blocker with partial β_2 agonist action, causes **rapid fall** in blood pressure **without** causing **reflex tachycardia**. It has an **established safety profile** in pregnancy so it is the drug of choice in hypertensive emergencies associated with pregnancy. **Hydralazine**

relaxes arteriolar smooth muscle, reduces peripheral vascular resistance and reduces blood pressure. Since it causes **severe postural hypotension**, reflex tachycardia and increases foetal heart rate it is not preferred.

7. *Clevidipine/Esmolol in perioperative hypertension.*

BACKGROUND

Antihypertensive drugs limit end organ damage in perioperative hypertension. Hypertension is a frequent complication of cardiac, carotid, abdominal and intraperitoneal surgeries and occurs during postoperative period. Acute pain stimulates sympathetic α receptor causing intense vasoconstriction. Hypothermia, hypoxia, volume overload are other reasons for increase in BP.

ESMOLOL

Esmolol is a β_1 selective ultrashort acting beta blocker. It has a very quick onset and short duration of action hence, useful in perioperative hypertension. It quickly brings down the increased heart rate, BP and cardiac output. Structurally it has an ester linkage and is metabolized by plasma and RBC esterase. Its duration of action is brief due to rapid metabolism. Action starts as early as 6 to 10 minutes and the effect terminates within 20 minutes. The main advantage of esmolol is the absence of reflex tachycardia mediated through blockade of cardiac β_1 receptors.

CLEVIDIPINE

It is a third generation calcium channel blocker, blocks L-type calcium channels. Similar to esmolol, it has a very quick onset and short duration of action. It is also metabolized by plasma esterase and therefore has short duration of action. It lowers BP by relaxing arterial smooth muscles and does not interfere with contractility and conductivity of heart. Although it has brief duration of action, it results in reflex tachycardia. This effect is secondary to rapid fall in peripheral resistance. Hence, clevidipine is not preferred in perioperative hypertension.

Drug of Choice: Esmolol

RATIONALE

Perioperative hypertensive emergency should be treated **immediately** to prevent end organ damage. Esmolol and clevidipine are both **short acting** drugs as they are metabolized by esterase. **Esmolol** is a β_1 **selective** blocker and **clevidipine** is a third generation **calcium channel blocker**. **Esmolol** blocks beta receptors of heart and **does not cause reflex tachycardia**, a physiological compensatory mechanism for the rapid fall in blood pressure. Clevidipine on the other hand, dilates arteries, inhibits peripheral resistance and causes reflex tachycardia. Hence, esmolol is preferred to clevidipine for perioperative hypertension.[86]

8. *Loop diuretics/Thiazide diuretics in mild hypertension.*

BACKGROUND

Prolonged hypertension leads to pathological changes in vasculature. Sustained increase in peripheral resistance results in left ventricular hypertrophy.

THIAZIDE DIURETICS

Thiazide diuretics are more frequently used in the management of mild hypertension. They effectively control hypertension through their renal and hemodynamic action reducing blood pressure initially by lowering plasma volume. In due course they reduce peripheral resistance and decrease BP. Thiazides block Na^+Cl^- symporter and favor the excretion of sodium and chloride. They inhibit carbonic anhydrase promoting excretion of bicarbonate and phosphate. They also have direct action on vasculature and reduce the peripheral resistance. Hydrochlorothiazide or chlorthalidone is preferred and given through oral route. Low dose effectively brings down BP and higher doses are seldom required. Thiazide diuretics are moderately potent and do not cause severe electrolyte depletion and are more suitable for long-term therapy. They are safe, well tolerated and dose titration is not required. In addition they are cost effective, have longer duration of action and their efficacy is comparable to other antihypertensives. Frequent adverse effects are hyponatremia, hypokalemia and hyperuricemia. They can also cause erectile dysfunction, altered lipid profile and glucose intolerance.

LOOP DIURETICS

Loop diuretics are high ceiling diuretics and cause significant natriuresis. Hence, they result in severe electrolyte depletion. They also result in intense volume depletion compared to thiazides. Besides they have shorter duration of action and require repeated administration. Frequent administration causes hyponatremia, hypokalemia, hypochloremia, hypomagnesemia, ototoxicity, hyperglycemia and hyperuricemia. Hence, loop diuretics are reserved only for patients with compromised renal function.

Drug of Choice: Thiazide Diuretics

RATIONALE

Prolonged therapy is required in the management of hypertension hence diuretic used should not result in severe volume depletion and electrolyte imbalance. **Thiazide** diuretics are **moderately potent**, have **both renal** and **direct vascular** effects. They are cost effective, long acting and do not result in excessive electrolyte and volume depletion. **Loop** diuretics are **cheaper** but require **frequent** administration, result in severe electrolyte depletion and volume constriction so, not preferred in management of hypertension.

9. *(Sodium Nitroprusside + Esmolol)/(Diazoxide + Esmolol) for management of hypertension following acute aortic dissection.*

BACKGROUND

Hypertension due to aortic dissection is an emergency situation. This situation requires immediate reduction of both preload and afterload.

SODIUM NITROPRUSSIDE

Sodium nitroprusside dilates both arterioles and venules through release of nitric oxide. Nitric oxide stimulates guanyl cyclase and increases cyclic GMP causing vasodilatation. It reduces preload through venous pooling and afterload by decreasing peripheral resistance. The action starts within 30 seconds after an intravenous infusion, reaching peak within two minutes and terminates within three minutes after stopping the infusion. Titration of dose is essential for nitroprusside to prevent unpredictable action and the infusion has to be monitored continuously. Since tachycardia occurs due to rapid fall in blood pressure, esmolol the cardioselective beta blocker is coadministered with nitroprusside to prevent reflex tachycardia.

DIAZOXIDE

Diazoxide was once used to manage hypertensive emergencies but no longer used now due to its potential adverse effects. It is an arteriolar dilator, inhibits peripheral resistance and reduces the preload. It is long acting with a half-life of about 24 hours resulting in significant hypotension and intense tachycardia that cannot be overcome by esmolol. Reflex tachycardia induced by diazoxide is often severe, resulting in angina. Hence, it is no longer used in hypertensive emergencies.

Drug of Choice: Sodium Nitroprusside + Esmolol

RATIONALE

Sodium nitroprusside reduces **both preload and afterload** as it dilates both arterioles and venules. It has **very quick onset** of action and **rapid termination** of effect thereby making it the **most effective** agent for treatment of hypertension due to aortic dissection. But **reflex tachycardia** is its troublesome side effect and can be effectively managed by coadministration of a selective beta blocker **esmolol. Diazoxide,** an arteriolar dilator, once preferred for treatment of hypertensive emergencies, is no more preferred as it causes severe reflex tachycardia that often results in angina.

CHAPTER 25

Drugs in Heart Failure

1. *Beta blockers/Calcium channel blockers in chronic heart failure as adjuvants to ACE inhibitors.*

BACKGROUND

Stimulation of sympathetic system is a compensatory mechanism in heart failure. It increases heart rate, augments cardiac contractility and increases cardiac output. Further, it causes peripheral vaso-constriction and activation of renin angiotensin pathway. In due course this leads to myocardial damage and ventricular dilatation. These physiological changes ultimately result in left ventricular hypertrophy and failure.

BETA BLOCKERS

Beta blockers inhibit heart rate, myocardial contractility and cardiac workload. They reduce left ventricular chamber size and improve ejection fraction. They also reverse left ventricular remodeling. Drugs like metoprolol improve exercise tolerance and beta blockers should be used only in 'stable' heart failure due to negligible volume overload in this condition. They do not act immediately and their actions are evident only after an interval. Therapy with beta blockers should be instituted gradually to prevent deterioration of symptoms. Carvedilol, a non-selective β blocker and selective α_1 blocker is approved for use. Metoprolol and bisoprolol, selective β_1 blockers are also approved.

CALCIUM CHANNEL BLOCKERS

Dihydropyridine calcium channel blockers reduce after load by dilating arterioles. They cause reflex tachycardia and worsen the cardiac status. Phenylalkylamine calcium channel blockers depress contractility of heart. This action may aggravate the cardiac failure. Besides, they do not rectify the main pathophysiology in heart failure since they do not block the sympathetic over activity. Hence, calcium channel blockers, in spite of their vasodilator action are better avoided.

Drug of Choice: Beta Blockers

RATIONALE

Since overactivity of sympathetic system is the main pathophysiology in heart failure, drugs that modulate adrenergic system are preferable. Beta blockers inhibit heart rate, myocardial contractility and reduce dilatation of left ventricle. They prevent cardiac remodeling, increase ejection fraction and improve exercise tolerance. On the contrary, calcium channel blockers increase the strain to already failing heart by causing reflex tachycardia and cardiac depression. Besides they do not interfere with sympathetic system over activity. Hence, beta blockers are preferred to calcium channel blockers in chronic heart failure.

2. *Metoprolol/Carvedilol in 'stable' heart failure.*

BACKGROUND

Chronic heart failure is a progressive condition which is due to inability of heart to adequately perfuse and oxygenate peripheral tissues. It is usually associated with pathologic ventricular remodeling which in due course causes ventricular dysfunction. Beta blockers prolong survival and cause 'reverse remodeling' of left ventricle. Therapy should be started at low dose and gradually increased to target dose. Carvedilol and metoprolol are both indicated in 'stable' heart failure.

CARVEDILOL

Carvedilol is a nonselective β blocker with an additional α_1 blockade. Carvedilol does not result in any intrinsic sympathomimetic activity.

By blocking α_1 receptors, it causes vasodilatation but does not cause tachycardia as β_1 receptors of heart are blocked. It is well tolerated and at a higher dosage blocks entry of calcium ions. It has an additional cardioprotective antioxidant action. Carvedilol also inhibits generation of free radicals. It should be started as 1/10th or 1/20th of its maximal dose. It is started at 3.125 mg orally twice daily for first two weeks. Dose is doubled every two weeks and the maximum permissible dose is 50 mg. It improves left ventricular ejection fraction and slows down progression of disease reducing overall mortality by 65%.

METOPROLOL

Metoprolol is a cardioselective beta blocker without any additional actions. It inhibits heart rate and cardiac contractility but does not have antioxidant action and does not block calcium entry. Extended release preparations of metoprolol increase ejection fraction. It improves exercise tolerance but reduces overall mortality only by 34%.

Drug of Choice: Carvedilol

RATIONALE

Beta blockers are indicated only in 'stable' heart failure and prolong survival through 'reverse remodeling'. Of the two most commonly used beta blockers, carvedilol is preferred because it blocks β_1, β_2, and α_1 receptors and mediates both cardiac and peripheral actions. It reduces cardiac workload, causes vasodilatation, blocks entry of calcium ions at high doses and exerts cardioprotective antioxidant actions. It slows progression of disease and reduces overall mortality by 65%. As a β_1 blocker, metoprolol inhibits cardiac contractility and heart rate. Unlike carvedilol, metoprolol does not result in additional benefits, although it improves exercise tolerance, it reduces overall mortality only by 34%. Therefore, carvedilol is preferred as a beta blocker in 'stable' heart failure.

3. *Dopamine/Dobutamine for CHF in patients with systolic dysfunction.*

BACKGROUND

In CHF, main therapy is focused on improvement of myocardial contractility. Dopamine and dobutamine are both positive inotropic agents and are used to improve cardiac contractility which offers short-term benefit.

DOBUTAMINE

Dobutamine is structurally similar to dopamine but acts only on α and β receptors and not on dopamine receptors. Inotropic effect of dobutamine is more prominent than its chronotropic action. It results in more or less uniform peripheral resistance which is due to α_1 mediated vasoconstriction and β_2 mediated vasodilatation. Hence, it does not cause reflex tachycardia. It does not alter heart rate or blood pressure. It increases stroke volume and cardiac output through positive inotropy. It has very rapid onset and very short half-life of about 2 minutes but tolerance develops if it is continued beyond four days.

DOPAMINE

Dopamine acts on dopamine D_1, α_1 and β_1 receptors. It has variable action at different dose levels. At low concentrations it stimulates D_1 receptors and results in vasodilatation of renal mesenteric and coronary arteries. At moderate dose levels, it results in positive inotropic action. Cardiac action is mediated through activation of β_1 receptors. Dopamine at high doses stimulates α_1 receptors that results in peripheral vasoconstriction and increases after load. Hence, dopamine is not preferred in CHF patients with systolic dysfunction.

Drug of Choice: Dobutamine

RATIONALE

Improved myocardial contractility is the main target in CHF patients with dysfunction of cardiac contractility. Dopamine and dobutamine are both positive inotropic agents and offer short-term benefit. **Dobutamine** does not alter peripheral resistance and does not increase after load. It is **preferred** because it increases stroke volume and cardiac output **without altering heart rate**. **Dopamine** increases peripheral resistance as it causes vasoconstriction. It increases after load and **deteriorates left ventricular performance**. Hence, it is not preferred in CHF patients with systolic dysfunction.

4. *Angiotensin converting enzyme (ACE) inhibitors/Angiotensin receptor blockers (ARB) in symptomatic left ventricular failure without edema.*

BACKGROUND

Angiotensin II increases peripheral resistance by direct vasoconstriction mediated through increased release of catecholamine. Angiotensin II stimulates proliferation of vascular endothelial cells increasing the production of extracellular matrix. It facilitates cardiac remodeling through matrix production by cardiac fibroblast. Hypertrophy of cardiac myocytes increases the size of heart.

ANGIOTENSIN CONVERTING ENZYME INHIBITORS

Angiotensin converting enzyme (ACE) inhibitors prevent progression of symptomatic left heart failure. They interfere with renin— angiotensin axis and inhibit the angiotensin converting enzyme. This action prevents the conversion of angiotensin I to angiotensin II. They also inhibit metabolism of bradykinin and increase the level of this potent vasodilator. Blockade of synthesis of angiotensin II leads to accumulation of angiotensin I increasing the synthesis of Ang (1-7), a vasodilator peptide. ACE inhibitors also increase the level of prostaglandins and nitric oxide which contribute to vasodilator action of ACE inhibitors. ACE inhibitors reduce after load, systolic wall stress but increase stroke volume. They increase cardiac output and improve renal blood flow. They reduce preload by decreasing pulmonary arterial and capillary wedge pressure. Long-term administration reduces left ventricular filling pressure. In heart failure patients, ACE inhibitors delay progression of disease hence, they improve survival and quality of life in such patients. They should be started with low dose to prevent initial hypotension but the dose is increased gradually till the clinical dose range is reached.

ANGIOTENSIN RECEPTOR BLOCKERS

Angiotensin receptor blockers (ARBs) block AT-1 receptors but do not have any additional mechanisms. They do not inhibit brady-kinin meta-bolism and do not enhance prostaglandins as well as nitric oxide levels. Hence, they are reserved only for patients who are unable to tolerate ACE inhibitors. They are indicated in patients who develop cough.

Drug of Choice: Angiotensin Converting Enzyme (ACE) Inhibitors

RATIONALE

Angiotensin II causes peripheral vasoconstriction, vascular and cardiac remodeling. ACE inhibitors and ARB block the actions of angiotensin II. ACE inhibitors block the synthesis of angiotensin II by inhibiting angiotensin converting enzyme. ARBs block AT-1 receptors. **ACE inhibitors** have **superior efficacy** as they act through additional mechanisms like increasing the level of bradykinin and synthesis of nitric oxide and prostaglandins which **potentiate** their **vasodilator** actions. **ARBs do not have** these **additional mechanisms** and are **less effective** when compared to ACE inhibitors. ACE inhibitors decrease preload, after load and improve cardiac output more effectively than ARBs and therefore preferred to ARBs.

5. *Inamrinone/Milrinone for short-term management in acute decompensated heart failure.*

BACKGROUND

Acute heart failure follows an acute attack of myocardial infarction and can also occur in patients suffering from chronic heart failure. The reasons are unaccustomed exertion, high salt intake or non-compliance to therapy. Short-term inotropic drug therapy in advanced heart failure has life-saving potential and can dramatically improve the functional status of the failing heart. Inamrinone and milrinone are both selective phosphodiesterase 3 inhibitors and inhibit this enzyme in cardiac and smooth muscle cells. They selectively suppress cyclic GMP—inhibited cyclic AMP phosphodiesterase elevating the levels of cyclic AMP. They are positive inotropic agents improving cardiac output and dilate resistance and capacitance vessels resulting in reduction of both pre and after load. They are approved for immediate short-term management to improve circulation in advanced CHF and are given parenterally. They result in direct myocardial contraction and potentiate myocardial relaxation. They reduce both systemic and pulmonary vascular resistance thereby reducing right and left ventricular filling pressures. As a consequence to these effects, they increase the cardiac output.

MILRINONE

Milrinone has long elimination half-life potentiating hypotension or arrhythmia even after discontinuation. Hence, maintenance dose instead of loading dose should be given whenever rapid hemodynamic responses are not required. Milrinone has greater selectivity to phosphodiesterase 3 and has a shorter half-life. Milrinone does not cause thrombocytopenia but it can cause QT prolongation and ventricular arrhythmia.

INAMRINONE

Inamrinone also has a long elimination half-life and even after discontinuation it can result in hypotension or arrhythmia. Maintenance dose is preferred to loading dose but inamrinone causes clinically significant thrombocytopenia in 10% of patients.

Drug of Choice: Milrinone

RATIONALE

Short-term parenteral administration of positive inotropic agents can be life-saving and can dramatically improve end organ function. Inamrinone and milrinone share the same pharmacological actions.

They reduce preload, after load and improve cardiac output. **Inamrinone** results in clinically **significant thrombocytopenia**. **Milrinone** is **short acting, does not cause thrombocytopenia** and has more **selectivity** toward phosphodiesterase 3 enzyme and so preferred. Since it can cause QT prolongation, long-term administration of milrinone is not advisable but it is preferred to inamrinone for short-term management.

6. *Loop diuretics/Thiazide diuretics in acute left-sided heart failure with pulmonary edema.*

BACKGROUND

Diuretics reduce edema due to volume overload in congestive heart failure and are given in acute left-sided heart failure with pulmonary edema.

LOOP DIURETICS

Loop diuretics are high ceiling diuretics and are preferred because this situation needs rapid and aggressive therapy. Loop diuretics act by inhibiting $Na^+K^+2Cl^-$ symporter, increase urinary excretion of sodium, potassium and chloride. They also result in direct vascular actions mediated through prostaglandins. They increase total renal blood flow (RBF) potentiating GFR which is directly proportional to RBF. Their vasodilatory action occurs prior to their renal action explaining their superiority in management of pulmonary edema. The loop diuretic, furosemide, decreases left ventricular filling pressure by increasing systemic venous capacitance. Intravenous infusion results in sustained natriuresis. Increased natriuresis decreases edema, reduces left ventricular filling pressure and relieves pulmonary edema. Hence, it is preferred to frequent intravenous bolus doses. Furosemide is started at 40 mg bolus dose followed by 10 mg per hour resulting in prompt reduction of preload. Risk of ototoxicity is lower if given by continuous infusion. On the contrary, repetitive, intermittent administration potentiates ototoxicity.

THIAZIDE DIURETICS

Thiazide group of diuretics are moderately potent diuretics. They have lower efficacy and are not preferred in this situation. Thiazides do not improve RBF or GFR. Hence, they cannot be used in acute situation. They are also not effective if GFR is less than 30 to 40 mL per minute. GFR is usually reduced in patients with acute heart failure. Thiazides may reduce the edema associated with heart failure but they do not improve RBF or GFR. They are not useful in this acute condition.

Drug of Choice: Loop Diuretics

RATIONALE

Therapy in acute left-sided heart failure with pulmonary edema should be rapid and aggressive as pulmonary congestion needs to be reduced quickly. **Loop diuretics**, the high ceiling diuretics cause **natriuresis** through inhibition of $Na^+K^+2Cl^-$ symporter and also result in **prostaglandin mediated increase in total blood flow and glomerular filtration rate**. They increase systemic venous capacitance and reduce the left ventricular filling pressure. Continuous intravenous furosemide causes very effective **natriuresis** and reduces pulmonary congestion and so is preferred. **Thiazide** diuretic is only **moderately potent** and causes only moderate natriuresis. They **do not provide any additional benefits** such as reduction of pulmonary edema. Hence, they are not preferred.

7. *Loop diuretics/Thiazide diuretics in severe heart failure without symptoms of pulmonary edema.*

BACKGROUND

Diuretics provide symptomatic relief in heart failure. Loop diuretics are preferred to thiazide diuretics in this condition.

LOOP DIURETICS

Oral therapy is sufficient and parenteral therapy is not required. Furosemide, torsemide and bumetanide are chosen for oral administration. Except torsemide, all other drugs have rapid onset of action and short duration of action. Hence, these drugs have to be repeated more than once per day. Edema responds quickly to loop diuretics even in patients with compromised renal function but electrolyte depletion and ototoxicity should be carefully monitored. They should be avoided in postmenopausal women since they promote calcium excretion and aggravate osteopenia.

THIAZIDE DIURETICS

Thiazide diuretics except metolazone and indapamide are ineffective if GFR falls below 30 to 40 mL per minute. They do not effectively reduce edema as they are only moderately potent. Hence, they are not preferred to loop diuretics in severe heart failure.

Drug of Choice: Loop Diuretics

RATIONALE

Loop diuretics are given orally and not parenterally in severe heart failure without symptoms of pulmonary edema as they are more potent and reduce edema effectively. They are also effective even if GFR falls below 30 to 40 mL per minute but overzealous therapy may result in severe natriuresis. Thiazide diuretics are moderately potent, but ineffective if GFR is less than 40 mL per minute.

CHAPTER

26

Antiarrhythmic Drugs

1. *Intravenous adenosine/Intravenous verapamil for terminating acute episodes of supraventricular tachycardia (SVT) due to re-entry with narrow QRS complex.*

BACKGROUND

Supraventricular tachycardia due to re-entry is more common than SVT due to accessory pathway. It occurs in two-thirds of patients suffering from SVT and is also known as *AV nodal re-entrant tachycardia* (AVNRT). The acute episodes need to be managed immediately. Therapy focuses on interruption of re-entry circuit which ensures blockade of abnormal conduction through AV node. Carotid massage, Valsalva maneuver can increase vagal tone but if these measures fail, rapidly acting intravenous drugs are preferred.

INTRAVENOUS ADENOSINE

Adenosine stimulates acetylcholine sensitive K^+ channels and causes hyperpolarization. It also inhibits sympathetic stimulation mediated increase in intracellular cyclic AMP inhibiting calcium currents. Inhibition of calcium currents increases refractoriness of AV node. It reduces SA nodal activity and inhibits AV conduction. It thereby shortens APD and slows down automaticity. It has shortest duration of action with half-life of less than 10 seconds. So, the drug must be given rapidly through intravenous route. It causes asystole for a very short period of less than 5 seconds and helps in the conversion of PSVT to sinus rhythm. Transient flushing or chest discomfort can occur in some. It can further delay the conduction in elderly and can promote bronchospasm.

These adverse effects are short lived as its action is terminated rapidly. Hence, it is preferred for terminating acute attacks.

INTRAVENOUS VERAPAMIL

The calcium channel blocker verapamil, blocks calcium channels in heart and decreases velocity of AV conduction, prolongs PR interval and AV nodal refractoriness. Intravenous verapamil formulation is an equal mixture of levo and dextro forms. Intravenous bolus administration of verapamil causes hypotension and sustained prolongation of PR interval. This effect is attributed to the levo isomer of verapamil which is a more potent and longer acting form of verapamil. Hence, verapamil should be avoided in ventricular tachycardia. It rapidly converts *paroxysmal supraventricular tachycardia* to sinus rhythm. Although it is superior to adenosine, it is not preferred due to the toxicity.

Drug of Choice: Intravenous Adenosine

RATIONALE

Therapy in acute episodes of *re-entrant supra ventricular tachycardia* is focused on interrupting the re-entrant pathway. Adenosine and verapamil are both equally effective. Adenosine is preferred to verapamil as it has very short half-life of less than 10 seconds and it stays in circulation for a very short period. Although it causes greater degree of side effects compared to verapamil, these effects are transient and so it is considered to be relatively safe. It should not be given in patients with bronchial asthma or COPD. Verapamil is cost effective but has a longer duration of action. This prolonged duration can potentiate hypotension and cause sustained prolongation of PR interval. Therefore, it should be avoided.

2. *Intravenous procainamide/Intravenous amiodarone in PSVT due to accessory AV pathway with widened QRS complex.*

BACKGROUND

Paroxysmal supraventricular tachycardia due to accessory pathways occur in one-third of patients with PSVT and this condition requires a different approach in therapy. In PSVT with wide QRS complex extra nodal or bypass pathway is common and this accessory pathway results in ventricular activation. Long acting AV nodal blocker verapamil is contraindicated in this condition. Verapamil causes paradoxical ventricular activation in accessory pathway with wide QRS complex resulting in tachycardia.

INTRAVENOUS PROCAINAMIDE

Procainamide is an amide derivative of local anesthetic procaine and is given intravenously to terminate acute attack. It blocks open sodium channels when frequency of channel activation is high and these channels have intermediate channel recovery time. It also blocks outward potassium current, prolonging action potential. Procainamide is better tolerated intravenously. It reduces automaticity, increases refractory period, prolongs the action potential and slows conduction. When given intravenously, it prolongs the refractoriness of bypass or accessory pathways facilitating termination of SVT. Eventhough hypotension and marked slowing of conduction are caused by procainamide, it is better tolerated as it is eliminated rapidly.

INTRAVENOUS AMIODARONE

Amiodarone blocks inactivated sodium channels, inhibits calcium and inward rectifier potassium currents. It is highly lipophilic and accumulates in many tissues. Since its excretion is extremely slow, it potentiates the intensity of its adverse effects. It is water insoluble so solvent dimethyl sulfoxide (DMSO) is used for injections. The solvent DMSO used in the preparation of intravenous formulation potentiates hypotension and inhibits myocardial contractility. It also augments cardiac depressant action of amiodarone. Besides, intravenous amiodarone is less effective in terminating the acute attack of PSVT.

Drug of Choice: Intravenous Procainamide

RATIONALE

The management of PSVT with wide QRS complex is different from PSVT with narrow QRS complex. Drugs prolonging AV nodal conduction like calcium channel blockers are contraindicated in this condition as they can cause paradoxical ventricular overactivity. Intravenous procainamide is well tolerated, prolongs refractoriness of accessory pathway, terminates the attack and so is preferred. The solvent used in intravenous amiodarone can potentiate hypotension and cardiac depression. Its higher lipophilicity can prolong its side effects. Moreover, it is less effective in controlling acute attacks. In view of the above, it is not preferred.

3. *Intravenous magnesium/Oral verapamil in automatic multifocal atrial tachycardia.*

BACKGROUND

Atrial tachycardia can arise from multiple supraventricular foci. Multiple ectopic foci in atria with enhanced automaticity also cause tachycardia. Heart rate ranges between 100 and 140 beats per minute. Marked irregular PP intervals occur in ECG. Since severe concomitant chronic obstructive pulmonary disease often coexists with this condition, beta blockers are contraindicated. Cardiomyopathy and left ventricular failure are reversed if tachycardia is controlled. In most patients, correction of precipitating factors such as acid-base and electrolyte disturbances revert tachycardia into sinus rhythm.

ORAL VERAPAMIL

If tachycardia persists, then drug therapy is required. Verapamil is the drug of choice for automatic multifocal atrial tachycardia. It alters atrial automaticity and reduces ventricular rate and cardiac response. It acts by blocking calcium mediated *late (delayed) after depolarizations* (DAD). It decreases velocity of AV node conduction. It is given orally at 240 to 480 mg daily in divided doses. This dose is effective in most patients with automatic multifocal atrial tachycardia.

INTRAVENOUS MAGNESIUM

Intravenous magnesium is effective even in those with normal serum magnesium level. It also acts by blocking calcium mediated *late (delayed) after depolarizations* (DAD). Higher dose is required and therapeutic benefit is short lived. Hence intravenous magnesium is not preferred.

Drug of Choice: Oral Verapamil

RATIONALE

Multiple ectopic foci in atria enhance automaticity of atria resulting in automatic *multifocal atrial tachycardia*. Since pathophysiology of this condition is more often due to pulmonary conditions, beta blockers are contraindicated. **Verapamil** is the **first line** of treatment. Verapamil decreases velocity of AV node conduction and inhibits calcium mediated DAD, **alters atrial automaticity** and **reduces ventricular rate**. It is effective **orally. Intravenous magnesium** also acts by blocking DAD but its **therapeutic benefit is short** and a high dose is required. Hence, magnesium is not preferred.

4. *Intravenous magnesium/Lignocaine in preventing recurrent episodes of torsades de pointes.*

BACKGROUND

Prolonged QT interval results in prolonged QT syndrome or *torsades de pointes*. It is a form of ventricular tachycardia and can progress to ventricular fibrillation. Ventricular fibrillation precipitates sudden cardiac death. QT prolongation predisposes to the development of *early after depolarization* (EAD). EAD triggers *re-entrant tachycardia*, a rare and lethal condition. It either occurs due to hypomagnesemia or due to coadministered drugs. Amiodarone, quinidine, procainamide, sotalol, erythromycin, ondansetron and domperidone cause *torsades de pointes*. Cisapride and terfenadine have been withdrawn from market due to this side effect. Such drugs should be discontinued before starting the treatment.

INTRAVENOUS MAGNESIUM

Intravenous magnesium sulfate is the first line drug. Magnesium when given intravenously prevents recurrent episodes. It probably acts by inhibiting calcium mediated inward current responsible for EAD but it does not shorten the QT interval. Magnesium sulfate 1 to 2 g mixed in 5% dextrose or normal saline is infused over a period of 5 to 60 minutes.

LIGNOCAINE

IV short acting beta blocker, esmolol is more effective in congenital QT syndrome but not effective in QT syndrome induced by drugs. Lignocaine is a class I-B antiarrhythmic agent and a local anesthetic. It blocks both open and inactivated sodium channels and reduces automaticity. It slightly shortens QT interval but does not prevent EAD. Hence, it is ineffective in preventing recurrent episodes of QT syndrome.

Drug of Choice: Intravenous Magnesium

RATIONALE

Prolonged QT syndrome or *torsades de pointes* may either be due to hypomagnesemia or due to coadministered drugs. It is a rare but potentially lethal condition. Before initiating treatment, the drug responsible should be stopped. **Intravenous magnesium sulfate** 1 to 2 g in 5% dextrose or normal saline infusion given over a period of 5 to 60 minutes **controls the episode effectively**. Even though it does not shorten QT interval, it acts by **inhibiting EAD. Intravenous lignocaine** shortens QT interval marginally but **does not reduce EAD**, the triggering factor in *torsades de pointes*. Hence, intravenous magnesium sulfate is preferred to intravenous lignocaine.

5. *Intravenous digoxin/Intravenous diltiazem as initial therapy for atrial fibrillation in hemodynamically stable patients.*

BACKGROUND

Antiarrhythmic drugs that restore sinus rhythm should not be given initially. Drugs that increase AV nodal refractoriness should be given first. Drugs that restore sinus rhythm decrease the number of impulses reaching AV node and suppress atrial conduction but, paradoxically AV node allows more impulses to reach ventricles. This in turn increases the ventricular response rate. Hence, drugs that prolong refractoriness of AV node should be given in initial therapy. This will effectively block the entry of impulses to ventricles.

INTRAVENOUS DILTIAZEM

Intravenous diltiazem suppresses automaticity. It prolongs the refractory period of AV node and slows down AV conduction. It is effective in controlling rapid ventricular rate temporarily in atrial fibrillation because, it causes dose dependent inhibition of ventricular rate. DAD mediated ventricular tachycardia responds well to intravenous diltiazem. Hence, diltiazem is preferred and administered intravenously. It is effective immediately, causes lesser degree of hypotension than verapamil. The incidence of bradycardia and myocardial depression is lesser than verapamil.

INTRAVENOUS DIGOXIN

Digoxin, the cardiac glycoside, slows down ventricular rate. It prolongs the refractoriness of AV node through its vagal action. Thus it helps in controlling ventricular response in atrial fibrillation. It should be used only in hemodynamically stable patients. Its onset of action is slow and often inadequate. Even after intravenous administration, it takes long time for a complete effect. The initial reduction in ventricular rate is evident within the first hour but total effect is delayed up to 24 to 48 hours. Atrial fibrillation due to thyrotoxicosis does not respond to digoxin because this condition is precipitated by increased adrenergic tone. Thyrotoxicosis induced atrial fibrillation potentiates digoxin automaticity and DADs. Digoxin clearance is also increased in thyrotoxicosis.

Drug of Choice: Intravenous Diltiazem

RATIONALE

The initial line of therapy in atrial fibrillation is aimed at increasing AV nodal refractoriness rather than quick restoration of sinus rhythm. Digoxin and diltiazem can both prolong the refractoriness of AV node when given parenterally but **digoxin** has a **narrow safety margin, results in inadequate, slower response** and is **capable** of **initiating arrhythmias**. Complete control of ventricular rate is achieved by **diltiazem** in atrial fibrillation. It **prolongs the refractory period of AV node** and is preferred for initial therapy in hemodynamically stable patients with atrial fibrillation.

6. *Amiodarone/Dronedarone for long term treatment in atrial fibrillation.*

BACKGROUND

Drugs that prolong refractoriness of AV node restore sinus rhythm in many patients. In case this does not happen, then treatment with type I or III agents is necessary. Amiodarone, dronedarone, sotalol, propafenone, flecainide and dofetilide are used. Only amiodarone and dronedarone are not proarrhythmogenic. The remaining four drugs are proarrhythmogenic and can cause arrhythmia. Amiodarone has greater efficacy but has lower safety profile. Dronedarone is less effective but has higher safety profile.

DRONEDARONE

Dronedarone is a non-iodinated derivative of amiodarone. Hence, it has similar pharmacodynamic actions. It prolongs APD and increases refractoriness. When refractory period is increased, conduction velocity is reduced. The intensity of side effects such as nausea, vomiting, diarrhea and asthenia are minimal. It is contraindicated in severe heart failure and should not be given to those with hemodynamic instability. Dronedarone also results in fewer rates of drug discontinuation and has improved compliance.

AMIODARONE

It has poor oral bioavailability. It is highly lipophilic and accumulates in many tissues delaying its onset of action by several weeks. Its metabolite desmethyl amiodarone is also active. Due to its tissue accumulation amiodarone results in cumulative toxicity. Pulmonary fibrosis, corneal micro deposits, photosensitivity or hepatotoxicity occur. It also alters level of thyroid hormones and induces peripheral neuropathy.

Drug of Choice: Dronedarone

RATIONALE

For restoration of sinus rhythm in patients with atrial fibrillation, drugs that restore sinus rhythm are indicated. Amiodarone and dronedarone can both prolong refractoriness and reduce conduction velocity. **Amiodarone** has **greater efficacy** but produces **more adverse effects**. **Dronedarone** is **less effective** but has **greater safety profile**. Amiodarone and its active metabolite result in cumulative toxicities that disappear slowly after discontinuation of drug. Although dronedarone is less effective, it is better tolerated with fewer side effects so it is preferred but it is contraindicated in severe heart failure and in patients with hemodynamic instability.

7. *Ibutilide/Dofetilide for cardio version in atrial fibrillation and flutter of recent episode.*

BACKGROUND

Restoration of sinus rhythm is safer only after three weeks of anticoagulant therapy. It is recommended for patients suffering from recent onset atrial fibrillation or flutter due to a known provocating factor. It is indicated in patients who remain symptomatic even after using rate control drugs. Cardioversion is conversion of atrial fibrillation or flutter to normal sinus rhythm. This is possible either electrically or pharmacologically. Disadvantages of cardioversion by drugs include less efficacy and more side effects. One such important side effect is *torsades de pointes*.

IBUTILIDE

Ibutilide is an activator of inward sodium current and is a blocker of rapid component of delayed rectifier current (I-kr). Rapid IV administration of 1 mg Ibutilide within ten minutes results in immediate cardioversion and is more effective for the conversion of flutter to sinus rhythm and very often converts fibrillation to flutter. It acts by prolonging APD and can result in *torsades de pointes* in 6% of patients.

DOFETILIDE

Dofetilide is a selective blocker of rapid component of delayed rectifier current (I-kr). It results in only cardiac and no extra cardiac actions but has limited efficacy in converting atrial fibrillation and flutter. Besides, dofetilide can cause *torsades de pointes*. It requires constant monitoring of dose depending on creatinine clearance in patients with renal dysfunction. Hence, it should be given only for the therapy of in-patients. Its availability is restricted only to those who know about its dosing procedures.

Drug of Choice: Ibutilide

RATIONALE

Three weeks of anticoagulant therapy is a pre-requisite before initiating pharmacological cardioversion in patients with atrial fibrillation or flutter of recent onset. Ibutilide and dofetilide block rapid component of delayed rectifier current, dofetilide being more specific. They are more effective in converting flutter to sinus rhythm than fibrillation but **dofetilide** is **less effective than ibutilide**. Although these drugs can cause *torsades de pointes* during cardio version, dofetilide is **more proarrhythmogenic**, needs **dose monitoring**, restricted only for **in-hospital treatment**. Hence, it is not preferred.

Diuretics and Antidiuretics

1. *Furosemide/Torsemide as diuretic for oral administration in severe heart failure and pulmonary edema.*

BACKGROUND

Furosemide and torsemide are both high ceiling loop diuretics. They are used in the treatment of heart failure and pulmonary edema. They are effective even in patients with impaired renal function with GFR below 30 to 40 mL per minute. They bind to plasma proteins extensively and not filtered through glomerulus but they are secreted by organic acid transport system. They block $Na^+K^+2Cl^-$ symporter in the thick ascending limb of loop of Henle.

TORSEMIDE

Torsemide is a sulfonylurea derivative. It is three times more potent than furosemide. It has a relatively reliable and better bioavailability of around 80%. It has a half-life of about three hours, has a longer duration action and results in sustained tubular levels. Hence, it need not be administered as frequently as furosemide thereby improving the quality of life and enhancing patient's compliance. It is administered once daily and balances cost differences with furosemide. Unlike furosemide, torsemide effectively controls blood pressure even at low doses. Hence, torsemide can also be an effective antihypertensive drug. It is more potent with a reliable oral absorption and long duration of action. So it is preferred to furosemide in heart failure and pulmonary edema.

FUROSEMIDE

Furosemide, in particular is more effective in pulmonary edema. It increases venous capacitance and reduces pressure symptoms. It is more effective than torsemide. Furosemide contains a sulphonamide moiety. The bioavailability of furosemide is unreliable and shows inter-individual variation and ranges between 10 to 100% averaging 65%. It is cheaper but less potent than torsemide. It has shorter half-life of 1.5 hours and short duration of action. Extended release preparations are not available so has to be administered two to three times a day. Frequent administration is needed to maintain adequate luminal concentration to prevent 'diuretic braking'. Adequate luminal level inhibits 'post diuretic sodium retention' or 'diuretic resistance' but leads to higher incidence of adverse effects of furosemide. Electrolyte disturbances, hyperglycemia and ototoxicity are a few such side effects.

Drug of Choice: Torsemide

RATIONALE

Furosemide and torsemide are both high ceiling loop diuretics. To prevent 'post diuretic sodium retention' that results in failure of treatment, it is necessary to maintain adequate concentration of the diuretic in the lumen. The **oral absorption** of **furosemide** is **variable** and it is **less potent**. It has **short half-life** resulting in **shorter duration** of action and has to be given frequently. **Torsemide**, on the other hand, is **more potent** with **good oral bioavailability**, has a **longer half-life** and longer duration of action requiring less frequent administration. Hence, it is **preferred** to furosemide, **in spite of the cost difference**, for the management of heart failure and pulmonary edema.

2. *Hydrochlorothiazide/Chlorthalidone in systemic hypertension.*

BACKGROUND

Hypertension is a predisposing factor for cardiac complication and ischemic stroke. The goal of treatment in hypertension is to effectively control blood pressure throughout the day to prevent complications. Hence, drugs having longer duration of action with once daily dosage are preferred. When compared to loop diuretics, thiazide diuretics are long acting. Therefore, they need not be administered as multiple daily doses and are widely used in the treatment of hypertension. They are either given as monotherapy or in combination with other drugs. They cause electrolyte depletion, hypercalcemia as well as glucose intolerance and result in erectile dysfunction on long-term administration. Thiazide diuretics have wide range of half-lives and variable protein binding. Their efficacy depends upon protein binding and tubular delivery of drugs.

HYDROCHLOROTHIAZIDE

Hydrochlorothiazide is equipotent to chlorthalidone. It is the least expensive drug among thiazides and has a short half-life of 2.5 hours. It has short duration of action and has to be administered more than once daily.

CHLORTHALIDONE

Chlorthalidone has a longer half-life of about 47 hours. The duration of action of chlorthalidone extends over 48 hours. Hence, chlorthalidone results in 24 hour control of blood pressure. Due to this reason, it is more suitable for effective control of blood pressure.

Drug of Choice: Chlorthalidone

RATIONALE

Effective control of blood pressure throughout the day is main goal of antihypertensive therapy. Thiazide diuretics are preferred to other classes of diuretics as they are inexpensive, well-tolerated and have effective control over blood pressure because they are long acting. **Chlorthalidone** in particular has a **long half-life of about 47 hours** and results in **sustained control** of blood pressure all through the day. Hence, it is preferred to hydrochlorothiazide which has a shorter duration of action.

3. *Metolazone/Hydrochlorothiazide for treatment of hypertension with concurrent kidney disease.*

BACKGROUND

Thiazide diuretics are preferred to loop diuretics in the treatment of hypertension because they do not result in severe electrolyte depletion. They inhibit sodium-chloride symporter in the early distal tubule. Therefore, they result in most consistent pharmacological effect and reduce blood pressure during early period through their diuretic action. Reduction of plasma volume contributes to their antihypertensive action but later on, they decrease BP mainly by reducing peripheral resistance through their direct vasodilatory action. Their diuretic and antihypertensive actions start at a lower dose but their metabolic actions require a much higher dose. Hence, they are more suitable for long-term therapy as only smaller doses are required for therapeutic benefit.

METOLAZONE

Metolazone is more effective than hydrochlorothiazide even at low doses and is ten times more potent. It is a thiazide diuretic that maintains its efficacy even when the GFR is low, around 20 to 30 mL per minute. So, it is preferred as antihypertensive in patients with concomitant kidney disease.

HYDROCHLOROTHIAZIDE

Hydrochlorothiazide is less potent than metolazone with a half-life of about 17 hours. It is given once daily to control hypertension. It is not effective in hypertension associated with kidney disease because it does not act effectively when GFR is low. Hydrochlorothiazide is much cheaper than metolazone.

Drug of Choice: Metolazone

RATIONALE

Except metolazone and indapamide, thiazide diuretics are not effective when the glomerular filtration rate is low. **Metolazone** the thiazide diuretic **acts even when the GFR** is around **20 to 30 mL per minute**. Metolazone is **ten times more potent but ten times costlier** than hydrochlorothiazide. Yet, metolazone is preferred to hydrochlorothiazide for treatment of hypertension associated with kidney disease.

4. *Mannitol/Furosemide in chronic congestive heart failure and pulmonary edema.*

BACKGROUND

Volume overload aggravates symptoms of chronic congestive heart failure causing pulmonary edema and its associated symptoms. The primary goal in CHF is rapid reduction of volume overload.

FUROSEMIDE

Furosemide increases venous capacitance and decreases preload effectively reducing the left ventricular filling pressure. It relieves the symptoms in patients with pulmonary edema. Its vascular actions start even before its diuretic action. The direct vascular effect of furosemide along with diuretic action rapidly relieves the symptoms of congestive heart failure and pulmonary edema. Therefore, furosemide is preferred in these conditions.

MANNITOL

Mannitol is an osmotic diuretic and an inert substance. So, it is not absorbed and is filtered completely by glomerulus. It draws water from intracellular compartments. This action of mannitol expands extracellular volume reducing blood viscosity thereby increasing the renal blood flow (RBF). Increased RBF increases glomerular filtration capacity of nephrons. In addition, it also inhibits renin release inhibiting sodium and water reabsorption. The sites of mannitol action are proximal convoluted tubule and thick ascending loop of Henle. It increases extracellular osmolality and extracts water from intracellular compartments. Therefore, it results in expansion of extracellular volume but increases work load of the failing heart and aggravates pulmonary congestion. Due to these actions mannitol worsens pulmonary edema. It is given as large dose that further expands plasma, causing volume overload. Therefore, mannitol is contraindicated in chronic congestive heart failure and pulmonary edema.

Drug of Choice: Furosemide

RATIONALE

Volume overload aggravates symptoms of chronic congestive heart failure and pulmonary edema. **Large quantity** of osmotic diuretic, **mannitol** is **required** to be given as infusion. It acts by expanding the extracellular volume resulting in **volume overload** and aggravates the symptoms of both conditions. **Furosemide** is helpful through its **direct vascular and diuretic actions**. It is the drug of choice as it rapidly relieves symptoms of chronic congestive heart failure and pulmonary edema.

5. *Spironolactone/Eplerenone in resistant hypertension due to primary hyperaldosteronism.*

BACKGROUND

Spironolactone and eplerenone are both aldosterone antagonists and potassium sparing diuretics. These drugs are mineralocorticoid receptor antagonists and act in late distal as well as collecting tubule. These diuretics competitively inhibit binding of aldosterone to its receptors. Their primary action is inhibition of aldosterone mediated physiological actions. By blocking aldosterone, they cause sodium excretion and potassium reabsorption and by promoting potassium reabsorption these drugs result in hyperkalemia.

EPLERENONE

Eplerenone is safe, effective and more specific to mineralocorticoid receptors. Unlike spironolactone it does not interact with steroid receptors. Hence, it does not cause gynecomastia, menstrual disturbances and hirsutism. It has a better safety profile and the main side effect is hyperkalemia. Eplerenone also results in gastrointestinal side effects. It has good oral bioavailability and its half-life is three times longer than spironolactone. It is preferred for resistant hypertension due to primary hyperaldosteronism.

SPIRONOLACTONE

Spironolactone shows higher affinity towards androgen and progesterone receptors. Hence, it interferes with the function of androgen and progesterone and cause gynecomastia, impotence, decreased libido and menstrual irregularities. Spironolactone blocks testosterone biosynthesis and so it is avoided in men. It is absorbed partially and has short half-life. It causes diarrhea, gastritis, peptic ulcer, drowsiness, headache and skin rashes. It is reported to be associated with breast cancer in rats but its capacity to induce tumors in humans is questionable.

Drug of Choice: Eplerenone

RATIONALE

Although spironolactone and eplerenone are both aldosterone antagonists and belong to the group of potassium sparing diuretics, they differ from each other in their bioavailability and safety profile. **Spironolactone** has partial absorption, undergoes extensive metabolism, has short half-life and results **in gynecomastia, hirsutism, decreased libido** and **menstrual irregularities**. **Eplerenone** has **more specific** action, **safe, effective** and has **good oral bioavailability**. It has moderate duration of action with **better safety profile** as it does not result in gynecomastia, hirsutism or menstrual irregularities. Hence, eplerenone is preferred to spironolactone.

6. *Furosemide/Hydrochlorothiazide in treatment of hypercalcemia in addition to isotonic saline.*

BACKGROUND

Hypercalcemia is associated with conditions such as hyperparathyroidism, acromegaly, thyrotoxicosis and pheochromocytoma. Hypercalcemia is also a frequent occurrence in most malignant conditions.

FUROSEMIDE

The $Na^+K^+2Cl^-$ symporter is present in thick ascending loop of Henle. It promotes the reabsorption of sodium, potassium and chloride. It transports these electrolytes into luminal epithelial cell. During this process, potassium is recycled back into lumen and chloride ions exit through basolateral membrane. This causes transepithelial potential difference with positivity towards luminal side. The transepithelial negativity is towards basolateral aspect. Lumen positivity repels positively charged divalent magnesium and calcium ions. Reabsorption of cations occurs through paracellular pathway into interstitial space. Furosemide inhibits this $Na^+K^+2Cl^-$ symporter. It abolishes transepithelial potential difference necessary for absorption of these ions inhibiting reabsorption of calcium and magnesium. It promotes the excretion of these divalent cations. Therefore, it is used in the treatment of hypercalcemia. It is administered with isotonic saline to prevent volume depletion.

HYDROCHLOROTHIAZIDE

Hydrochlorothiazide has variable effect in calcium excretion during initial therapy but markedly reduces its excretion on chronic administration. Therefore, it reduces the level of calcium ions in tubular lumen preventing formation of calcium stones. Hydrochlorothiazide exacerbates hypercalcemia because it increases serum calcium level. So, it should be avoided in hypercalcemia. It is preferred for the treatment of calcium nephrolithiasis.

Drug of Choice: Furosemide

RATIONALE

Furosemide promotes excretion of **calcium** by abolishing luminal transepithelial potential difference. The **effect** of **hydrochlorothiazide** on calcium excretion is **variable** during initial period of treatment but on **chronic** administration, it **reduces calcium excretion**. Hence, it should be avoided in hypercalcemia as it increases serum calcium level. **Hydrochlorothiazide** is **used** for prevention of **calcium nephrolithiasis** while **furosemide** is preferred in the treatment of **hypercalcemia**.

7. *Acetazolamide/Spironolactone in ascites due to hepatic cirrhosis, along with furosemide.*

BACKGROUND

The hydrostatic pressure increases in portal hypertension but the oncotic pressure falls due to hypoalbuminemia. This pressure difference causes ascites in cirrhosis. It is potentiated by nitric oxide mediated splanchnic and systemic vasodilatation as well as elevated renin and angiotensin levels. As liver function is compromised it is unable to metabolize aldosterone increasing sodium and water retention, aggravating edema. Treatment options are minimal as ACE inhibitors and ARBs should be avoided. Vasopressin receptor antagonists are expensive, not very effective and cause thirst.

SPIRONOLACTONE

The drug of choice spironolactone, if given alone delays the therapeutic benefit. The clinical benefit is delayed by 14 days hence, it is combined with furosemide. Furosemide augments diuresis but it may also increase the risk of volume contraction because it is a very potent diuretic. Spironolactone is started with 100 mg daily dose and gradually increased every 3 to 5 days up to 400 mg per day.

ACETAZOLAMIDE

Acetazolamide is a weak diuretic and acts by inhibiting carbonic anhydrase, the enzyme present in proximal convoluted tubule and collecting duct. Normally ammonia combines with hydrogen ions and excreted as ammonium ions. The hydrogen ions required are available through exchange with sodium ions and this process is mediated by sodium hydrogen antiporter. Acetazolamide inhibits the availability of hydrogen ions preventing the excretion of ammonia. It also diverts ammonia of renal origin from urine in to systemic circulation. Normally ammonia gets detoxified to urea by liver but the cirrhotic liver is unable to detoxify ammonia. The excess ammonia either induces or worsens hepatic encephalopathy causing delirium or drowsiness. Acetazolamide is contraindicated in ascites due to cirrhosis of liver.

Drug of Choice: Spironolactone

RATIONALE

Treatment options are minimal in ascites due to hepatic cirrhosis. **Spironolactone does not provide immediate benefit** if given alone as the **onset** of action is **evident** only **after 14 days**. Similarly the risk of **volume contraction** is high, **if furosemide is given alone**. Hence, these diuretics are combined together. **Acetazolamide** diverts ammonia to systemic circulation and causes hepatic encephalopathy. Hence, it is **contraindicated** in ascites due to liver cirrhosis.

8. *Mannitol/Acetazolamide in reducing high altitude cerebral edema.*

BACKGROUND

Cerebral edema may occur due to brain trauma or due to non traumatic causes. Ischemic stroke or inflammation can lead to cerebral edema. Ascent to high altitudes without proper acclimatization induces cerebral hypoxia. Hypoxia not only causes but also aggravates cerebrovascular edema.

ACETAZOLAMIDE

Acetazolamide, a carbonic anhydrase inhibitor, modulates CSF production. It is effective in cerebral edema due to high altitude. Therefore, it is the drug of choice. It is given prophylactically to provide symptomatic relief in mountain sickness and prevent high altitude cerebral edema but the mechanism of its prophylactic action is unclear and may be due to its capacity to induce metabolic acidosis. It can result in paresthesia, drowsiness, polyurea and myopia.

MANNITOL

The osmotic diuretic mannitol is given IV as a 15 to 20% solution. At a dose of 0.25 to 2 g/kg it can reduce cerebral edema but it is ineffective in cerebral edema due to high altitude. It is effective in cerebral edema due to other causes. In cerebral edema, by removing water from extracellular compartment into vasculature it helps in reducing intracranial volume improving intracranial compliance and perfusion. Mannitol is inert, nontoxic and relatively stable with a half-life of 4 to 6 hours. It does not accumulate in brain and has minimal systemic side effects. It is contraindicated in active intracranial bleeding and can cause rebound cerebral edema after it is terminated. Pulmonary edema, low blood volume and electrolyte disturbances can also occur.

Drug of Choice: Acetazolamide

RATIONALE

Cerebral edema can occur due to traumatic and nontraumatic causes. If it occurs due to high altitude, the treatment pattern is different. The osmotic diuretic mannitol is effective in cerebral edema due to other causes but only carbonic anhydrase inhibitor, **acetazolamide** is **helpful in relieving** the symptoms of **high altitude cerebral edema**. The effect of acetazolamide may be due to its **capacity to induce metabolic acidosis**.

9. *Desmopressin/Hydrochlorothiazide in nephrogenic diabetes insipidus (DI) along with indomethacin.*

BACKGROUND

In nephrogenic diabetes insipidus the renal absorption of water is compromised due to defect in renal tubules. Inspite of normal or high level of vasopressin, polyurea persists in these patients because the primary defect occurs in kidney. Hypercalcemia and hypokalemia can induce diabetes insipidus. Lithium, clozapine and demeclocycline are a few drugs that can induce this condition. Desmopressin is the drug of choice for central diabetes insipidus.

HYDROCHLOROTHIAZIDE

Hydrochlorothiazide is the first line of therapy for nephrogenic DI. It helps in reducing polyurea causing extracellular fluid volume contraction due to natriuresis stimulating compensatory proximal tubular reabsorption of sodium chloride. Hydrochlorothiazide reduces the amount of urine formed by 50% due to reduction in volume of fluid delivered to distal tubule. Indomethacin acts by decreasing the prostaglandin mediated GFR and urinary volume. Combined therapy of hydrochlorothiazide with indomethacin is more effective.

DESMOPRESSIN

Desmopressin is an analog of the antidiuretic hormone vasopressin. It has more selectivity to antidiuretic than vasopressor activity. Its antidiuretic capacity is 3000 times greater than vasopressin. Desmopressin is more effective in central DI and not in nephrogenic DI because the main cause of central DI is vasopressin deficiency.

Drug of Choice: Hydrochlorothiazide

RATIONALE

Nephrogenic DI is due to a primary defect in renal tubules with normal or elevated serum vasopressin level. **Hydrochlorothiazide**, a moderately **potent diuretic** is effective in the treatment of nephrogenic diabetes insipidus. This paradoxical action of hydrochlorothiazide is due to its capacity to **inhibit** the amount of **urine formation** by 50%, helping to reduce polyurea. Hydrochlorothiazide is more effective when given with indomethacin. **Desmopressin**, a vasopressin analog is effective in the treatment of central DI and not nephrogenic DI because it has **more selective antidiuretic action than vasopressor action**.

10. *Vasopressin/Terlipressin in the management of esophageal varices.*

BACKGROUND

Esophageal varices are common in patients with portal hypertension. This occurs due to dilatation of submucosal veins and when pressure gradient between portal vein and inferior vena cava is high. If gradient exceeds 10 mm Hg instead of 2 to 6 mm Hg varices are formed. Vasopressin V_1 receptors mediate vasopressin actions but antidiuretic action is mediated by Vasopressin V_2 receptors. Stimulation of V_1 receptors causes contraction of vascular smooth muscle. Intense vasoconstriction helps to reduce bleeding.

TERLIPRESSIN

Terlipressin is a V_1 receptor agonist and causes vasoconstriction of splanchnic arterial vessels. It decreases blood flow to portal system thereby reducing portal pressure. This decreases bleeding in esophageal varices, so terlipressin is effective. Terlipressin is given through intravenous route and causes significant and sustained reduction in portal and variceal pressure. It does not alter renal perfusion significantly. Terlipressin has an orphan drug status. It is given to prevent hemorrhage in portal hypertension during abdominal surgery. It should be avoided in cerebral, coronary or peripheral vascular disease.

VASOPRESSIN

Vasopressin stimulates both V_1 and V_2 receptors. Its pharmacological actions are similar to terlipressin. It decreases portal pressure and reduces bleeding of esophageal varices. Vasopressin is no longer used in this condition due to its marked side effects. It is given IV and avoided in cerebral, coronary or peripheral vascular disease. It causes severe cutaneous vasoconstriction resulting in facial pallor. It is also capable of causing severe coronary vasoconstriction. It increases intestinal motility due to stimulation of intestinal muscles. Hence, it causes nausea, abdominal cramps, belching and urge to defecate.

Drug of Choice: Terlipressin

RATIONALE

Portal hypertension is a common cause for esophageal varices. Vasopressin and terlipressin act by stimulating V_1 receptors. **Terlipressin** is **more selective** V_1 agonist, **highly effective**, results in **sustained, significant reduction** in portal hypertension and prevents bleeding in esophageal varices through vasoconstriction. Vasopressin is more toxic causes more severe side effects such as increased intestinal motility, facial vasoconstriction and pallor. They are both contraindicated in coronary and peripheral vascular disease.

11. *Tolvaptan/Conivaptan in the treatment of hyponatremia associated with syndrome of inappropriate secretion of ADH (SIADH).*

BACKGROUND

SIADH occurs due to inappropriate secretion of vasopressin leading to reduced excretion of water causing hyponatremia and hypo-osmolality. SIADH can occur due to malignant conditions, stroke and tuberculosis. SSRIs, chlorpropamide, carbamazepine cyclophosphamide, vinca alkaloids and TCAs also cause SIADH. Tolvaptan and conivaptan, the V_2 receptor antagonists block the actions of vasopressin. These 'Aquaretics', are mainly used in the treatment of SIADH as they increase water excretion without affecting excretion of electrolytes. Hence, they are very useful in hypervolemic and euvolemic hyponatremia. They do not interfere with reabsorption of sodium, so they do not trigger the feedback mechanism for increased sodium reabsorption.

TOLVAPTAN

Tolvaptan is a selective V_2 antagonist. It has 29 times more selectivity for V_2 rather than V_{1a}. V_2 receptors mediate the antidiuretic effect of vasopressin. So, selective V_2 antagonists inhibit vasopressin action in SIADH. Nonselective vasopressin antagonists are not so effective. Hence, the selective V_2 antagonist, tolvaptan, is preferred. Tolvaptan can be given orally at 15 mg daily but has to be administered under supervision. Tolvaptan has black box warning against rapid correction of hyponatremia.

CONIVAPTAN

Conivaptan acts on both V_2 and V_{1a} receptors. Being a nonselective antagonist, conivaptan is less effective in SIADH. Conivaptan is associated with multiple drug interactions and it has to be infused into different veins every time. This mode of administration prevents infusion site reaction. It should be given only through intravenous route. It is given initially at a 20 mg bolus dose followed by 20 mg over 24 hours. It is later repeated at 20 mg per day by continuous infusion for 3 days.

Drug of Choice: Tolvaptan

RATIONALE

SIADH occurs due to multiple reasons and is usually treated with vasopressin antagonists. Although tolvaptan and conivaptan are both vasopressin antagonists, **tolvaptan** is preferred as it is a **selective V$_2$ antagonist**. Since V$_2$ receptors mediate the antidiuretic action of vasopressin, the selective V$_2$ antagonists are more useful in this condition. Besides, **conivaptan** is prone for **multiple drug interactions** as it is metabolized by CYP3A4 and has to be infused through different veins every time. This makes it more **unsuitable** for long-term therapy. Tolvaptan however should only be given under supervision to prevent too rapid correction of hyponatremia, which can be fatal.

CHAPTER
28
Anticoagulants, Thrombolytics and Antiplatelets

1. *Heparin/Low molecular weight heparins (LMWH) as initial therapy in venous thromboembolism.*

BACKGROUND

Venous thromboembolism is associated with cancer, trauma, major surgery in lower limbs and hypercoagulable states. A rapid acting anticoagulant with warfarin is most preferable for treatment. Heparin and LMWHs dalteparin, enoxaparin and tinzaparin act rapidly but low molecular weight heparins (LMWHs) are preferred.

LOW MOLECULAR WEIGHT HEPARINS

LMWHs act mainly on factor Xa, but have minimal effect on factor IIa. They have no effect on thrombin inhibition by antithrombin. Hence, they do not affect activated partial thromboplastin time (aPTT). Due to this advantage they do not require continuous monitoring. LMWHs are equally effective as compared to heparin but they have many pharmacokinetic advantages over heparin. LMWH have better subcutaneous bioavailability (90%). They have more predictable anticoagulant action and no antiplatelet action. This minimises the hemorrhagic complications. LMWHs have longer biological half-life independent of the dose administered. They result in lower incidence of thrombocytopenia and osteoporosis.

HEPARIN

Heparin acts by binding to antithrombin. It potentiates antithrombin inhibition on clotting factors. Intrinsic and common pathways are both involved. Factors IXa, Xa, XIa, XIIa, XIIIa and IIa are inhibited but the main target factors are only Xa and IIa. Bioavailability of heparin after subcutaneous administration is only 30%. The half-life of heparin is dose dependent. Heparin results in higher incidence of thrombocytopenia and osteoporosis. It causes plasma lipemic clearance and 'rebound hyperlipemia' after discontinuation.

Drug of Choice: Low Molecular Weight Heparins (LMWHs)

RATIONALE

LMWHs are preferred to heparin as anticoagulants because they do not affect thrombin function so do not need constant monitoring of aPTT. They do not have antiplatelet action and do not result in hemorrhagic complications. They have better subcutaneous bio-availability, more predictable anticoagulant action, have longer biological half-life independent of dose administered and lower incidence of side effects.

2. *Enoxaparin/Fondaparinux as anticoagulant in patients with ST segment elevated myocardial infarction (STEMI) undergoing primary percutaneous coronary intervention (PCI).*

BACKGROUND

Fondaparinux is a synthetic pentasaccharide. Enoxaparin, the LMWH, is a natural agent from animal source. They are anticoagulants which mainly act by inhibiting factor Xa.

ENOXAPARIN

Enoxaparin has a minimal action on factor IIa. It does not require monitoring of aPTT as it does not affect thromboplastin time. It directly inhibits the activity of thrombin and has minimal inhibition on thrombin (factor IIa). It can be safely administered without the risk of catheter thrombosis and does not stimulate clotting mechanism through intrinsic pathway.

FONDAPARINUX

Fondaparinux has 100% bioavailability when given as subcutaneous injection because it is absorbed completely from the site of administration. It does not require aPTT monitoring and can be given at a fixed dose once daily. It does not bind to plasma proteins but binds to antithrombin specifically. Fondaparinux does not undergo metabolism and is excreted unchanged. It binds to anti-thrombin reversibly and does not affect thrombin. It selectively inhibits factor Xa while preserving the regulatory functions of thrombin. Fondaparinux should not be given in patients with STEMI undergoing PCI. If given, it can cause catheter thrombosis because it promotes catheter induced stimulation of factor XII stimulating the clotting mechanism mediated through intrinsic pathway. Hence, fondaparinux should be avoided during PCI.

Drug of Choice: Enoxaparin

RATIONALE

Fondaparinux selectively inhibits factor Xa and does not interfere with the regulatory functions of factor IIa (thrombin). Besides, it also results in catheter-induced activation of factor XII, the factor responsible for inducing the intrinsic pathway of clotting mechanism. Hence, if given in patients with STEMI undergoing PCI, it causes catheter thrombosis. **Enoxaparin inhibits** factor **Xa**, has minimal inhibition on thrombin and **does not** result in catheter induced stimulation of factor XII or **catheter thrombosis** hence, preferred as anticoagulant during PCI.

3. *Lepirudin/Argatroban for initial treatment in patients with heparin-induced thrombocytopenia.*

BACKGROUND

Heparin causes 50% reduction in pre-treatment value of platelets. Incidence is only around 5% but still is significant because of the drastic reduction. Thrombocytopenia occurs usually around 5 to 10 days after the initiation of therapy. IgG antibodies and heparin-platelet factor complexes binds to platelets activating them leading to thrombocytopenia and life-threatening thrombosis. Platelet transfusion is not required for correction of thrombocytopenia. An anticoagulant should be given initially till platelet counts recovers. Direct thrombin inhibitor inhibits thrombosis and should be given immediately. Lepirudin and argatroban, the direct thrombin inhibitors bind to different sites. They are titrated based on aPTT target 1.5 to 3.0 times the normal.

ARGATROBAN

Argatroban binds reversibly only to the catalytic site of thrombin. When given intravenously, action starts immediately but has a short half-life of 40 to 50 minutes. It causes modest bleeding risk and is cheaper compared to lepirudin. Hence, argatroban is preferred to lepirudin. It is chiefly metabolised by liver and is excreted through bile. So, dose reduction for argatroban is necessary in hepatic insufficiency.

LEPIRUDIN

Lepirudin binds to both sites of thrombin. They are catalytic site and extended substrate recognition site of thrombin. Lepirudin needs daily monitoring of aPTT because it can cause paradoxical increase in aPTT. The dose of lepirudin should be reduced in renal failure.

Drug of Choice: Argatroban

RATIONALE

Heparin-induced thrombocytopenia occurs in around 5 to 10 days after initiation of therapy. After discontinuation of heparin, an anticoagulant is preferred than platelet transfusion in this condition. Immediate administration of a direct thrombin inhibitor is required till platelet counts recover. Argatroban as well as lepirudin are titrated based on aPTT target of 1.5 to 3.0 times the normal value. **Argatroban** is preferred as it has **immediate onset** of action with a very short half-life, causes **modest bleeding risk** and is **cheaper**.

Lepirudin can result in paradoxical increase in aPTT, needs to be monitored daily. Hence, it is not preferred.

4. *Enoxaparin/Warfarin for initial management of patients with acute coronary syndrome without ST segment elevation.*

BACKGROUND

An antiplatelet agent along with an anticoagulant is preferred in acute coronary syndrome without ST segment elevation. Fibrinolytic therapy is usually avoided in this condition because thrombosis does not pose a problem in majority of patients.

ENOXAPARIN

Enoxaparin is a low molecular weight heparin. It is given subcutaneously every 12 hours at the dose of 1 mg/kg. The rate of absorption of enoxaparin is uniform after subcutaneous administration and results in predictable therapeutic benefit. Since it has rapid onset of action, it is preferred for the initial treatment. It is given in combination with an antiplatelet agent. Enoxaparin is started with warfarin and continued for five days.

WARFARIN

Vitamin K epoxide is the oxidized form and vitamin K hydroquinone is the reduced form of vitamin K. Warfarin inhibits conversion of epoxide to hydroquinone thereby decreasing the synthesis of vitamin K dependent clotting factors. It also diminishes biological activity of these clotting factors. The half-lives of these clotting factors are variable. The shortest acting is factor VII that acts for six hours. The longest acting is prothrombin which acts for 50 hours. The complete effect of warfarin appears only after a few days because it takes several days for plasma clotting factors to disappear. Therefore, warfarin is not suitable for initial therapy, as an immediate anticoagulant action is needed in the management of acute coronary syndrome without ST segment elevation. Hence, warfarin is coadministered with enoxaparin. Enoxaparin is effective initially and effect of warfarin starts later.

Drug of Choice: Enoxaparin

RATIONALE

Initial management of acute coronary syndrome without ST segment elevation requires treatment with an anticoagulant and an antiplatelet agent. **Enoxaparin** is given subcutaneously, has more uniform bioavailability, **immediate onset** of action, **predictable therapeutic benefit** and so it is preferred. The therapeutic benefit of warfarin, the oral anticoagulant, **starts** only **after a few days** as it **acts indirectly** by inhibiting the synthesis of vitamin K dependent clotting factors. Hence, it is unsuitable for initial monotherapy as immediate anticoagulant action is required in the management of acute coronary syndrome without ST segment elevation.

5. *Dalteparin/Warfarin as anticoagulant in pregnancy.*

BACKGROUND

An anticoagulant with high molecular weight does not cross placenta. Hence, such an anticoagulant does not induce fetal malformations. Drugs with smaller molecular weight freely cross placental barrier and are unsafe in pregnancy.

DALTEPARIN

Dalteparin is a low molecular weight heparin compared to heparin. Its molecular weight is 5000 daltons and is derived from animal tissue. It is a large molecule and does not cross placenta so it is safe in pregnancy and does not cause fetal malformations, fetal mortality or prematurity. Dalteparin belongs to pregnancy category B and has predictable and uniform bioavailability. Hence, it can be given once daily as subcutaneous administration. Besides, it does not require frequent laboratory monitoring as it results in low incidence of thrombocytopenia and osteoporosis.

WARFARIN

Warfarin is a smaller molecule and crosses placental barrier. So, it is teratogenic in nature and causes either abortion or fetal malformations. If given during first trimester, it typically causes 'Warfarin syndrome' which is characterized by hypoplasia of nose and epiphyseal calcifications. When given during second and third trimesters, it causes abnormalities of CNS. The risk of fetal or neonatal hemorrhage is high with warfarin. The incidence is high inspite of normal values of maternal prothrombin time. It belongs to pregnancy category X and it is absolutely contraindicated as an anticoagulant during pregnancy.

Drug of Choice: Dalteparin

RATIONALE

Dalteparin and other LMWH are drugs of choice in pregnancy as they **do not cross placenta** due to their **large molecular size**. **Warfarin** is **teratogenic** and causes **'warfarin syndrome'** in fetus. It results in fetal malformations, fetal hemorrhage and abnormalities of fetal central nervous system. It belongs to pregnancy category X and is absolutely contraindicated during pregnancy.

6. *Protamine sulfate/Vitamin K in heparin overdose.*

BACKGROUND

Bleeding is the main problem in overdose of heparin and causes hemorrhages. The incidence is around 1 to 5% in patients administered with intravenous heparin. Mild bleeding stops after effect of drug wanes off and does not require antidote. In case of life-threatening hemorrhage, an antidote is essential to save life.

PROTAMINE SULFATE

Protamine sulfate is a mixture of basic polypeptides. It is isolated from sperms of salmon fish. In heparin overdose, it binds tightly to heparin and neutralises its action. It is more selective for heparin overdose and not effective for LMWH as it binds only with long heparin molecules. Protamine itself can act as an anticoagulant as it directly interacts with fibrinogen, platelets and other plasma proteins. So, only a minimal dose should be given for reversing the action of heparin. The usual recommended dose is 1 mg for every 100 units of heparin given intravenously over a period of 10 minutes. Maximum permitted dose is 50 mg. Protamine quickly reverses the anticoagulant effect of heparin. Hence, it is given for heparin overdose following cardiac and other vascular surgeries. Anaphylaxis, hypertension, neutropenia and right ventricular dysfunction can occur.

VITAMIN K

Vitamin K helps in activation of clotting cascade. It does not bind to or block heparin. Vitamin K is more specific to warfarin overdose. Hence, it is not indicated in heparin reversal.

Drug of Choice: Protamine Sulfate

RATIONALE

In case of hemorrhage due to heparin overdose, **protamine** sulfate **quickly** reverses its effect by binding and neutralising its effect. Since protamine itself can act as anticoagulant it should be started with a **minimal dose**. It is also given to neutralise the effect of heparin following cardiac or vascular surgeries. **Vitamin K** is used to treat the overdose of warfarin and does not help in heparin overdose as it does not bind to heparin.

7. *Dabigatran etexilate/Warfarin as oral anticoagulant in atrial fibrillation.*

BACKGROUND

Anticoagulants are given in atrial fibrillation to reduce the risk of stroke. They also effectively prevent systemic embolism in chronic atrial fibrillation.

DABIGATRAN ETEXILATE

Dabigatran etexilate is a prodrug, gets converted by serum esterase to dabigatran. It reversibly binds with active site of thrombin and acts as a potent, direct inhibitor of thrombin. It results in more predictable anticoagulant action. Dabigatran does not need regular monitoring. Its half-life is around 12 to 14 hours. Hence, twice daily dosing has better anticoagulant effect. Dabigatran is an alternative to warfarin. It is more effective in the prevention of stroke in patients with atrial fibrillation. It does not result in intracranial hemorrhage in such patients so, it is preferred.

WARFARIN

Warfarin is very effective but it increases the risk of intracranial hemorrhage. Older patients are more sensitive to anticoagulant action of warfarin. It is 99% bound to plasma albumin and it competes for plasma protein binding sites with coadministered drugs leading to a number of drug interactions. In hereditary warfarin resistance, synthesis of vitamin K dependent clotting factors is inhibited. The international normalized ratio (INR) should be maintained between 2.0 to 3.0 during warfarin therapy to prevent bleeding. Hence, frequent laboratory monitoring is required in patients receiving warfarin. It can unmask gastrointestinal bleeding diatheses. It commonly causes bruising of arms as well as legs including skin necrosis.

Drug of Choice: Dabigatran Etexilate

RATIONALE

Although warfarin is very effective in preventing the occurrence of stroke in patients with atrial fibrillation, it can increase the risk of intracranial hemorrhage in these patients. Besides, older patients are more sensitive to action of warfarin. It has very minimal action in patients with hereditary resistance. It is highly bound to plasma proteins and results in drug interactions. Further, it requires frequent laboratory monitoring. **Dabigatran** has more **predictable** anticoagulant **action, does not need** regular **monitoring** and does not cause intracranial hemorrhage.[87] Hence, it is preferred.

8. *Reteplase/Tenecteplase as fibrinolytic agent for acute myocardial infarction with ST elevation (STEMI).*

BACKGROUND

Fibrinolytic therapy reduces the size of infarct. It prevents mortality in patients with acute MI with ST segment elevation (STEMI).

Fifty percent reduction in mortality is reported if they are given during the first three hours but benefit declines thereafter with increase in incidence rates.

TENECTEPLASE

Reteplase and tenecteplase are recombinant variants of tissue plasminogen activator. Tenecteplase acts a little longer with a half-life of 20 minutes. Hence, there is no necessity for repeating the bolus dose. First 30 minutes is critical period in the management of STEMI. Administration of tenecteplase as a single bolus dose is more convenient and can be given even while transporting the patient and starting treatment early is advantageous. It has an additional superiority of having higher fibrin sensitivity and is relatively more resistant to inhibition due to plasminogen activator inhibitor-1. Besides, it has comparable efficacy to tissue plasminogen activator (t-PA). So, it results in significantly lesser noncerebral bleeding. It is costlier than reteplase and has higher incidences of reocclusion. It is also prone for minimal allergic reactions compared to reteplase.

RETEPLASE

Since reteplase has a plasma half-life of only about 15 minutes, the bolus dose has to be repeated again as it is deactivated quickly. Although reteplase has equal efficacy, it has to be given as two bolus doses because it is short acting and has lesser specificity to fibrin. It is cheaper than tenecteplase and causes lesser reocclusions.

Drug of Choice: Tenecteplase

RATIONALE

Fibrinolytic therapy forms an essential component while treating myocardial infarction with ST segment elevation and has to be administered within the first 30 minutes. Newer recombinant tissue plasminogen activators are preferable due to their efficacy and lack of immunogenic reactions compared to older thrombolytic agents.

Tenecteplase is **preferred** more as it has **longer half-life** and is effective as a **single bolus dose**. It has higher fibrin sensitivity and resistant to inhibition by PAI. Reteplase has to be **given twice, has lesser specificity, not so resistant to inhibition by PAI**. Hence, tenecteplase is preferred to reteplase as a thrombolytic agent.

9. *Ticlopidine/Clopidogrel as antiplatelet agent in combination with aspirin in patients with unstable angina.*

BACKGROUND

Antiplatelet agents like aspirin should be given during acute stage of MI. This should be done irrespective of fibrinolytic therapy given in acute MI. Ticlopidine and clopidogrel are antagonists of puriner- gic receptors (P_2Y). They are combined with aspirin as maintenance for secondary prevention. The ADP mediated purinergic receptor P_2Y_1 changes shape of platelets. Irregular shape of platelets poten- tiates platelet aggregation. P_2Y_{12} also inhibits cyclic AMP mediated inhibition of platelet activation facilitating platelet aggregation. Although platelet aggregation is promoted through activation of both receptors it is prevented if either one of receptors is inhibited. Ticlopidine and clopidogrel are both irreversible inhibitors of P_2Y_{12} and prevent platelet aggregation effectively.

CLOPIDOGREL

Clopidogrel has slow onset of action but is more potent. It is asso- ciated with less frequent episodes of thrombocytopenia. Hence, it is preferred in the prevention of recurrent attacks of ischemia. Clopidogrel exerts synergistic effect with aspirin. Hence, it is com- bined with aspirin in patients with unstable angina.

TICLOPIDINE

Ticlopidine is a 'hit and run' drug with a short half-life but prolonged effect. The maximal effect is seen only after eight days of starting therapy. The antiplatelet effect persists for a few days after cessa- tion of therapy besides it is associated with life-threatening blood dyscrasias. It results in severe neutropenia and fatal agranulocytosis with thrombocytopenia. Hence, the therapy requires constant monitoring.

Drug of Choice: Clopidogrel

RATIONALE

Clopidogrel and ticlopidine are both antiplatelet agents and act through inhibition of P_2T_{12}. **Ticlopidine** has **prolonged** effect **but** maximum benefit occurs **only after eight days** and its effect persists for few days after discontinuation of drug but it results in **life threatening blood dyscrasias. Clopidogrel** has **more potent** action and **does not result in blood dyscrasias**, exhibits synergistic action with aspirin so it is preferred.

10. *Clopidogrel/Ticagrelor in acute coronary syndrome.*

BACKGROUND

Ticagrelor is a reversible inhibitor of P_2Y_{12}. Clopidogrel is an irreversible inhibitor of P_2Y_{12}.

TICAGRELOR

It results in more predictable inhibition of ADP mediated platelet aggregation and is not a prodrug, causes 90% inhibition of platelet aggregation within first two hours. Therefore, it has quick onset of action and its action terminates rapidly within three days. It is more effective than clopidogrel in preventing ischemic events. Hence, it prevents cardiovascular deaths in patients with acute coronary syndrome. It is less susceptible to drug interaction, not influenced by genetic polymorphisms but it is more expensive and has to be given twice daily. It results in higher overall risk for minor bleeding but the incidence of major bleeding is much lower. The higher cost of ticagrelor poses major restriction in its use.

CLOPIDOGREL

The platelet aggregation mediated by clopidogrel is more unpredictable. It is a prodrug and gets converted to active drug. Clopidogrel has slow onset of action but its action terminates only after three days.

The delay in termination of action is due to its irreversible blockade. It is less effective in preventing ischemic events and cardiovascular deaths. Thirty percent people show resistance to clopidogrel due to genetic polymorphisms. It is affordable, in usage for a long time and can be given once daily. It has variable response and causes more drug interactions.

Drug of Choice: Ticagrelor

RATIONALE

Clopidogrel is an irreversible inhibitor of P_2Y_{12} with delay in termination of action. Hence, it is unsuitable for patients requiring surgery. It shows difference in response due to wide **inter-individual variations**, causes **more drug interactions** and influenced by genetic polymorphisms compared to ticagrelor. **Ticagrelor** prevents cardiovascular deaths more effectively and is associated with **lesser** events of major **bleeding episodes** than clopidogrel.[88] Although clopidogrel is time tested and more affordable, ticagrelor is preferred.

Hypolipidemic Drugs

1. *Atorvastatin/Rosuvastatin as hypolipidemic drug for hypercholesterolemia.*

BACKGROUND

Statins are competitive inhibitors of beta-hydroxy beta-methyl glutaryl-coenzyme A (HMG-CoA) reductase and act by inhibiting an early, rate limiting step in cholesterol biosynthesis. They enhance the synthesis of low-density lipoprotein (LDL) receptors and stimulate transcription of LDL gene. They also inhibit the degradation of LDL receptors. Statins reduce total cholesterol, low-density lipoprotein cholesterol (LDL-C) and very low-density lipoproteins cholesterol (VLDL-C) levels and at higher dosage they also reduce triglycerides but they differ in their capacity to increase high-density lipoproteins cholesterol (HDL-C) level. They also augment nitric oxide mediated vasodilatation, maintain plaque stability and reduce lipoprotein oxidation. In addition, they also have anti-inflammatory action. All statins except atorvastatin and rosuvastatin should be taken in the evening because cholesterol synthesis by liver is highest between midnight and 2.00 AM. The major adverse effects of these statins are almost similar. They cause myopathy, rhabdomyolysis and hepatotoxicity. They result in tenfold increase in serum creatinine kinase (CK) levels.

ROSUVASTATIN

Rosuvastatin is given at the dose of 5 to 40 mg. It can be taken at any time of the day and undergoes extensive first pass metabolism. It is not lipophilic, metabolized by CYP2C9/P2C19 to its active metabolite. It has an elimination half-life of about 13 to 20 hours. Eighty-eight percent of rosuvastatin binds to plasma proteins and has long half-life. Therefore, it effectively reduces cholesterol level. Since the risk of adverse effects is proportional to its dose and plasma concentration, rosuvastatin results in lower incidence of myopathy. It has an additional advantage of antiplatelet action as it reduces platelet aggregation and prevents deposition of platelet thrombi. Rosuvastatin results in 43% reduction in venous thromboembolic events. It also inhibits fibrinogen levels and preferred to atorvastatin. Rosuvastatin results in very few drug interactions.

ATORVASTATIN

Atorvastatin is effective in the dose range between 10 and 80 mg. It can also be administered at any time of the day. It is lipophilic metabolized by CYP3A4 to its active metabolite. It has an elimination half-life of about 7 to 14 hours. The plasma protein binding capacity of atorvastatin is much higher. 96% of atorvastatin binds to plasma proteins and its longer half-life is responsible for its greater efficacy. Since it is metabolized by CYP3A4 it results in many drug interactions. Coadministered drugs potentiate its capacity to induce myopathy because they compete with each other for the same enzyme site in metabolism.

Drug of Choice: Rosuvastatin

RATIONALE

Statins act by increasing LDL receptor synthesis and inhibiting LDL receptor degradation. They reduce plasma cholesterol, LDL-C, VLDL-C and triglycerides. They also result in other pleiotropic actions like improvement of endothelial function, plaque stability, anti-inflammatory action and reduce lipoprotein oxidation. Atorvastatin and rosuvastatin exert a prolonged control over cholesterol levels due to their long duration of action and can be administered at any time of the day. **Rosuvastatin** has **additional antiplatelet action** and **inhibits fibrinogen** levels. It is also used at much **lower dose** range than atorvastatin hence result in **lower**

incidence of myopathy as this side effect is directly proportional to its dose and plasma concentration. Rosuvastatin is not metabolized by CYP3A4 so does not result in many drug interactions.

2. *Fibrates/Niacin in hypertriglyceridemia.*

BACKGROUND

High level of triglycerides increases the risk of pancreatitis. Niacin and fibrates are both effective in reducing triglycerides. Niacin is a water-soluble vitamin B with activity on lipid levels.

FIBRATES

Fibrates like fenofibrate and gemfibrozil lower lipoprotein levels and also raise HDL-C levels. They act on peroxisome proliferator activated receptor-α (PPAR-α). These receptors are mainly present in liver and brown adipose tissue. They modulate PPAR-α mediated fatty acid oxidation, increase plasma lipoprotein lipase (LPL) action and reduce the expression of apolipoprotein C-III (apoC-III). Fibrates reduce triglycerides by increasing LPL levels and LPL enhances clearance of triglyceride rich lipoproteins, VLDL-C and chylomicrons. They inhibit synthesis of apoC-III and enhance the clearance of VLDL-C. They increase HDL-C through stimulation of apo A-I and apo A-II. They reduce triglycerides level by 50% and increase HDL-C by 15%. Fibrates may also increase the level of LDL-C by 10%. They are well tolerated but cause myopathy as an occasional side effect. Fibrates can increase the lithogenicity of bile.

NIACIN

Niacin decreases the synthesis of triglycerides by liver. It acts by inhibiting production and esterification of fatty acids. Niacin increases LPL activity, potentiating clearance of triglycerides. Niacin also increases the clearance of chylomicrons as well as VLDL-C and inhibits diacylglycerol acyltransferase-2, the rate limiting enzyme involved in the synthesis of triglycerides. It does not stimulate HDL-C synthesis but increases its level due to decreased clearance of apo A-I. It causes hepatotoxicity, dyspepsia and prostaglandin mediated flushing. Niacin increases uric acid levels and stimulates insulin resistance in diabetics. The side effects of niacin make it unsuitable to be the first line drug.

Drug of Choice: Fibrates

RATIONALE

Fibrates reduce triglycerides by increasing LPL levels, potentiating LPL mediated clearance of triglycerides. Niacin acts by increasing LPL activity. They also increase HDL-C levels. **Fibrates** are **well tolerated** and result in **infrequent side effects**. Niacin causes many side effects such as flushing, hepatotoxicity, hyperuricemia and insulin resistance. Hence, it is considered as second line drug in treating hypertriglyceridemia.

3. *Gemfibrozil/Fenofibrate in hypertriglyceridemia associated with high LDL-C levels with statins.*

BACKGROUND

Gemfibrozil and fenofibrate are both fibric acid derivatives. They have similar mechanism of action and act by stimulating and modulating PPAR-α receptors. Gemfibrozil is a nonhalogenated fibrate. Fenofibrate is a halogenated second generation fibrate. They inhibit coagulation and enhance fibrinolysis. They result in antithrombotic activity. They reduce fatal and nonfatal coronary artery disease (CAD) events but increase the lithogenicity of bile. Oral absorption is 99% when combined with meal. Absorption is relatively less when given on empty stomach.

FENOFIBRATE

Fenofibrate has prolonged half-life of 20 hours. Fenofibrate is long acting and given once daily at 145 mg. Fenofibrate does not increase but decreases LDL-C levels by 15 to 20%. It is less likely to cause myopathy when combined with statins because both are glucuronidated by different enzymes. So, it is more suitable for combination therapy with statins but fenofibrate displaces anticoagulants from their binding sites. Hence, it has to be monitored for prothrombin time if given with anticoagulants.

GEMFIBROZIL

Gemfibrozil has a short half-life of 1 hour and has to be given at high dose of 600 mg twice a day. Since it increases LDL-C levels in patients with hypertriglyceridemia, it has to be combined with statins. When so combined, it reduces the hepatic uptake of statin by inhibiting the anionic transporter and increasing its plasma level. It further increases statin level by competing for the same glucuronyl transferase preventing its excretion. Hence, when administered with statins, gemfibrozil potentiates myopathy.

Drug of Choice: Fenofibrate

RATIONALE

Fibrates are the drugs of choice in treatment of hypertriglyceridemia. Gemfibrozil increases LDL-C levels in patients with triglyceridemia. Hence, gemfibrozil has to be combined with statins to prevent the elevation of LDL-C levels. The second generation halogenated fibric acid derivative **fenofibrate, does not increase LDL-C levels**. **Gemfibrozil** increases plasma level of statins by inhibiting its uptake by liver and by preventing its excretion, **potentiating the myopathy induced by statins**. Fenofibrate does not increase plasma statins levels. Therefore, it is preferred to gemfibrozil.

4. *Statins/Niacin in dyslipidemia associated with diabetes mellitus.*

BACKGROUND

Dyslipidemia is a disorder of lipoprotein metabolism. Diabetes mellitus is a common cause of this condition. It is characterized by high levels of total cholesterol, LDL-C and triglycerides but HDL-C is low. The smaller dense LDL-C in diabetes mellitus is more atherogenic but the large buoyant forms are not atherogenic. Every 1% reduction in LDL-C is responsible for 1% reduction in CAD risk and every 1% increase in HDL-C results in 2% risk reduction.

STATINS

In patients with good glycemic control, statins are most preferred drugs in CAD because they are well tolerated and very effective. Statins reduce the synthesis of hepatic cholesterol thereby decreasing LDL-C by 20 to 50% and increasing HDL-C by 10%. Higher doses of statins are required to reduce triglycerides. They are effective even when triglyceride level exceeds above 250 mg/dL. Pleiotropic effects of statins offer additional cardioprotective benefits in diabetics. Elevated transaminases level is uncommon in nonalcoholic fatty acid disease. It is more commonly associated with diabetes mellitus. It may cause 10% increase in risk for development of diabetes mellitus but still statins are found to be comparatively safer in such patients. Diabetics with insulin resistance benefit from statins as they reduce CAD risk. Hence, diabetics can safely be treated with statins. Renal impairment associated with diabetics can augment the risk of myopathy because excretion of statins is delayed thereby increasing their plasma level. The risk of rhabdomyolysis is also increased in renal impairment.

NIACIN

Niacin decreases LDL-C levels by 20 to 30%. It decreases triglycerides by 35 to 45% and increases HDL-C by 30 to 40%. It is the only currently available hypolipidemic agent that reduces LPA levels but it induces insulin resistance and can cause severe hyperglycemia. So niacin therapy requires constant blood glucose monitoring. It results in frequent changeover from oral hypoglycemic agents to insulin. This indicates loss of diabetic control in many patients. Hence, it should be avoided in diabetic patients.

Drug of Choice: Statins

RATIONALE

Statins are the drugs of choice in diabetic patients with dyslipidemia. They are very effective, well tolerated and can safely be given in diabetics. **Niacin** reduces LDL-C, triglycerides, increases HDL-C and lowers LPA but **potentiates hyperglycemia** as it causes **insulin resistance**. Hence, niacin is not preferred in the treatment of dyslipidemia associated with diabetes mellitus.

5. *Colesevelam/Colestipol as adjuvant in primary hypercholesterolemia.*

BACKGROUND

Bile acid sequestrants or bile acid binding resins act by binding to intestinal bile acids. They reduce LDL-C by 12 to 28% and increase HDL-C by 4 to 5%. Colestipol is an anion exchange resin. It is a mixture of tertiary and quaternary diamines. It is hygroscopic and available as chloride salt that is insoluble in water. Colesevelam is a polymer and available as a hard capsule. Since it is hydrophilic, it forms a gel in intestine on absorption of water. They are usually combined with either statins or niacin in hypercholesterolemia and this combination results in better reduction of LDL-C. Since they are not absorbed, their side effects are mostly related to gastrointestinal tract (GIT).

COLESEVELAM

Colesevelam is a hard capsule and absorbs water. It becomes a soft gel and causes lesser GIT irritation. The incidence of dyspepsia, bloating and constipation is infrequent with colesevelam. Unlike colestipol, it does not interfere with the absorption of fat soluble vitamins. Colesevelam does not interfere with absorption of most of the drugs; still, the drugs should be given either before or after its administration.

COLESTIPOL

Colestipol is available as both powder to be mixed in water or as tablet. In powder form it is highly unpalatable, due to gritty sensation. It is devoid of gritty sensation in tablet form but causes similar GIT irritation. Dyspepsia and bloating occurs even if it is suspended for many hours in water. All other drugs have to be given one hour before or three hours after administration of colestipol. Concomitant administration of other drugs is not advisable to prevent interference of colestipol in their absorption.

Drug of Choice: Colesevelam

RATIONALE

Among the bile acid sequestrants, **colesevelam** is preferred to colestipol as it is **better tolerated and improves compliance**. Colesevelam is available as a hard capsule that absorbs water to become a soft gel, devoid of gritty feeling when administered unlike colestipol which is highly unpalatable. Colesevelam **does not cause dyspepsia, bloating** or constipation, **does not interfere with absorption of fat soluble vitamins A, D, E and K**. Unlike colestipol, it does not interfere with absorption of many coadministered drugs.

6. *Statins/Niacin in hypercholesterolemia.*

BACKGROUND

Hypercholesterolemia is usually associated with hyperthyroidism, nephrotic syndrome and acute intermittent porphyria. Thiazides, progestins, beta blockers and sirolimus increase plasma cholesterol levels.

STATINS

Statins are highly preferred in the treatment of hypercholesterolemia. They are not only very effective but also well tolerated. They act by inhibiting HMG-CoA reductase, the rate limiting enzyme in the synthesis of cholesterol. They reduce triglycerides, LDL-C and improve HDL-C level but do not affect LPA levels. They are most potent LDL-C lowering agents as they reduce its synthesis and increase its catabolism. Other beneficial actions are antiplatelet, anticoagulant and antithrombotic effects. They maintain plaque stability and inhibit production of matrix metalloproteinase improving the vascular endothelial cell function. Statins cause dose related myopathy which can be minimized by starting with a low dose. They are very effective in hypercholesterolemia and have better compliance.

NIACIN

Niacin exerts favorable action on all lipid parameters but it has limited use due to its side effects. It reduces LDL-C, triglycerides, LPA and increases HDL-C but its effect on triglycerides is more prominent than LDL-C. It induces prostaglandin mediated flushing and pruritus at the beginning of therapy. Hence, niacin is usually coadministered with aspirin. It has to be given as a large dose for effective therapy. Such high dose potentiates dyspepsia. Flushing and dyspepsia limit the compliance in patients treated with niacin. It also results in insulin resistance and hyperuricemia and causes toxic amblyopia, toxic maculopathy and atrial tachyarrhythmia.

Drug of Choice: Statins

RATIONALE

Statins are more effective in reducing LDL-C levels and niacin is more effective in controlling triglycerides level. Statins related myopathy can be managed by starting the therapy with a low dose. **Niacin** has to be given at a **large dose**, resulting in **flushing** and dyspepsia that interferes with patient's compliance. It can cause other side effects such as **insulin resistance** and **hyperuricemia**. Hence, statins are preferred to niacin for the treatment of hypercholesterolemia.

7. *Niacin/Fenofibrate in patients with low HDL-C levels.*

BACKGROUND

Low HDL-C by itself is a strong independent risk predictor of coronary artery disease (CAD). HDL-C less than 40 mg/dL is considered to be a risk factor. Usually this condition occurs due to malnutrition, obesity and physical inactivity. It is common in patients with insulin resistance. Anabolic steroids and progestins can also lead to low HDL-C levels.

NIACIN

Niacin inhibits lipoprotein lipase as well as lipolysis and reduces synthesis of triglycerides. Niacin is started with a low dose to minimize flushing and dyspepsia. The dose has to be increased gradually for an effective control. Low dose niacin is sufficient to increase HDL-C levels. Higher doses are required to reduce LDL-C levels. It increases HDL-C levels by 30 to 40% by inhibiting its catabolism through selective inhibition of hepatic metabolism of HDL apolipoprotein A. Niacin is preferred to fenofibrate to increase HDL-C levels. At higher doses it results in more serious hepatotoxicity or hyperuricemia but it is required only at low doses for increasing HDL-C. Hepatotoxicity due to niacin is potentiated through sustained release preparations. Hence, such preparations should be avoided. Immediate release preparations are more effective than sustained release preparations.

FENOFIBRATE

Fenofibrate reduces triglycerides more effectively by interacting with PPAR-α but it increases HDL-C only by 15%. Hence, it is less suitable than niacin for treating low HDL-C levels.

Drug of Choice: Niacin

RATIONALE

Low HDL-C, by itself is a strong risk predictor of coronary heart disease. Even at a **low dose**, **niacin increases HDL-C** more effectively than fenofibrate. Although it causes unpleasant **side effects** such as flushing and dyspepsia, they rarely require discontinuation of therapy and are **minimized by** starting at a **low dose** and then gradually increasing the dose. Niacin sustained release preparations potentiate the hepatotoxicity and should be avoided.

8. *Niacin/Fibrates in familial type III hyperlipoproteinemia.*

BACKGROUND

Familial type III hyperlipoproteinemia, also known as familial dys-betalipoproteinemia occurs due to mutant apoE. It often presents with yellow discoloration of palms and digital creases. Cutaneous xanthomas are common occurrence in this condition. It leads to premature or early onset atherosclerosis involving coronary, internal carotid and other peripheral arteries. Mutation in APOE, the ligand receptor for chylomicrons, intermediate-density lipoprotein cholesterol (IDL-C) and VLDL-C is apo E prevents binding of these remnants to hepatic surface resulting in defective metabolism of these lipid particles. Accumulation of cholesterol within macrophages potentiates atherosclerosis. The plasma level of triglycerides is elevated in type III hyperlipoproteinemia. Remnant lipoproteins like chylomicrons and IDL-C are also increased.

FIBRATES

Type III lipoproteinemia patients respond more effectively to fibrates than to niacin. Fibrates dramatically reduce triglyceride and remnant lipoprotein level. They reduce hepatic production of apoC-III and enhance the clearance of triglycerides and VLDL-C. Fibrates result in regression of tuberous or tuberoeruptive cutaneous xanthomas. Symptoms of CAD and intermittent claudication improve immediately after starting therapy with fibrates.

NIACIN

Niacin is effective in reducing type III lipoproteinemia but its safety profile is inferior to fibrates. So, it is not preferred.

Drug of Choice: Fibrates

RATIONALE

Mutant apo E in familial type III hyperlipoproteinemia causes improper hepatic binding of remnant lipoproteins resulting in elevated levels of triglycerides and remnant lipoproteins. Patients usually present with cutaneous xanthomas or early onset atherosclerosis. Fibrates inhibit hepatic production of apoC-III and increase clearance of triglycerides and VLDL-C. **Niacin** is **effective only at high doses** while **fibrates** have **better safety profile**. Therefore, fibrates are preferred.

CHAPTER

30

Pharmacotherapy of Shock

1. *Dopamine/Norepinephrine in the management of cardiogenic shock with signs and symptoms of shock.*

BACKGROUND

Cardiogenic shock is characterized by systemic hypoperfusion. Decreased cardiac performance causes overall reduced perfusion. Filling pressure is elevated but systolic arterial hypotension is sustained. In persons with shock renal function should be preserved otherwise the patient will end up with renal failure.

DOPAMINE

The pharmacodynamic actions of dopamine are concentration dependent. At a low dose of 2 µg/kg/min, it stimulates vascular D_1 receptors, causes dilatation of splanchnic and renal blood vessels. Dopamine also has prodiuretic effect on renal tubules, contributing to volume reduction. The renal perfusion and GFR are highly compromised whenever BP falls drastically between 70 and 100 mm Hg. Hence, dopamine is the drug of choice in cardiogenic shock with signs and symptoms of shock. Hypovolemia should be corrected before dopamine is administered in such patients. Higher doses stimulate myocardial contractility causing peripheral vasoconstriction. Therefore, only low dose of dopamine should be administered. Lower dose adequately preserves renal function in shock. The main side effects of dopamine infusion are nausea and vomiting.

NOREPINEPHRINE

Being alpha agonist norepinephrine leads to intense vasocon-striction. Norepinephrine also increases cardiac work index tre-mendously worsening the already compromised cardiac function. Further, it decreases splanchnic and renal blood flow. It is not sui-table as it does not improve renal function.

Drug of Choice: Dopamine

RATIONALE

Cardiac performance declines causing systemic hypoperfusion in cardiogenic shock. Improving renal performance is the most important goal in cardiogenic shock. Low dose **dopamine** stimulates vascular D_1 receptors resulting in **dilatation of renal blood vessels**. Its **diuretic** action further augments volume reduction, decreasing **the strain on heart** but volume correction is required before administration of dopamine. **Norepinephrine increases cardiac workload** and **reduces renal blood flow**. Hence, dopamine is preferred to norepinephrine in cardiogenic shock with signs and symptoms of shock.

2. *Dopamine/Norepinephrine as the initial vasopressor in patients with septic shock.*

BACKGROUND

Septic or bacteremic or endotoxic shock is the most common type of shock. It is the main cause for vasodilatory or distributive shock. There is overall reduction of peripheral resistance and intense vasodilatation. Profound vasodilatation reduces cardiac output and causes hypoperfusion of tissue. Gram-positive, gram negative or polymicrobial organisms can cause septic shock.

NOREPINEPHRINE

Norepinephrine reduces mortality in septic shock. Hence, it is preferred as initial vasopressor agent. As a potent alpha stimu-lant, it counteracts peripheral vasodilatation resulting in intense vasoconstriction. It increases systolic, diastolic, mean arterial and mean pulmonary pressure. Norepinephrine increases coronary blood flow and splanchnic blood flow. It does not stimulate heart and does not cause tachycardia and tachyarrhythmias. Hence, norepinephrine is preferred as the initial vasopressor in septic shock.

DOPAMINE

Large dose of dopamine is required to maintain heart rate and blood pressure but it should not be given before appropriate volume correction in shock. Peripheral resistance is usually unchanged at moderate dose. It causes profound stimulation of sympathetic system at higher doses. It increases heart rate and causes tachyarrhythmias. So, it is not preferred.

Drug of Choice: Norepinephrine

RATIONALE

A potent vasopressor is most essential agent required in any vasodilatory shock. **Norepinephrine** is a **potent vasoconstrictor** and counteracts vasodilatation in septic shock, a type of distributive shock. It stimulates blood pressure, increases coronary and splanchnic circulation. It **does not stimulate heart** and **does not result in tachyarrhythmias**. Hence, it is preferred as an initial agent. Dopamine should not be administered before appropriate volume correction, as it can cause sympathetic stimulation, and increase tachyarrhythmias.

3. *Epinephrine/Antihistamines in anaphylactic shock.*

BACKGROUND

Drugs, insects, venoms and food can induce IgE mediated response causing severe Type I anaphylactic reaction. Mediators such as histamine are released from mast cells. Histamine is one of the main mediators of systemic manifestations of anaphylactic shock. Intense vasodilatation leads to hypotension and bronchoconstriction. Further aggravation causes angioedema, urticaria and smooth muscle contraction. Anaphylactic shock is a medical emergency and unless treated quickly, it can be fatal. The drug used to treat this condition should reverse hypotension quickly and should also relieve the bronchoconstriction effectively.

EPINEPHRINE

Epinephrine is a physiological antagonist of histamine and reverses the physiological actions to histamine. It results in potent vasoconstriction and bronchodilatation. It has different site of action and does not interact with histamine receptors but its clinical effects on similar physiological parameters are different. Epinephrine reverses vasodilatation through α receptors mediated vasoconstriction. It increases blood pressure reversing the potent vasodilatation induced by histamine. It causes bronchodilatation through stimulation of β_2 receptors. Hence, epinephrine is the drug of choice in anaphylactic shock.

ANTIHISTAMINES

Antihistamines have limited efficacy in management of anaphylactic shock because, apart from histamine other mediators are also involved in the pathogenesis. When compared to epinephrine, antihistamines do not result in immediate onset of action and do not reverse hypotension and bronchospasm as effectively as epinephrine. Since both H_1 and H_2 receptors are present in the vasculature, blockade of both receptors are essential to antagonize the action of histamine completely. A nonselective H_1H_2 blocker is not available to reverse its action.

Drug of Choice: Epinephrine

RATIONALE

Anaphylactic shock is a medical emergency and has to be managed quickly. It is characterized by intense vasodilatation and bronchoconstriction. The effect of antihistamines is limited as they do not reverse bronchoconstriction and vasodilatation effectively.

Epinephrine is a **physiological antagonist** of histamine causes rapid, **intense vasoconstriction** and **bronchodilatation**. Since it is a life-saving drug in this condition, it is the drug of choice in anaphylactic shock.

4. *Dextran/Hydroxyethyl starch products as plasma expanders in hypovolemic shock.*

BACKGROUND

Dextran and hydroxyethyl starch products are colloidal plasma expanders. They have high molecular weight and remain in circulation over a long period. Their main pharmacological action is to increase the blood volume. They increase the oncotic pressure secondary to their effect on blood volume.

HYDROXYETHYL STARCH PRODUCTS

Hetastarch is a hydroxyethyl starch product. It has similar colloidal properties to plasma albumin. Unlike dextran-70 it does not cause allergy or anaphylaxis and does not interfere with anticoagulant and antiplatelet action. It has a prolonged elimination half-life of about 17 days and maintains blood volume for a longer period. It does not interfere with renal performance. It is preferred to dextran due to its advantages.

DEXTRAN

Dextran is isolated from beet root and available as dextran 70 and dextran 40. Their oncotic pressure is similar to plasma proteins. They have a long half-life of about 24 hours. Intravascular expansion is directly proportional to amount of dextran administered. They improve microcirculation by preventing rouleaux formation. Dextran preparations do not interfere with blood typing but their main disadvantage is their anticoagulant and antiplatelet action. They cause severe bleeding and hemorrhage on account of this. Since it is filtered rapidly by glomerulus, it can clog in renal tubules and can cause oliguria. Higher molecular weight dextran 70 is more prone for allergy. Dextran 70 can also result in anaphylactic reactions.

Drug of Choice: Hydroxyethyl Starch Products

RATIONALE

Colloidal plasma expanders increase oncotic pressure and are therefore used to improve blood volume. The level of intravascular expansion that occurs after infusion of dextran is proportional to the amount infused. It interferes with coagulation, platelet function, causes allergic reactions and anaphylaxis hence, it is not preferred. **Hydroxyethyl starch** products **do not interfere with coagulation, do not cause bleeding**, maintains blood volume for a long period, are devoid of allergic reactions, do not interfere with renal function hence, they are preferred.

5. *Normal saline/Hypertonic saline in traumatic head injury.*

BACKGROUND

Restoration of blood supply and maintenance of both systemic and cerebral circulation is vital in traumatic head injury. Crystalloid plasma expanders are used for resuscitation of blood volume. Normal saline and hypertonic saline are both crystalloid plasma expanders. They contain salts of soluble substances that dissolve in water. Their actions are not limited to vessels as they can freely enter interstitial tissue.

NORMAL SALINE

The osmolality of normal saline is identical to plasma and increases blood volume and blood pressure. Since it is isotonic with plasma, it does not result in cellular damage. Hence, it is comparatively safer to veins and for intravenous infusion. So, it is preferred to hypertonic saline in traumatic head injury.

HYPERTONIC SALINE

Hypertonic saline can cause rapid expansion of intravascular compartment due to transfer of fluid from intracellular space. It lowers intracranial pressure rapidly and improves perfusion of vital organs.

Since hypertonic saline reduces blood viscosity it improves cerebral blood flow, increases cerebral oxygenation effecting auto regulatory vasoconstriction. Cerebral vasoconstriction helps in reducing intracranial pressure but hypertonic saline induced hypernatremia can cause sudden fluid shifts resulting in cellular crenation and cellular damage. Higher osmolality can damage peripheral veins. Hence, hypertonic saline can also result in hyperchloremic acidosis. It has no superior efficacy over normal saline and the therapeutic benefit is similar in both forms of sodium chloride.

Drug of Choice: Normal Saline

RATIONALE

Crystalloid plasma expanders enter freely into the interstitial tissue and unlike colloid plasma expanders, their action is not limited to vessels. **Hypertonic saline** can rapidly reduce intracranial pressure secondary to reduction of blood viscosity and improvement of cerebral blood flow but it causes **cellular crenation and damage**. **Normal saline** is **equally effective** and being **isotonic** with plasma it **does not result in cellular damage**. Therefore, it is preferred.

Hematopoietic Agents

1. *Ferrous salts/Ferric salts preferred for oral therapy of iron deficiency anemia.*

BACKGROUND

Either low iron stores or higher iron requirement increases iron absorption. Iron is absorbed mainly in duodenum and proximal jejunum and absorbed only in ferrous form and not in ferric form. Heme iron, present in meat hemoglobin and myoglobin is absorbed as such. It does not get converted to elemental iron before absorption. Non-heme iron present in vegetables and grains is in ferric form. This should be reduced by ferrireductase to ferrous form for absorption. Side effects of low dose oral iron therapy are heart burn, constipation and diarrhea. Nausea and gastritis are more commonly related to high dosage.

FERROUS SALTS

Ferrous iron binds to divalent metal transporter-1, a mucosal protein. This bound form is transported into mucosal cell and gets internalized where the iron is oxidized to ferric form, binds to ferritin for temporary storage. When iron is released from mucosal cell, it is again reduced to ferrous state. It is then reoxidized to ferric state by ceruloplasmin and bound to transferrin. Hence, orally administered ferrous salts are preferred to ferric salts for therapy. Intestinal absorption of all ferrous salts is three times more than ferric salts. Various ferrous salts are sulphate, gluconate, fumarate, succinate and aspartate. They have minimal differences in their bioavailability. The dose of all these types of salts is based on their iron content.

FERRIC SALTS

Inorganic ferric salts can be absorbed only after reduction to ferrous salts. They should be reduced by ferrireductase to ferrous form before absorption. Besides, ferric salts have poor bioavailability and are not absorbed completely.

Drug of Choice: Ferrous Salts

RATIONALE

Iron is mainly absorbed from duodenum and proximal jejunum. Ferric salts have to be reduced by ferrireductase to ferrous form for better absorption. Hence, iron salts when given as **ferrous form** have **greater bioavailability**. Ferrous salts have **three times** greater absorption than ferric form and bioavailability increases proportionately for higher dosages. The degree of absorption for various types of ferrous salts is almost similar with minimal variations. Higher doses result in nausea and gastritis most frequently, while lower doses commonly produce constipation, diarrhea and heart burn.

2. *Iron dextran/Sodium ferric gluconate for intravenous administration in parenteral iron therapy.*

BACKGROUND

Parenteral iron therapy is indicated when serum iron stores are very low. It is also indicated in persons who are unable to tolerate oral iron. It is required in patients with ulcerative colitis or kidney disease.

SODIUM FERRIC GLUCONATE

Sodium ferric gluconate does not require processing by macrophages. Hence, it has quick onset of action. Within 24 hours, 80%

of sodium ferric gluconate is delivered to transferrin. It has a lower risk of inducing anaphylaxis. It is also devoid of other hypersensitivity reactions. It has to be administered every week as a fixed dose till iron values improve.

IRON DEXTRAN

Iron dextran is a colloidal solution of iron and dextran. It can be administered by either intravenous or deep intramuscular routes. Iron dextran can be given as a total dose one time infusion to replace iron stores. The plasma half-life of iron dextran through intravenous route is about 6 hours. Iron cleaved from dextran is stored in reticuloendothelial cells. It can also be transported to bone marrow by transferrin. It is gradually released from its stores and may take months for complete delivery. Iron dextran can cause anaphylaxis and other hypersensitivity reactions and can also result in cardiovascular instability. Hence, test injection with undiluted iron dextran is necessary every time, before administering iron dextran intravenously.

Drug of Choice: Sodium Ferric Gluconate

RATIONALE

Iron dextran and sodium ferric gluconate are indicated for parenteral iron therapy. **Sodium ferric gluconate** acts quickly as it is **delivered** to **transferrin within 24 hours** and has **a lower risk** for **anaphylaxis** or **hypersensitivity** reactions. **Iron dextran** is delivered to transferrin very **gradually** over a period of weeks and has a comparatively **lower safety profile** causing anaphylactic or **hypersensitivity** reactions. Hence, sodium ferric gluconate is preferred to iron dextran for parenteral therapy.

3. *Cyanocobalamin/Folic acid for megaloblastic anemia with neurological signs.*

BACKGROUND

Hydroxocobalamin and cyanocobalamin are inactive forms of vitamin B_{12}. They have to be converted to their active forms, deoxyadenosylcobalamin and methylcobalamin. Deficiency of both vitamin B_{12} and folic acid results in megaloblastic anemia. Additionally, B_{12} deficiency can cause irreversible damage to nervous system. Normally homocysteine is converted to methionine in the presence of cofactor methylcobalamin. Disruption of this pathway in B_{12} deficiency causes neurological manifestations as homocysteine accumulates due to nonavailability of methyl-cobalamin. Neurological manifestations are swelling of myelin sheaths, demyelination and neuronal cell death leading to paresthesia and alteration of position senses and progression to psychosis.

CYANOCOBALAMIN

Cyanocobalamin, the inactive form of B_{12} can correct megaloblastic anemia by favoring the conversion of homocysteine to methionine. This helps to prevent neurological manifestations due to excess homocysteine. Hence, cyanocobalamin and not folic acid is necessary to treat megaloblastic anemia. Cyanocobalamin should never be given through intravenous route because it can result in anaphylaxis though rare in incidence.

FOLIC ACID

Large doses of Folic acid can correct peripheral picture in mega-loblastic anemia. It is due to 'methyl folate trap', the biochemical step that links B_{12} and folic acid. Folic acid gets reduced to tetrahy-drofolate that takes part in one carbon reactions that are necessary for purine synthesis. This may mask the deficiency of B_{12} through improvement of megaloblastic anemia but this does not correct the neurological manifestations due to B_{12} deficiency.

Drug of Choice: Cyanocobalamin

RATIONALE

B_{12} and **folic acid** are **linked** through **'methyl folate trap'** where folic acid supplements for the deficiency of B_{12} in the synthesis of tetrahydrofolate but **folic acid does not help in the conversion of**

homocysteine to methionine. Hence in B_{12} deficiency, homocysteine accumulates leading to **irreversible neurological manifestations**. Folic acid can correct only the peripheral blood picture of megaloblastic anemia due to B_{12} deficiency but not its neurological manifestations. Hence, cyanocobalamin and not folic acid is required in the treatment of megaloblastic anemia with neurological signs.

4. *Parenteral cyanocobalamin/Oral cyanocobalamin + hog intrinsic factor for treatment of megaloblastic anemia with intrinsic factor deficiency.*

BACKGROUND

Intrinsic factor, a glycoprotein, is secreted by gastric parietal cells. Vitamin B_{12} forms a complex with intrinsic factor that is mainly absorbed in distal ileum. In the absence of intrinsic factor, absorption of B_{12} is negligible. Defective secretion of intrinsic factor from gastric cells results in pernicious anemia. Schillings test shows defective absorption of radiolabeled B_{12} in pernicious anemia.

PARENTERAL CYANOCOBALAMIN

Parenteral cyanocobalamin overcomes the necessity for intestinal absorption of B_{12}. Parenteral therapy also effectively reverses B_{12} deficiency. So, intramuscular cyanocobalamin is preferred. It has better reliability than the combination of oral cyanocobalamin and hog intrinsic factor.

ORAL CYANOCOBALAMIN + HOG INTRINSIC FACTOR

Since the primary defect is lack of intrinsic factor, it can be corrected. External administration of intrinsic factor can correct the deficiency. Hog intrinsic factor is available for use in patients with pernicious anemia. It can be given together with oral B_{12} preparations but clinical improvement is totally unreliable. On prolonged administration patients become refractory to hog intrinsic factor probably due to development of antibodies against hog protein.

Drug of Choice: Parenteral Cyanocobalamin

RATIONALE

Intrinsic factor is necessary for absorption of orally administered vitamin B_{12}. It forms a complex with B_{12} and promotes its absorption in distal ileum. Although administration of intrinsic factor, such as **hog intrinsic factor** with cyanocobalamin appears to be a proper clinical approach, it does not work on long-term. Due to **development** of **antibodies** to hog intrinsic factor, patients fail to respond to such therapy after some time. Hence, **parenteral cyanocobalamin** is **preferred** to hog intrinsic factor-cyanocobalamin combination in the treatment of megaloblastic anemia due to intrinsic factor deficiency.

5. *Natural granulocyte colony stimulating factor (G-CSF)/Pegfilgrastim as granulocyte colony stimulating factor in cancer chemotherapy induced neutropenia.*

BACKGROUND

Most of the anticancer drugs result in severe bone marrow depression. Hence, bone marrow stimulants are indicated in such patients. Since specific depression of leucocytes particularly granulocytes occurs, G-CSF and pegfilgrastim stimulate colony forming units of granulocytes (CSF-G). These drugs increase the production of neutrophil. Natural G-CSF is purified from cultured human cell lines.

PEGFILGRASTIM

Pegfilgrastim is a recombinant human G-CSF. It is a polyethylene glycol and a conjugated covalent product of filgrastim. It also enhances the phagocytic and cytotoxic actions of neutrophils. It is used in chemotherapy induced neutropenia. Pegfilgrastim increases neutrophil counts. Therefore, it reduces the incidence of febrile neutropenia. It has a longer half-life and can be given once during each chemotherapy cycle. It is given less frequently and reduces the period of severe neutropenia effectively. It is little more effective than G-CSF. Pegfilgrastim causes reversible bone pain.

NATURAL GRANULOCYTE COLONY STIMULATING FACTOR (G-CSF)

It promotes differentiation and proliferation of neutrophils as it selectively stimulates CSF-G of neutrophil lineage. It increases concentration of hematopoietic stem cells in peripheral blood. It is effective in the treatment of cancer chemotherapy induced severe neutropenia. G-CSF has a shorter half-life and needs to be given once daily but its clinical efficacy in increasing neutrophil count is lower than pegfilgrastim. It causes reversible bone pain that disappears once the drug is stopped.

Drug of Choice: Pegfilgrastim

RATIONALE

Anticancer drugs cause bone marrow depression. They cause severe neutropenia. These drugs effectively increase the level of neutrophils. Pegfilgrastim has a longer half-life and administered during each chemotherapy cycle but G-CSF has shorter half-life and has to be given daily. The clinical improvement by pegfilgrastim is better than G-CSF. Therefore, it is preferred.

6. *Pegfilgrastim/Sargramostim as bone marrow stimulant in treating neutropenia following cancer chemotherapy.*

BACKGROUND

Unexplained fever, sore throat and ulceration occur due to neutropenia and the patients are susceptible to infection. The mortality rate due to neutropenia is around 20% and fever can lead to death.

PEGFILGRASTIM

It is a pegylated recombinant human granulocyte colony stimulating factor (G-CSF). It is well-tolerated by most patients and reduces episodes of febrile neutropenia after chemotherapy. It also effectively reduces the duration of chemotherapy induced neutropenia. Pegfilgrastim is given as a single dose. The main adverse effect is reversible bone pain but can cause fever, malaise, myalgia, arthralgia and infrequent allergic reactions. It increases capillary permeability causing pleural and pericardial effusions and increases the incidence of peripheral edema.

SARGRAMOSTIM

It is a recombinant human granulocyte macrophage colony stimulating factor. Sargramostim at lower doses selectively increases neutrophil count. Flushing, hypotension, dyspnea and vomiting occurs following administration of first dose in some patients. Although it reduces duration of chemotherapy induced neutropenia, sargramostim by itself can induce fever. Hence, it has limited role in reducing the episodes of febrile neutropenia. Besides, it has a lesser safety profile and causes many side effects.

Drug of Choice: Pegfilgrastim

RATIONALE

At lower doses **sargramostim** increases neutrophils **selectively**. Although it reduces the duration of chemotherapy induced neutropenia, it does not reduce episodes of febrile neutropenia and **can cause fever by itself**. Besides, it has to be given **daily** and causes severe side effects. **Pegfilgrastim** is **well-tolerated, reduces duration** of chemotherapy induced neutropenia, reduces **episodes** of febrile neutropenia and causes only reversible bone pain. Hence it is preferred.

7. *Oprelvekin/Romiplostim for thrombocytopenic purpura.*

BACKGROUND

Thrombocytopenia is a less frequent complication. Thrombocytopenia induces the risk of spontaneous bleeding. Increased destruction and decreased production of platelets are the important causes.

ROMIPLOSTIM

Romiplostim is a small molecular form of recombinant thrombopoietin. It belongs to 'Peptibody', peptide group with important biological activity. Antibody fragments are bound covalently to the peptide increasing its half-life. It is safe, nonimmunogenic and well-tolerated. It results in durable improvement of platelet counts. It has variable half-life depending on platelet counts. Half-life is longer, if platelet count is low and shorter, if the count is high. Romiplostim is more effective in increasing platelet counts than oprelvekin. Romiplostim causes only mild headache during initiation of therapy.

OPRELVEKIN

Oprelvekin is a recombinant form of Interleukin-11. It is approved for the treatment of idiopathic thrombocytopenic purpura. It has a half-life of 7 hours and stimulates thrombopoiesis in 5 to 9 days. Oprelvekin causes fatigue, headache, blurred vision, paresthesia, dizziness, hypokalemia and transient atrial arrhythmias. It causes dyspnea due to fluid accumulation in lung and anemia due to hemodilution. It has a lower safety profile when compared to romiplostim.

Drug of Choice: Romiplostim

RATIONALE

Romiplostim is a **'peptibody',** a peptide bound covalently to antibody fragments that helps to increase its half-life. It has variable half-life, shorter, if platelet counts are higher, longer, if platelet counts are lower. It is **nonimmunogenic**, safe causing only headache, **well-tolerated**, causes durable improvement in platelet count and so preferred. **Oprelvekin** is a recombinant Interlukin-11, has only **moderate efficiency** with **lower safety profile**. Hence, it is not preferred.

SECTION 4

Chemotherapy

32

General Principles of Antimicrobial Therapy

1. *Streptomycin/Penicillin preferred for infrequent dosing schedule.*

BACKGROUND

The concentration and time determine efficacy of an antibiotic and optimal therapeutic benefit occurs by modifying the concentration-time curve. Minimum inhibitory concentration (MIC) is lowest effective antibiotic concentration. The efficacy of antibiotics is determined by MIC and the duration of exposure.

STREPTOMYCIN

The action of aminoglycosides depends on its peak concentration. Persistence of concentration has no relevance in determining its action. Persistent concentration above MIC alone does not improve its efficacy. Intermittent dosing is adequate to achieve clinical efficacy of streptomycin. Hence, once daily dosage is more effective than thrice daily divided dose administration.

PENICILLIN

The efficacy of penicillin is determined by concentration-time curve. Duration of exposure plays a greater role than the concentration. Longer duration of therapy and concentrations above MIC improve its efficacy. If duration of overall therapy is reduced the efficacy of penicillin is reduced. Increase in concentration alone beyond 4 to 6 times the MIC is ineffective. Merely increasing concentration and not the time does not improve its action because peak plasma concentration is secondary to duration of therapy in determining its efficacy. Persistence of plasma concentration is more relevant determinant of its action.

Drug of Choice: Streptomycin

RATIONALE

Concentration-time curve determines the efficacy of an antibiotic and some antibiotics are dependent on persistent concentration for its efficacy. They need to achieve a concentration above MIC for a longer duration to be effective against the microorganisms. **Penicillin** action is dependent on the **persistence** of its **plasma concentration** hence, has to be administered frequently. **Aminoglycosides** like streptomycin are dependent on the **peak concentration** for maximum efficacy and their action is not dependent on duration of exposure. Hence, streptomycin can be **dosed infrequently**. A **higher dose** of streptomycin given **once** a day is **more effective** than **lower doses** given **three** times a day.

2. *Penicillin G/Levofloxacin for pulmonary infections.*

BACKGROUND

In pulmonary infections the drug used should achieve higher concentration in lung. The alveolar capillary endothelium is extremely thin. Inflammation of lung facilitates paracellular transport of hydrophilic solutes. Disruption of epithelial and endothelial barrier increases permeability and hyper-permeability promotes transport of hydrophilic drugs.

LEVOFLOXACIN

Fluoroquinolones are well absorbed and widely distributed. Peak plasma concentration is reached within 3 hours. Its concentration in lung, kidney, prostate and macrophages is high. The concentration of 'respiratory fluoroquinolones such as levofloxacin in lung is higher than plasma concentration and epithelial lining-to-plasma ratio of levofloxacin is >1:1. Hence, levofloxacin is preferred to penicillin.

PENICILLIN G

In pulmonary infections such as pneumonia, the drug should reach epithelial lining fluid because the pathogenic organisms are usually found in this fluid. Epithelial lining fluid-to-plasma ratio determines the efficacy of drug. Penicillin G is widely distributed throughout the body but its concentration in tissues is variable. Its concentration in kidney, liver, joint fluid and lymph is significant. Its concentration in lung is relatively lesser because epithelial lining fluid-to-plasma ratio of penicillin G is only 0.1:1 indicating that the concentration in lung is one tenth its plasma level.

Drug of Choice: Levofloxacin

RATIONALE

In case of pulmonary infection pulmonary epithelial and endothelial barrier is disrupted increasing its permeability. Although most drugs can enter lung in infection due to this hyper permeability, **epithelial lining-to-plasma ratio** is the main determinant. When compared to 'respiratory fluoroquinolone', levofloxacin, penicillin G does not reach adequate concentration in lung. The concentration of **penicillin G** is **lower** than its plasma concentration as its ratio is 0.4 to 1. **Levofloxacin** achieves **a higher** concentration than plasma and its ratio is >1:1. Hence, levofloxacin is preferred.

CHAPTER
33
Sulfonamides, Trimethoprim, Quinolones, Chemotherapy of Urinary Tract Infection and Urinary Antiseptics

1. *Sulfamethoxazole/Sulfisoxazole for otitis media in children along with erythromycin.*

BACKGROUND

Most organisms have developed resistance to sulfonamides, so it is no longer used as monotherapy. Sulfisoxazole is short acting and sulfamethoxazole is intermediate acting sulfonamides. In otitis media, sulfonamides are more effective if combined with erythromycin.

SULFISOXAZOLE

Sulfisoxazole is the most preferred agent among sulfonamides due to its excellent antibacterial activity. It has high solubility and extensive plasma protein binding. It is tasteless, hence preferred for oral administration in children. The incidence of crystalluria is minimal due to its high solubility but still adequate fluid supplementation is required during therapy.

SULFAMETHOXAZOLE

Sulfamethoxazole is closely related to sulfisoxazole. Its absorption and elimination are a little slower. Its acetylated form is insoluble in urine resulting in higher incidence of crystalluria.

Drug of Choice: Sulfisoxazole

RATIONALE

Sulfonamides are **rarely** given as **monotherapy** because many microorganisms have developed **resistance**. Sulfamethoxazole and sulfisoxazole are both short acting sulfonamides. The **acetylated** form of **sulfamethoxazole** is highly **insoluble** in urine leading to higher incidence of **crystalluria**. **Sulfisoxazole** is highly **soluble**, excreted freely, safe, as it is **devoid** of **crystalluria**. Besides, it is tasteless and preferred in children **but adequate fluid** intake during its administration is advisable.

2. *Sulfisoxazole/Sulfadiazine for UTI by susceptible organisms.*

INRODUCTION

Sulfonamides are not the drug of first choice in urinary tract infection (UTI) as many organisms have developed resistance. Although trimethoprim-sulfamethoxazole combination or quinolones are preferred in UTI, sulfonamides may still be used if the organisms are sensitive. Sulfonamides inhibit the incorporation of PABA into bacteria. However, they should be avoided in those at risk of developing bacteremia due to pyelonephritis.

SULFISOXAZOLE

Sulfisoxazole reaches peak plasma concentration within 2 to 4 hours and the concentration in urine exceeds its plasma concentration. Hence, it is bactericidal to microorganisms in urine and so preferred in UTI. Besides, it is highly soluble and its acetylated form is freely excreted. The incidence of severe adverse effects is minimal, less than 0.1%. Crystalluria and hematuria occur only in 0.2 to 0.3% of patients on therapy.

SULFADIAZINE

Sulfadiazine is excreted both in free and acetylated forms. The acetylated form is excreted more promptly than its free form.

It is excreted within a period of 30 minutes. Initially the excretion is rapid but becomes slow afterwards. The urine output should be maintained at 1.2 liters to prevent the risk of crystalluria. Coadministration of sodium bicarbonate increases its excretion.

Drug of Choice: Sulfisoxazole

RATIONALE

Although **not the first line drug** in UTI, sulfonamides are **still preferred** for the treatment of UTI if the **organisms** are **sensitive**. The **concentration** of **sulfisoxazole** in **urine exceeds** that of **plasma** and is **bactericidal** in urine. It is highly soluble, excreted freely decreasing the risk of crystalluria and hematuria. Hence, sulfisoxazole is preferred. Sulfadiazine is excreted in both free and acetylated forms. Although its acetylated form is more promptly excreted than the free form, the **risk** of **crystalluria** is a **little higher necessitating** the **co-administration** of **sodium bicarbonate** to **accelerate** its **excretion** and to prevent its reabsorption. Therefore, sulfadiazine is not preferred.

3. *Sulfasalazine/Mesalamine in ulcerative colitis and regional enteritis.*

BACKGROUND

Inflammatory bowel disease is idiopathic and chronic condition. It is broadly divided into two subtypes. They are ulcerative colitis involving colon and regional enteritis or Crohn's disease affecting any part of intestine. Therapy is aimed at reducing exacerbations and for maintenance of remissions.

MESALAMINE

Mesalamine is the drug of first choice for mild to moderate ulcerative colitis. It is a salicylate but its clinical benefit is not related to suppression of prostaglandins. Specific mechanism of action is yet to be identified but inhibits lipoxygenase pathway and production of TNF-α. It also acts as an antioxidant and inhibits production of inflammatory mediators. It provides symptomatic improvement in around 75% of patients. Interstitial nephritis is its main side effect and it rarely causes nephrotoxicity. Hence, mesalamine is preferred in ulcerative colitis and regional enteritis.

SULFASALAZINE

Sulfasalazine is a poorly soluble sulfonamide, active in bowel lumen. It consists of 5-aminosalicylic acid (5-ASA) linked by an azo bond to sulfapyridine. Sulfasalazine is not absorbed in upper gastrointestinal tract (GIT) and reaches distal GIT because colonic bacteria alone can cleave the azo bond to release sulfapyridine minimizing the systemic absorption of sulfapyridine thereby reducing its adverse effects. The active component of sulfasalazine is 5-ASA that provides relief of symptoms but, the toxic effects are mediated through sulfapyridine which causes hemolysis in G-6PD deficient individuals, arthralgia, fever and rashes. Its clinical efficacy is comparable to mesalamine but toxic effects limit its use in these conditions.

Drug of Choice: Mesalamine

RATIONALE

Sulfasalazine is a combination of 5-aminosalicylic acid and sulfa-pyridine. The **active component** of sulfasalazine is **5-ASA**. The therapeutic **efficacy** of sulfasalazine is **similar** to **mesalamine** but the **side effects** are **higher** hence, not preferred. The toxic effects are due to its inactive component sulfapyridine. Mesalamine is a 5-ASA with a probable mechanism of inhibiting synthesis of leuko-trienes, TNF-α and other inflammatory mediators. Mesalamine has a better safety profile, so preferred.

4. *Sulfacetamide/Sulfadiazine as eye drops.*

BACKGROUND

Sulfonamides are used in the treatment of ocular infections such as conjunctivitis. They are also used in other superficial infections but their lack of efficacy and risk of sensitization limit their use. Aqueous solubility of ocular sulfonamide determines its topical use.

SULFACETAMIDE

Sulfacetamide is an acetyl substituted derivative of sulfanilamide. It has aqueous solubility ratio of 1:140, 90 times higher than sulfadiazine. Sodium sulfacetamide is used as eye drops for ocular infections. Aqueous preparations of sodium sulfacetamide are nonirritant to eye. It is available in variable strengths as 1%, 10%, 15%, and 30% and effective in susceptible infections. Although its pH at 30% concentration is 7.4, others are more alkaline. Since its ocular penetration is high, it achieves adequate level in ocular fluids and tissues. It causes rare sensitivity reactions but still is preferred to other sulfonamides.

SULFADIAZINE

Sulfadiazine is an intermediate acting drug with a good solubility. Its serum half-life extends to 10 hours but its aqueous solubility ratio is 90 times lesser than sulfacetamide. Hence, it is not suitable in the treatment of ocular infections.

Drug of Choice: Sulfacetamide

RATIONALE

Sulfonamides are not used as first line drugs in the treatment of ocular infections due to their **lack of efficacy** and **high** incidence of **hypersensitivity** reactions. Among sulfonamides, **sodium sulfacetamide** is still preferred for **conjunctivitis** and other **superficial infections** as it has an **aqueous solubility** ratio of **1:140** which is **90 times higher** than **sulfadiazine**. It achieves **higher concentration** in **ocular fluids**. It is a **nonirritant**, available as eye drops with an **alkaline pH** and causes rare sensitivity reactions. Hence, it is preferred.

5. *Silver sulfadiazine/Mafenide in burns.*

BACKGROUND

Silver sulfadiazine and mafenide are effective as topical agents in burns. They prevent microbial colonization on surface of wounds thereby reducing the incidence of infection in burns but they should be avoided in the treatment of deep infections due to the possibility of superinfection.

SILVER SULFADIAZINE

Silver sulfadiazine is the drug of choice for prevention of burns infection. This preparation slowly releases silver ions, which are highly toxic to the microorganisms. The advantage of this preparation is silver mediated selective toxicity to microorganisms but little metal may be absorbed into systemic circulation. Although infrequent, it can cause burning, itching and rashes.

MAFENIDE

Mafenide acetate is acetate salt of α-amino-p-toluene sulfonamide which is absorbed into systemic circulation. It is converted into para-carboxylbenzene sulfonamide. The drug and its metabolite can both inhibit carbonic anhydrase enzyme causing metabolic acidosis and hyperventilation. Allergic reactions and intense pain at the site of application are the main side effects. Mafenide is not preferred due to these side effects.

Drug of Choice: Silver Sulfadiazine

RATIONALE

Silver sulfacetamide and mafenide are both used for topical application in burns. Silver sulfacetamide releases silver slowly. **Silver ions inhibit microorganisms** on the surface of burns but little metal is absorbed causing **infrequent itching** and **burning**. **Mafenide** is **equally effective but** it gets **absorbed** from the site of application. Higher systemic concentration of mafenide inhibits enzyme carbonic anhydrase inducing **metabolic acidosis**. The side effects of mafenide limit its use.

6. *Sulfisoxazole/Sulfadiazine in nocardiosis.*

BACKGROUND

Nocardia causes pulmonary and systemic nocardiosis. Trimethoprim-sulfamethoxazole and imipenem are effective and preferred.

Sulfonamides are also effective in the treatment of nocardiosis. They can be combined with other antibiotics for better clinical outcome but therapy should be extended for many months until symptoms disappear. Sulfisoxazole and sulfadiazine are both effective in nocardiosis. Sulfisoxazole and sulfadiazine are absorbed quickly and excreted freely. They are given at a high dose of about 4 to 6 g per day.

SULFISOXAZOLE

Sulfisoxazole has excellent antibacterial activity and only less than 0.1% of patients suffer from severe adverse effects. It is highly soluble and relatively safe. Its high solubility results in minimal incidence of crystalluria.

SULFADIAZINE

Sulfadiazine is absorbed rapidly, reaches peak plasma concentration within 6 hours but incidence of crystalluria is higher than sulfisoxazole.

Drug of Choice: Sulfisoxazole

RATIONALE

Trimethoprim-sulfamethoxazole and imipenem are preferred to sulfonamides in the treatment of nocardiosis. The short acting **sulfisoxazole**, and intermediate acting **sulfadiazine**, are preferred among the sulfonamides. They are both **equieffective** but **toxic effects** of **sulfadiazine** are **higher** than sulfisoxazole. Since the incidence of serious toxic effects of sulfisoxazole is less than 0.1%, it is preferred. It is highly soluble and so excreted quickly reducing the incidence of crystalluria and hematuria but adequate fluid intake is necessary to prevent crystallization.

7. *Trimethoprim-sulfamethoxazole/Ciprofloxacin in shigellosis.*

BACKGROUND

Shigella species induced bacillary dysentery characterized by bloody diarrhea with mucus and abdominal colic is often mild and self-limiting. Most strains of *shigella* have developed resistance to amoxicillin. Trimethoprim-sulfamethoxazole and fluoroquinolones are equally effective.

CIPROFLOXACIN

Norfloxacin, ciprofloxacin and levofloxacin are the fluoroquinolones used. Ciprofloxacin acts by inhibiting DNA gyrase of *Shigella* as it is a gram-negative organism. Although well tolerated, it can result in nausea and vomiting. It is costlier but has lesser side effects. Therefore, it is preferred.

TRIMETHOPRIM-SULFAMETHOXAZOLE

Shigella species is susceptible to the combination of sulfonamide and trimethoprim. It acts through a mechanism that causes 'sequential blockade' inhibiting consecutive steps in the synthesis of tetrahydrofolic acid. Currently available preparations contain sulfamethoxazole and trimethoprim in the ratio of 5:1 to achieve optimal plasma concentration of 20:1. It can cause dermatological reactions, blood dyscrasias and cholestatic jaundice. Even though it is cheaper and effective it causes many adverse effects so, not preferred.

Drug of Choice: Ciprofloxacin

RATIONALE

Fluoroquinolones and trimethoprim-sulfamethoxazole are used in the treatment of shigellosis as they are equieffective. **Trimethoprim-sulfamethoxazole** combination acts by inhibiting the synthesis of tetrahydrofolic acid. It is **cheaper** but causes many side effects. Fluoroquinolones, **ciprofloxacin**, norfloxacin and levofloxacin are all indicated in shigellosis. Although costlier than trimethoprim-sulfamethoxazole, ciprofloxacin is **well tolerated** with **minimal side effects** so, preferred as the drug of first choice in shigellosis.

8. *Sulfadiazine/Sulfadoxine in the treatment of toxoplasmosis along with pyrimethamine and folinic acid.*

BACKGROUND

The incidence of toxoplasmosis in developing countries is higher than 80%. Therapy may not be required in individuals with good immune status as the condition is often self-limiting. If infection is severe or persistent, therapy is indicated for a period of 1 month. Sulfonamides are combined with pyrimethamine and folinic acid for therapy. A loading dose of 200 mg of pyrimethamine is followed by a daily dose of 1 mg/kg. This combination (sulfonamides +pyrimethamine) causes sequential blockade in the synthesis of folic acid. Bone marrow suppression induced by this combination can be prevented by folinic acid. Sulfadiazine and sulfadoxine are both clinically effective. Sulfadiazine is intermediate acting and sulfadoxine is long acting drug.

SULFADIAZINE

Sulfadiazine and pyrimethamine coadministration is the first line therapy. However, adequate fluid intake is essential to maintain 1.2 liters of urine output to prevent crystalluria.

SULFADOXINE

Sulfadoxine is a congener of sulfanilamide with a long plasma half-life. Its half-life is 7 to 9 days and is due to its high degree of protein binding. It is combined with pyrimethamine for treatment of malaria and toxoplasmosis. It is particularly effective in chloroquine resistant *Plasmodium falciparum* malaria. It may cause severe fatal Stevens-Johnson syndrome so, not preferred.

Drug of Choice: Sulfadiazine

RATIONALE

Severe persistent infection requires therapy in toxoplasmosis. **Sulfadiazine** is **intermediate** acting while sulfadoxine is long acting drug. **Sulfadoxine** can cause severe **Stevens-Johnson syndrome** and so **not preferred**. However, **adequate intake of fluids** is essential during sulfadiazine treatment to prevent crystalluria.

9. *Trimethoprim-Sulfamethoxazole/Pentamidine in pneumocystosis.*

BACKGROUND

Pneumocystosis and *Pneumocystis jirovecii* pneumonia are synonymous. It presents as interstitial plasma cell pneumonia and occurs in 80% of AIDS patients. X-Ray chest shows diffuse pulmonary interstitial infiltration, consolidation and cavities of lung.

TRIMETHOPRIM-SULFAMETHOXAZOLE

Trimethoprim-sulfamethoxazole (TMP-SMZ) is preferred due to its low cost and excellent bioavailability. Sulfamethoxazole prevents incorporation of PABA into folic acid and trimethoprim prevents the synthesis of tetrahydrofolate or folinic acid. It may cause hypersensitivity reactions in susceptible individuals and can be either given orally or as intravenous infusion.

PENTAMIDINE

Pentamidine is an aromatic diamine and an alternative agent in this condition. It is a reserve drug for those who cannot tolerate TMP-SMZ or any other drug. It is administered intravenously daily as 4 mg/kg for 21 days as intramuscular injection and is associated with abscess at the site of administration. It is given as 5 to 10% aerosolized form for prophylaxis at 300 mg monthly dose. Although convenient, it is less efficient against other opportunistic infections. When given as IV it causes hypotension, headache and life threatening hypoglycemia. It is not preferred as it is highly toxic and not well tolerated by many patients.

Drug of Choice: Trimethoprim-Sulfamethoxazole (TMP-SMZ)

RATIONALE

In pneumocystosis due to *Pneumocystis jirovecii* **TMP-SMZ** is the **preferred** drug. It is **cheaper**, very **effective** with **excellent**

bioavailability and **limited side effects** when compared to penta-midine. **Pentamidine** is highly toxic and **reserved** for those who are unable to tolerate other drugs or in whom TMP-SMZ is ineffective.

10. *Trimethoprim-Sulfamethoxazole/Nitrofurantoin for UTI due to E. coli.*

BACKGROUND

Urinary tract infection is commonly caused by gram-negative organisms. *E. coli* is the common organism for majority of infections. Drugs used should be effective against causative organisms and should also be able to reach adequate concentration in urine. High urinary concentration is very effective and offers better therapeutic benefit against susceptible organisms.

TRIMETHOPRIM-SULPHAMETHOXAZOLE

A single dose of TMP-SMZ is effective in uncomplicated lower UTI. Generally a three day course is effective in acute uncomplicated UTI. It attains adequate concentration in vaginal secretions in women, suppressing *E. coli* present around urethra and thus reducing the ascending infection. Hence, it is effective in recurrent chronic infection in women.

NITROFURANTOIN

Nitrofurantoin is used in prevention as well as treatment of UTI. It acts by forming highly reactive intermediates which are toxic to bacterial DNA. Its urinary concentration is higher than plasma as it is excreted rapidly. Nausea, vomiting and diarrhea are common and it colors urine brown. Hypersensitivity reactions, hepatitis, pulmonary fibrosis and pneumonitis occur. Besides, its therapeutic efficacy is inferior to TMP-SMZ and its toxicity is more. Hence, nitrofurantoin is reserved as a second line agent in the treatment of UTI.

Drug of Choice: Trimethoprim-Sulfamethoxazole

RATIONALE

Trimethoprim-sulphamethoxazole and nitrofurantoin are both indicated in the treatment of uncomplicated UTI due to susceptible *E. coli* organisms. The **concentration** of **TMP-SMZ** and **nitrofurantoin** is **high** in **urine**. TMP-SMZ attains **high concentration** in **vaginal** fluid reducing ascending urinary infection by inhibiting the organisms around the urethral orifice. **Nitrofurantoin** can only be used as a **second** line drug as it is less effective and more toxic.

11. *Methenamine/Nalidixic acid as urinary antiseptic.*

BACKGROUND

Therapeutic agents that concentrate maximally in renal tubules are known as 'urinary antiseptics' and used in prophylaxis of UTI because they inhibit the growth of many bacterial species in urine. These compounds do not attain higher concentration in plasma. They are useful in chronic, resistant urinary infection but are ineffective in treating systemic infections.

METHENAMINE

Methenamine is a pro-drug and degrades into formaldehyde in urine which mediates its antibacterial action by inhibiting microorganisms. It is more effective in acidic urine because low pH favors formaldehyde release. Since the decomposition to formaldehyde is slow, it takes 3 hours for 90% of its action. It mainly inhibits *E. coli* but can also suppress other sensitive organisms. It is not effective in infection due to urea splitting organism like *Proteus vulgaris* as these organisms prevent maintenance of acidic urinary pH below 5.5.

NALIDIXIC ACID

Nalidixic acid is a less potent, less effective fluoroquinolone with limited spectrum. Its urinary concentration is 50 times higher than plasma concentration but development of resistance is rather rapid. Hence, it is not used in active infections and it is only a second line urinary antiseptic. It causes neurological, GIT side effects and contraindicated in infants.

Drug of Choice: Methenamine

RATIONALE

Agents that attain **higher concentration** in **urine** compared to their plasma concentration are **effective** in treatment of **UTI**. Methenamine and nalidixic acid act as prophylactic agents in chronic resistant infection due to susceptible organisms. **Methenamine** is a prodrug and **releases formaldehyde** at **acidic pH**, hence may require acidification of urine. The antibacterial activity of methenamine is due to formaldehyde. It is not effective in infections due to urea splitting organisms like *Proteus* which interfere with urinary pH. The urinary concentration of **nalidixic acid** is **50 times higher** than its plasma concentration yet it can be used only as a second line drug as many organisms develop rapid resistance.

12. *Phenazopyridine/NSAIDs as urinary analgesic.*

BACKGROUND

Inflammation of urinary tract is the most common cause of dysuria. Painful urination or dysuria also occurs due to infection or auto-immune disorders. Dysuria commonly occurs due to prostatitis in elderly and urethritis in young men. In women, the most common cause of dysuria is cystitis.

PHENAZOPYRIDINE

Phenazopyridine is an azo dye and a locally acting urinary analgesic. It is excreted in urine and exerts topical analgesic action and provides symptomatic relief from pain and burning as well as urinary frequency and urgency. Dose is 200 mg thrice daily but therapy should not be continued for more than 2 days. It colors urine reddish orange and patient should be warned about the same. Phenazopyridine eliminates the need for systemic analgesics.

NSAIDs

Nonsteroidal anti-inflammatory drugs (NSAIDs) are potent analgesics but do not act selectively in urinary tract. Since the pain arises mainly in urinary tract, any drug acting selectively at this site is preferred. NSAIDs are systemic analgesics and their concentration in plasma and other tissues is higher. They interfere with prostaglandin synthesis reducing renal blood flow (RBF) and glomerular filtration rate (GFR). Since they are devoid of local action they can cause other unwanted side effects. Hence, NSAIDs are not preferred to phenazopyridine as urinary analgesic.

Drug of Choice: Phenazopyridine

RATIONALE

Phenazopyridine is an azo dye attaining **higher urinary concentration**. It is **effective** as urinary analgesic since it provides **symptomatic relief** from pain, dysuria, frequency and urgency. It is preferred to NSAIDs as it exerts a **local action** and **devoid** of **systemic actions**. It colors **urine orange or red**. Nausea and epigastric distress are a few side effects. NSAIDs are not preferred as they do not have selective action in urinary tract.

13. *Trimethoprim-Sulfamethoxazole/Ciprofloxacin in chronic prostatitis due to susceptible organisms.*

BACKGROUND

Gram-negative rods and gram-positive *Enterococcus* are the causative organisms. Chronic bacterial prostatitis is difficult to cure and causes recurrent episodes because very few antibacterial agents attain therapeutic concentration in prostate. Hence, a drug which reaches high intraprostatic concentration is preferable but the causative organisms should not have developed resistance to that drug.

TRIMETHOPRIM-SULFAMETHOXAZOLE

Bacteria that synthesize their own para-aminobenzoic acid (PABA) are susceptible to TMP-SMZ which causes 'sequential blockade'.

SMZ and TMP are given in conventional dose ratio of 800:160 mg because this dose attains the ideal plasma concentration of 20:1. Trimethoprim is 20 times more potent than sulfamethoxazole which is due to its higher lipid solubility. Hence, therapeutic concentration of 20:1 results in clinical benefit similar to sulfamethoxazole. Trimethoprim is a weak base and at therapeutic dose concentrates in acidic prostatic and vaginal fluid. Hence, TMP-SMZ combination is more effective in chronic prostatitis provided the causative organism is susceptible to TMP-SMZ.

CIPROFLOXACIN

Ciprofloxacin is also used in the treatment of chronic prostatitis. It is given for a period of 4 to 6 weeks in the treatment of this condition. The concentration of ciprofloxacin in prostate is higher than its serum level. Still, it is reserved for those who do not tolerate or respond to TMP-SMZ.

Drug of Choice: Trimethoprim-Sulfamethoxazole

RATIONALE

Most antibacterial agents do not attain adequate therapeutic concentration in prostate. **TMP-SMZ** is very effective in chronic prostatitis if the **causative organism** has **not developed resistance**. The **concentration** of trimethoprim in **prostatic fluid** is much **higher** than its plasma level. Hence, TMP-SMZ is very effective. **Ciprofloxacin** is a **second line drug** reserved for those unable to tolerate or resistant to TMP-SMZ. The serum concentration of ciprofloxacin is lower than its prostatic concentration.

14. *Ofloxacin/Trimethoprim-sulfamethoxazole in acute pyelonephritis.*

BACKGROUND

Pyelonephritis is an inflammatory disease involving renal pelvis and parenchyma. It is caused primarily by gram-negative organisms such as *E. coli. Proteus, Klebsiella, Pseudomonas*. Less frequently gram positive *Staphylococcus* and *Enterococcus* are involved. Generally in pyelonephritis, infection from lower urinary tract ascends upwards and involves kidneys but in case of *Staphylococcus aureus* the infection spreads from systemic circulation.

OFLOXACIN

Ofloxacin has an excellent antibacterial activity against gram-negative organisms. It inhibits the DNA gyrase enzyme and also has moderate to good activity against gram-positive organisms. The concentration of ofloxacin in urine is higher than its plasma concentration. The oral bioavailability of ofloxacin is very high and around 95%. It is extremely well tolerated but contraindicated in children and during pregnancy.

TRIMETHOPRIM-SULFAMETHOXAZOLE

Trimethoprim-sulfamethoxazole selectively inhibits bacterial dihydrofolate reductase. Individually these drugs are bacterostatic and the combination is bactericidal but drug resistance by microorganisms is the major problem. Besides, when compared to ofloxacin the combination is less effective. Since acute pyelonephritis is associated with fever and other constitutional symptoms, sulfonamides should be avoided for patients at risk of bacteremia and shock.

Drug of Choice: Ofloxacin

RATIONALE

Acute pyelonephritis is caused mainly by gram-negative organisms. **Ofloxacin** has a superior antibacterial activity against gram-negative organisms. Many microorganisms are still susceptible to ofloxacin. It is **well tolerated, has 95% bioavailability** and attains **high urinary concentration**. Therefore, it is preferred. Trimethoprim-sulfamethoxazole combination is less effective since most organisms have already developed resistance. Sulfonamides should be avoided in patients with acute pyelonephritis who are at risk of developing bacteremia and shock. Hence, ofloxacin is preferred.

15. *Ciprofloxacin/Norfloxacin in acute cystitis.*

BACKGROUND

Cystitis or bladder infection is more common in women than in men. Cystitis in men indicates infected calculus, prostatitis or urinary retention. Urinary urgency, frequency, dysuria and suprapubic discomfort are common symptoms. Common causative organisms are *E. coli* and occasionally it is caused by *Enterobacter*. Short-term therapy up to 9 days is indicated in women with uncomplicated cystitis. TMP-SMZ is mostly ineffective due to rapid emergence of resistance. Ciprofloxacin and norfloxacin are second generation fluoroquinolones. Food does not delay absorption or interfere with their bioavailability but it interferes with time taken for peak plasma concentration. Antacids, di and trivalent cations interfere with their absorption. Since clinical efficacy of fluoroquinolones is concentration-time dependent, the required AUC to MIC ratio should be above 25 to 30 for better therapeutic benefit.

CIPROFLOXACIN

Ciprofloxacin is the most potent among first generation fluoroquinolones. It is bactericidal to many gram-negative bacteria at higher concentrations. Ciprofloxacin has a higher oral bioavailability of around 95%. The common causative organism *E. coli* is highly susceptible to ciprofloxacin. It has long postantibiotic effect on *Enterobacter*, an infrequent causative organism. Hence, it is preferred to norfloxacin in the treatment of acute cystitis.

NORFLOXACIN

Norfloxacin is the least effective agent among fluoroquinolones. It is less effective against both gram positive and gram-negative organisms. The required minimum inhibitory concentration (MIC) is four to eight times higher than ciprofloxacin. The oral bioavailability of norfloxacin is only around 80%. It is mainly used in UTI due to susceptible organisms.

Drug of Choice: Ciprofloxacin

RATIONALE

Cystitis occurs more commonly in women than in men. Gram-negative-bacteria are the main causative organisms and occasionally gram positive *Enterobacter* species may be involved. Fluoroquinolones are indicated in the therapy of acute cystitis but **norfloxacin** is **less potent**, has minimal effect on both gram negative and positive organisms, so not preferred. **Ciprofloxacin** is **very effective**, exerts **potent antibacterial** effect on causative organisms, and has **good bioavailability**, so preferred.

16. *Ciprofloxacin/Norfloxacin in chronic osteomyelitis.*

BACKGROUND

Osteomyelitis occurs either due to systemic bacterial dissemination or due to local infection. Inadequate treatment often results in chronic osteomyelitis. Sudden onset fever with chills, local tenderness and pain can occur during acute attacks. *Salmonella*, *Staphylococcus*, *Pseudomonas* or *Serratia* are the common causative pathogens. Prolonged therapy with antibiotics is required with necrotic bone debridement. An antibiotic should be well tolerated but has to be effective against causative bacteria. When compared to serum concentration, the concentration of fluoroquinolones is lower in bone.

CIPROFLOXACIN

The commonest causative bacteria *Salmonella* is highly sensitive while *Staphylococcus* and *Pseudomonas* are moderately sensitive to ciprofloxacin. It attains adequate concentration in bones and joints. The recommended dose is 500 mg twice daily and in severe conditions, 750 mg twice a daily. Prolonged therapy for 6 to 8 weeks results in clinical cure rate of 75%. Since it is very well tolerated it is more suitable for prolonged therapy. Anorexia, nausea, dizziness, photosensitivity and hypersensitivity are a few side effects.

NORFLOXACIN

Norfloxacin does not reach adequate concentration in bone and joints. When compared to ciprofloxacin, norfloxacin is less effective against the causative organisms. Many organisms have developed resistance to the antibacterial activity of norfloxacin.

> **Drug of Choice: Ciprofloxacin**

RATIONALE

The common causative organisms in osteomyelitis are *Salmonella, Staphylococcus, Pseudomonas* and *Serratia.* **Ciprofloxacin** is very effective against the common pathogen **Salmonella** and moderately effective against *Staphylococcus* and *Pseudomonas.* It attains **adequate concentration** in **bones and joints, well tolerated** and most **suitable** for **prolonged therapy.** Norfloxacin achieves relatively lower concentration in bone and only minimally effective against causative organisms. Hence, ciprofloxacin is preferred.

17. *Amoxicillin/Ciprofloxacin for prophylaxis and treatment of anthrax.*

BACKGROUND

Strains of *Bacillus anthracis* are used as tools in 'bioterrorism.' Anthrax starts as nonspecific respiratory symptoms that rapidly progresses to dyspnea. It presents in three forms cutaneous, inhalational and gastrointestinal types. Inhalational form occurs either within 10 days or after 6 weeks of exposure and progresses to fulminant stage. Gastrointestinal type causes ulcerative lesions resulting in blood tinged emesis and malena. After exposure to anthrax spores, cutaneous form occurs within 2 weeks. Bacillus is resistant to cephalosporins and penicillins as it expresses the enzyme β-lactamase.

CIPROFLOXACIN

Ciprofloxacin is the drug of choice for both prophylaxis and the treatment of anthrax infection. It is indicated as monotherapy for prophylaxis particularly in those exposed to anthrax spores. Coadministration of doxycycline is essential for disseminated disease. Prognosis in cutaneous infection is excellent while failure rate in other forms is around 85%. Duration of therapy for pro-phylaxis may extend from 60 to 100 days. Being a well-tolerated agent, ciprofloxacin is most suitable for long-term therapy.

AMOXICILLIN

Amoxicillin is amino penicillin and a congener of ampicillin. It is acid resistant but not penicillinase resistant and has extended spec-trum activity. β-lactamase or penicillinase producing organisms are resistant to amoxicillin. *Anthrax bacillus* is resistant to amoxicillin as it expresses β-lactamase. Hence, amoxicillin is not preferred as monotherapy in disseminated anthrax.

Drug of Choice: Ciprofloxacin

RATIONALE

Bacillus anthracis strains are used in **'bioterrorism'**. To prevent reinfection due to spores, prophylaxis may extend from 60 to 100 days. **Ciprofloxacin** is indicated as **monotherapy** for **prophylaxis**. **Coadministration** of **doxycycline** is required for the treatment of **active** disease. Amoxicillin is acid resistant but not penicillinase resistant. Since the **organism expresses** β-**lactamase** it is **resis-tant** to **amoxicillin**. Ciprofloxacin is well tolerated and so suited for prolonged therapy. It results in excellent prognosis in cutaneous anthrax but has a failure rate of 85% in inhalational and GIT forms.

18. *Norfloxacin/Moxifloxacin in UTI due to E. coli.*

BACKGROUND

Gram-negative *E. coli* is the most common organism causing acute UTI. Acute infection is usually self-limiting but chronic UTI requires therapy. The drug used should attain adequate concentration in urine to be clinically effective.

NORFLOXACIN

Norfloxacin is a second generation fluoroquinolone that achieves a higher concentration in urine. Hence, it is effective in the treatment of UTI due to susceptible *E. coli* infection. In case of chronic UTI, it is given for a period of 8 to 12 weeks.

MOXIFLOXACIN

Moxifloxacin is a long acting second generation fluoroquinolone. It has a wide spectrum of activity but is ineffective in UTI because it achieves relatively low concentration in urine. Moxifloxacin is predominantly metabolized in liver. It is unique as its primary route of excretion is non-renal. Hence, norfloxacin is preferred to moxifloxacin in UTI.

Drug of Choice: Norfloxacin

RATIONALE

Most common organism causing UTI is *E. coli*. Although **moxifloxacin** has a **wide spectrum** of activity it is not effective in UTI because its **urinary concentration** is **minimal**. It is **mainly metabolized in liver** and follows **nonrenal route of excretion**. **Norfloxacin** is very effective against *E. coli* as its urinary concentration is high.

19. *Moxifloxacin/Norfloxacin for respiratory tract infections.*

BACKGROUND

Fluoroquinolones are very effective in the treatment of respiratory tract infections. Although most agents are effective against common respiratory pathogens such as *H. influenzae, M. pneumoniae, Chlamydia pneumoniae* and *Legionella*, earlier second generation fluoroquinolones are ineffective against *S. pneumoniae*.

MOXIFLOXACIN

Few newer fluoroquinolones such as moxifloxacin, levofloxacin and gemifloxacin have excellent activity against *S. pneumoniae*. They are therefore called as 'respiratory fluoroquinolones' as they are effective even against resistant respiratory infections. The bioavailability of moxifloxacin is very high and above 85%. It has a long duration of action with half-life of about 10 hours. Hence, it can be conveniently given at once daily dosage. The concentration of moxifloxacin in lung is higher than its serum level as it has wide volume of distribution. Besides, its dose need not be adjusted in renal dysfunction as it is primarily metabolized in liver and excreted through bile.

NORFLOXACIN

Norfloxacin has poor *in vitro* activity on *S. pneumonia* and anaerobic bacteria. Besides, the concentration of norfloxacin in lung is very poor. Hence, it is not effective in respiratory tract infections. Its bioavailability is lower than moxifloxacin and its half-life is shorter. Hence, it requires twice daily administration.

RATIONALE

Microorganisms such as *S. pneumoniae* and anaerobes are resistant to earlier second generation fluoroquinolones like norfloxacin but not to recent quinolones like moxifloxacin. While the **concentration** of **norfloxacin** in **lung** is **low**, moxifloxacin attains **higher** and **sustained concentration** hence it is long acting. Moxifloxacin is also called as **'respiratory fluoroquinolone'**. The dose of moxifloxacin need not be reduced in patients with compromised renal function but it should be reduced in liver dysfunction.

34 Beta Lactam Antibiotics (Penicillins, Cephalosporins and Carbapenems)

1. Penicillin G/Ampicillin in gram-negative infection.

BACKGROUND

Penicillin G is highly effective against susceptible gram-positive cocci and bacilli. Ampicillin, the amino penicillin, is extended spectrum penicillin. It is also effective against a few gram-negative microorganisms. Penicillin acts by inhibiting the cell wall synthesis. These drugs inhibit the synthesis of peptidoglycan that provides rigid mechanical stability for cell wall, by binding to penicillin-binding proteins (PBP) which serve as targets for binding. The cell wall of gram-positive bacteria is 50 to 100 molecules thick but that of gram-negative bacteria is only 1 to 2 molecules thick. The cell wall of gram-negative is more complex than gram-positive bacteria. The inner membrane is similar to cytoplasmic membrane of gram-positive bacteria but is surrounded by an outer membrane, a lipopolysaccharide and a capsule. This capsule is impenetrable to many antibiotics.

AMPICILLIN

'Porins', the aqueous channels are present in outer capsule of gram-negative bacteria permitting the diffusion of small hydrophilic antibiotics. Ampicillin rapidly and significantly diffuses through 'porins' and its rate of diffusion is faster than penicillin G. Hence, it is more effective than penicillin G against gram-negative organisms. Various gram-negative bacteria differ in the size and number of 'porins'. Since this determines the sensitivity of organisms, ampicillin is effective only against a few gram-negative bacteria.

PENICILLIN G

In gram-positive bacteria peptidoglycan is present nearer to the cell surface. It binds freely to PBP of sensitive gram-positive organisms but unable to penetrate the layers of gram-negative organisms. Hence, penicillin G is not useful in the treatment of gram-negative infection.

Drug of Choice: Ampicillin

RATIONALE

The cell wall of gram-negative bacteria is thin but complex when compared to thick cell wall of gram-positive organisms. The cytoplasmic layer in gram-negative bacteria is surrounded by lipopolysaccharide layer and a capsule that contains aqueous pores called 'porins'. **Penicillin G** is **unable** to **penetrate** into **capsule** but **ampicillin diffuses significantly** and **rapidly** through the pores, hence effective against gram-negative infection. The number and size of pores vary in different bacteria and they determine intracellular concentration of various antibiotics and the susceptibility of bacteria to antibiotics. This forms the basis of decreased susceptibility of many gram-negative bacteria to ampicillin.

2. *Penicillin G/Penicillin V for oral administration.*

BACKGROUND

Penicillin G and V are both effective against gram-positive bacteria. *Streptococci* are sensitive *Enterococci* and *Corynebacterium* are less sensitive and most anaerobic organisms including *Clostridia* are highly sensitive. Many organisms have developed resistance to these penicillins because they are hydrolysed by penicillinase expressed by bacteria.

PENICILLIN V

Penicillin V is more acid stable than penicillin G and not inhibited by gastric acid. Therefore, bioavailability is high resulting in 2 to 5 times higher plasma concentrations than penicillin G. Hence, it is better suited for oral administration.

PENICILLIN G

Penicillin G is 5 to 10 times more effective against *Neisseria* organisms. Only one third of total oral dose of penicillin G is absorbed. The absorption is reduced and incomplete in gastric acidic medium. Besides, food particles get adsorbed to penicillin G reducing its absorption but the rate of absorption is rapid and peak concentration is reached within 30 minutes. It should be given on empty stomach either 30 minutes before or 2 hours after food. As age advances, the intestinal absorption of penicillin G is enhanced due to reduced gastric acid secretion increasing its oral bioavailability.

Drug of Choice: Penicillin V

RATIONALE

Although penicillins have similar spectrum of activity, penicillin G is more effective on *Neisseria* species but it is unsuitable for oral administration. The **bioavailability** of **penicillin G** is low because of **lesser absorption in acidic medium**. Even though the absorption is incomplete, the **rate of absorption** is **rapid** resulting in **peak concentration** within 30 minutes. Food particles are adsorbed with drug further reducing its absorption. The absorption increases as age advances because of reduced acid secretion in older age group. **Penicillin V** is more **stable** and **achieves a higher plasma concentration**. Hence, it is more suited than penicillin G for oral administration.

3. *Procaine penicillin G/Benzathine penicillin G as intramuscular injection for prophylaxis of pharyngitis due to group A β-hemolytic streptococci.*

BACKGROUND

A test dose of penicillin is required before parenteral administration. It is required to prevent severe hypersensitivity reactions such as anaphylaxis and angioedema. Low persistent concentration of penicillin is effective in prophylaxis of pharyngitis. Penicillin G reaches peak plasma level within 30 minutes following intramuscular injection but the concentration declines rapidly creating difficulty in maintenance of plasma level due to its very short half-life of 30 minutes. Probenecid reduces excretion of penicillin and is helpful in maintaining its plasma concentration. To reduce the frequency of administration and to prolong the action, preparations like procaine or benzathine penicillin are used. Such repository preparations delay its absorption increasing the duration of action and reduce the need for frequent administration decreasing cost of overall therapy.

BENZATHINE PENICILLIN G

It is an aqueous suspension of ammonium base and penicillin in the ratio 1:2 that releases penicillin slowly resulting in prolonged plasma concentration. A dose of 1.2 MU reaches high plasma concentration that declines gradually resulting in low but persistent plasma concentration of the antibiotic. Benzathine penicillin G maintains the therapeutic level for approximately 26 days. Therefore, it is very effective for prophylaxis when given as once a month injection. It is a pain free preparation and its local anethetic effect is similar to procaine penicillin G.

PROCAINE PENICILLIN G

The peak concentration after procaine penicillin G is reached within 3 hours but is much lower than the concentration achieved by benzathine penicillin G. The maximum duration of effect persists only for about 24 hours and it has to be administered thereby daily increasing the cost of therapy.

Drug of Choice: Benzathine penicillin G

RATIONALE

Low persistent concentration of an antibiotic is **effective** in prophylaxis of pharyngitis due to *group A β-hemolytic streptococci.* An antibiotic having a prolonged duration is preferred for prophylaxis as it reduces the frequency and cost of therapy improving the compliance. **Repository** preparations such as **benzathine penicillin G** and **procaine penicillin G** are preferred as they **reduce** the **absorption** of penicillin from injected site. 1.2 MU of **benzathine penicillin G elevates** its plasma **concentration quickly** then **declines gradually** maintaining a low level of drug for approximately 26 days. The **duration** of action of **procaine penicillin G** is much **shorter** when comparable to benzathine penicillin G so, not preferred.

4. *Ampicillin/Amoxicillin for oral administration in upper respiratory tract infection (URI).*

BACKGROUND

Ampicillin and amoxicillin are aminopenicillins and are bactericidal in action. They are effective against both gram-positive and gram-negative infections. Penicillin resistant organisms expressing β lactamases are generally resistant to aminopenicillins. Amoxicillin and ampicillin are both acid resistant and are stable in acid medium. They are effective against organisms responsible for URI. *S. pneumoniae, S. pyogenes* and *H. influenzae* are susceptible and are the most common upper respiratory tract pathogens. So, ampicillin and amoxicillin are effective in sinusitis, epiglottitis, otitis media and bronchitis.

AMOXICILLIN

Amoxicillin is very effective against penicillin sensitive and resistant *S. pneumoniae*. Hence, amoxicillin is more effective than ampicillin in upper respiratory infection (URI). It is absorbed more completely and rapidly resulting in reduced incidence of diarrhea. Since food does not interfere with absorption, its bioavailability is absolute. The duration of action of amoxicillin is two times longer than ampicillin but it is less effective in shigellosis.

AMPICILLIN

Although ampicillin is stable in acid environment, its absorption is incomplete. Food interferes with absorption of ampicillin and oral administration induces diarrhea. It is more effective than amoxicillin in shigellosis due to incomplete absorption, favoring local action in gastrointestinal tract (GIT).

Drug of Choice: Amoxicillin

RATIONALE

The aminopenicillins, ampicillin and amoxicillin have almost similar spectrum of activity. They are both very effective against the common upper respiratory tract pathogens such as *S. pneumoniae, S. pyogenes* and *H. influenzae*. In addition, amoxicillin is more effective in treating penicillin sensitive and resistant *S. pneumoniae* so, is preferred. The **incidence** of **diarrhea** is **minimal** with **amoxicillin** as it is completely absorbed but amoxicillin is **less effective in shigellosis**. Ampicillin is more effective in **shigellosis** as it exerts **local action** in GIT due to its incomplete absorption.

5. *Nafcillin/Oxacillin in penicillin G resistant S. aureus infection.*

BACKGROUND

Nafcillin and oxacillin are effective against penicillin resistant *Staphylococcal aureus* because they are not hydrolysed by penicillinase produced by these organisms. They are not effective against methicillin resistant strains of *S. aureus* and are also not a replacement for penicillin as their spectrum of activity is smaller.

NAFCILLIN

Nafcillin is extremely resistant to penicillinase and slightly more active than oxacillin in penicillin resistant *S. aureus* infection. Nafcillin is the most effective agent among the penicillinase resistant penicillins but its efficacy is inferior to penicillin G. It is 90% bound to plasma proteins, attains adequate level in CSF hence, effective in staphylococcal meningitis. The plasma and biliary concentration of nafcillin are similar.

OXACILLIN

Oxacillin is relatively stable in acid medium yet it is inadequately absorbed after oral administration. Food interferes with absorption reducing its bioavailability. Hence, it is preferably given on empty stomach. It is very potent against penicillinase producing *S. aureus* but less effective against other organisms susceptible to penicillin.

Drug of Choice: Nafcillin

RATIONALE

Nafcillin and oxacillin are penicillinase resistant, effective against penicillin resistant *S. aureus* but are not substitutes for penicillin as their spectrum of activity is low. **Nafcillin** is more **potent**, absorbed **better**, **more effective** against penicillinase resistant organisms, attains **adequate level** in CSF. **Oxacillin** is **less effective** against *S. aureus*, **incompletely absorbed** and **less potent**. Hence, nafcillin is preferred.

6. *Piperacillin/Ticarcillin in Pseudomonas and other severe gram-negative infection.*

BACKGROUND

Piperacillin and ticarcillin are antipseudomonial penicillins but they are susceptible to β-lactamase expressed by microorganisms. Ticarcillin is carboxypenicillin and piperacillin is ureidopenicillin.

PIPERACILLIN

Piperacillin has superior efficacy to nafcillin on *Pseudomonas aeruginosa*. It is also effective against non β-lactamase producing *Enterobacteriaceae*, *Bacteroides* species and *E. faecalis*. It is also effective in many other serious infections caused by gram-negative bacteria. Patients with neutropenia as well as impaired immune response who are most susceptible for *Pseudomonas* infections, respond better to piperacillin. So, it is used for bacteremia, pneumonia and UTI caused by resistant organisms.

TICARCILLIN

Among carboxypenicillins, ticarcillin is very potent and highly effective. Although it is two to four times more potent against

Pseudomonas infection its overall efficacy is less because it does not share other advantages of piperacillin. Hence, it is inferior to piperacillin in the treatment of serious gram-negative infections.

Drug of Choice: Piperacillin

RATIONALE

Piperacillin and ticarcillin are both effective against *Pseudomonas aeruginosa*. Microorganisms expressing β-lactamase are resistant to these drugs but **piperacillin** is **more potent** and has **higher efficacy** against *Pseudomonas* species. It is also effective in severe gram-negative infections in neutropenic patients with impaired immune responses. **Ticarcillin** is less effective against *Pseudomonas* organisms, **not effective** against **serious gram-negative** infections. Due to its advantages, piperacillin is preferred.

7. *Penicillin V/Dicloxacillin in erysipelas due to Group A β-hemolytic Streptococci.*

BACKGROUND

Skin infections occur due to colonization of *Group A β-hemolytic Streptococci*. Streptococcal infections may occur in two forms namely erysipelas or impetigo. Impetigo is a focal infection and may present as vesicular or pustular lesion. Erysipelas is superficial lesion presenting as painful cellulitis. It is erythematous, edematous and spreads to other areas. It often occurs in face or lower limb affecting areas with impaired lymphatic drainage. Any skin abrasion or lesion may be the site of entry of organisms and improper treatment promotes further spread causing severe systemic infection. Parenteral therapy is required in case of systemic spread.

PENICILLIN V

A seven day oral therapy of 250 mg of penicillin V is effective against *Group A β-hemolytic Streptococci* and *Staphylococci*. Diabetic patients who are at risk for *Staphylococcus* infection are benefited. Penicillin V is distributed widely with variable concentrations at different sites. 60% is reversibly bound to plasma proteins and released when its plasma level falls. Significant concentration of penicillin V accumulates in lymph and lymph nodes preventing spread of organisms through lymphatic circulation.

DICLOXACILLIN

Dicloxacillin, 250 mg for 7 days is given as an alternative to penicillin V. It is penicillinase resistant penicillin more effective against *Staphylococci* but less effective against other organisms. Since, it has inferior clinical efficacy it is not preferred.

Drug of Choice: Penicillin V

RATIONALE

Erysipelas is painful cellulitis with a risk for systemic spread if not treated promptly. The organism responsible is mostly *Group A β-hemolytic Streptococci* but *Staphylococci* may also play a role. In case of systemic spread parenteral penicillin G is preferred. Otherwise a seven day course of oral antibiotic is preferred. Penicillin V is drug of choice for oral therapy as it is better absorbed than penicillin G. When compared to dicloxacillin, it has wider distribution and attains higher concentration in lymphatic system which may prevent the spread of organisms. Dicloxacillin has lesser spectrum of activity, has no clinical superiority to penicillin V and has minimal efficacy. Hence, it is not preferred.

8. *Penicillin V/Azithromycin in scarlet fever.*

BACKGROUND

The most common cause of bacterial pharyngitis is *Group A β-hemolytic Streptococci*. Erythrogenic toxin of *Group A β-hemolytic Streptococci* causes 'scarlet fever'. Pharynx, soft palate and tonsils become red and oedematous with sudden onset of fever, sore throat, pain on swallowing and malaise. The erythematous rash is diffuse with red papules often seen in groin and axilla. Strawberry tongue or enlarged red coated tongue is a classic feature.

PENICILLIN V

It is available as potassium salt called potassium phenoxymethyl penicillin V. Oral administration of penicillin V 500 mg four times daily for 10 days is effective. The risk of subsequent rheumatic fever is reduced by penicillin V. On oral administration, its plasma concentration is 4 to 5 times higher than penicillin G. It is acid resistant and freely soluble in water. Its concentration in infected, inflamed area is high so, it is effective.

AZITHROMYCIN

Macrolide antibiotics are less effective against scarlet fever. Azithromycin 500 mg once daily is effective if the organism is sensitive. It is an alternative to penicillin and used in patients unable to tolerate penicillin.

Drug of Choice: Penicillin V

RATIONALE

Streptococcal pharyngitis if not treated promptly can increase the risk of subsequent rheumatic fever. *Streptococcus* is highly sensitive to penicillin V and oral administration of 500 mg four times a day for 10 days is effective. The **concentration** of **penicillin V** in **inflamed areas** is very high and therefore it is effective. **Azithromycin** is less effective in scarlet fever and is an **alternative** to penicillin.

9. *(IV Penicillin G + IV Clindamycin)/IV Immunoglobulin in streptococcal toxic shock syndrome.*

BACKGROUND

The causative organism for streptococcal toxic shock syndrome is Group A *streptococci*. It is characterized by necrotizing fasciitis, acute respiratory distress syndrome and renal failure. It is due to erythrotoxin produced by *Streptococci*. The toxin or antigen releases massive amounts of inflammatory cytokines that are responsible for shock and organ failure.

PENICILLIN G + CLINDAMYCIN

Penicillin G is the drug of choice because it is effective against the causative organism. Since this condition is life threatening, therapy is aimed at toxin reduction. Hence, clindamycin, a lincosamide, effective against *streptococci* is added to reduce toxin production. It binds to 50S ribosomal subunit inhibiting the protein synthesis and is given IV at the dose of 600 mg every 8 hours in toxic shock syndrome. It is effective and has the potential to reduce the toxin production.

IMMUNOGLOBULIN

IV immunoglobulin is given as a specific antibody against streptococcal erythrotoxin to reduce the immune reactions but its therapeutic benefit is inferior and unproven.

Drug of Choice: Penicillin G + Clindamycin

RATIONALE

Sudden onset of high fever, due to bacteremia induced by pyrogenic erythrotoxin eloborated by *streptococci* causes streptococcal toxic shock syndrome. Since this **toxin induces immunological reactions** the treatment is aimed at **inhibiting both causative organism and production of toxin**. Coadministration of IV **penicillin** and IV **clindamycin** is **more effective** than IV immunoglobulin. **Penicillin G inhibits** *streptococci* while **clindamycin inhibits** the **production of toxin**. Immunoglobulin is given as an antibody to counteract the antigen erythrotoxin but its effect is inferior and unproven.

10. *Cefazolin/Cephalexin for prophylaxis before surgery with risk of infection from contaminated skin.*

BACKGROUND

Skin and soft tissue infections are commonly caused by gram-positive bacteria. *Staphylococcus aureus* and *Group A β-hemolytic*

Streptococci are most common. While *Group A β-hemolytic Streptococci* causes non purulent infections, *Staphylococcus aureus* cause purulent skin infections. Antibiotics reduce the organisms below critical level and prevent infections.

CEFAZOLIN

Cefazolin is a parenterally acting agent and most preferred among the first generation cephalosporins. *Streptococci* and *Staphylococci* organisms are both susceptible to cefazolin. Hence, it is very effective against skin and soft tissue infections. Unlike other first generation drugs it is effective against *Enterobacter* organisms. Intravenous or intramuscular administration is well tolerated. It attains good plasma concentration and is highly plasma protein bound. It does not cross blood-brain barrier (BBB) and so cannot be used in meningitis. It has a long half-life and therefore a single dose is adequate for prophylaxis. Cefazolin is preferred where the skin flora is likely to be the source of infection.

CEPHALEXIN

It is orally effective and acts against *Streptococci* and *Staphylococcus aureus* but not effective against penicillinase producing *Staphylococcus aureus*. So, it is not suitable for prophylaxis before surgery for those with risk of infection from contaminated skin.

Drug of Choice: Cefazolin

RATIONALE

Prophylaxis is required to avoid contamination from skin pathogens prior to surgery for those with high risk. The common pathogens causing skin infections are *Staphylococcus aureus* and *Group A β-hemolytic Streptococci*. Cefazolin and cephalexin are first generation cephalosporins. **Cefazolin** is **parenteral** while **cephalexin** is **orally** acting cephalosporin. They are both effective against organisms causing skin infections but **cephalexin is not effective** against **penicillinase** producing *Staphylococcus aureus*. **Cefazolin is long acting** and so even a **single** intramuscular **dose** is **effective** as prophylaxis. Due to its higher efficacy and the advantage of a single dose, cefazolin is preferred.

11. *Cephalexin/Cefadroxil for UTI due to E. coli and Proteus.*

BACKGROUND

Treatment of UTI is mainly aimed at eradicating infections. Prevention and treatment of recurrence also forms part of the goal. Cephalexin and cefadroxil are orally acting first generation cephalosporins. They are effective against UTI due to *E. coli* and *Proteus*. They are bactericidal and are more effective than sulfonamides in *E. coli* infection.

CEFADROXIL

Cefadroxil is para-hydroxy analog of cephalexin. It has similar spectrum of activity but its urinary concentration is higher than cephalexin. Hence, it is preferred in UTI due to susceptible *E. coli* and *Proteus*. Probenecid inhibits the urinary excretion of cefadroxil.

CEPHALEXIN

The urinary concentration of cephalexin is very high because it is not metabolized and around 70 to 100% is excreted unchanged mainly through glomerular filtration and tubular secretion. Probenecid interferes with its excretion by competing for tubular secretion.

Drug of Choice: Cefadroxil

RATIONALE

The **first generation** cephalosporins are effective in UTI due to susceptible *E. coli* and *Proteus*. They are **bactericidal**, more suitable than sulfonamides provided the **organisms** have **not developed resistance**. Since, the **urinary concentration** of both drugs is **higher** than their plasma or tissue concentration, they are effective. **Cefadroxil** has **similar spectrum** but attains much **higher urinary level** than cephalexin. Hence, cefadroxil is preferred.

12. *Cefoxitin/Cefuroxime for anaerobic and mixed aerobic-anaerobic infections.*

BACKGROUND

Cefoxitin and cefuroxime are both parenteral second generation cephalosporins. Their utility has declined and they are used only in selected conditions. Third generation agents have superseded their use as they are more effective.

CEFOXITIN

Cefoxitin is less active on gram-positive organisms but effective against few β-lactamase expressing gram-negative organisms. It is very effective against anaerobes particularly *B. fragilis*. Hence, it is specifically indicated in anaerobic and mixed infections. So, it is used in pelvic and intraabdominal infections involving anaerobic organisms.

CEFUROXIME

Cefuroxime has a broader spectrum of activity moderately resistant to β-lactamase. Even gram-negative organisms such as *Enterobacter* and *Citrobacter* are susceptible. Though it is very effective against anaerobes it lacks activity against *B. fragilis* hence, it is less effective against aerobic and mixed aerobic-anaerobic organisms.

Drug of Choice: Cefoxitin

RATIONALE

Second generation cephalosporins have **limited** utility as they are superseded by third generation agents. However, **cefoxitin** has a **special role** in the treatment of **anaerobic** or **mixed aerobic-anaerobic** infections. Since it is **particularly** effective **against** *B.fragilis* it is useful for **pelvic** and **intraabdominal infections** due to anaerobic and mixed infections. Although effective against anaerobes, cefuroxime does not inhibit *B.fragilis*. Hence, it is not preferred.

13. *Cefditoren pivoxil/Ceftibuten in pharyngitis and tonsillitis.*

BACKGROUND

The characterestic features in pharyngitis and tonsillitis are sore throat, fever and cervical lymphadenopathy commonly due to *S. pneumoniae* and *Group A β-hemolytic Streptococci.* Although cephalosporins are more effective than penicillins, resistant strains of *S. pneumoniae* pose difficulty in antibiotic selection.

CEFDITOREN PIVOXIL

Cefditoren pivoxil is a prodrug and third generation cephalosporin, hydrolysed by esterases to yield the active drug. It is effective against methicillin sensitive *S. aureus* and penicillin sensitive *S. pneumoniae, S. pyogenes, Moraxella catarrhalis* and *H. influenzae.*

CEFTIBUTEN

Ceftibuten is orally acting cephalosporin and less effective against many organisms. Its spectrum of activity is smaller than cefditoren pivoxil and *S. pneumoniae, S. pyogenes* and *H. influenzae* are less susceptible. Hence, it is less useful than cefditoren pivoxil in tonsillitis and pharyngitis.

Drug of Choice: Cefditoren pivoxil

RATIONALE

Common organisms causing tonsillitis and pharyngitis are *S. pneumoniae* and *Group A β-hemolytic streptococci.* **Cefditoren pivoxil** is a prodrug that gets converted to cefditoren by plasma esterases. Since **S. pneumoniae** is **highly susceptible** to cefditoren it is very effective in **tonsillitis** and **pharyngitis** but **S. pneumoniae** is **less susceptible** to ceftibuten.

14. *Ceftriaxone/Cefuroxime in H. influenzae meningitis.*

BACKGROUND

A bactericidal drug reaching concentration above minimum inhibitory concentration (MIC) in cerebrospinal fluid (CSF) is preferred in *H. influenza* meningitis. β-lactamase producing strains of *H. influenzae* are less common in adults in whom meningitis usually coexists with sinusitis or otitis media. 10 to 14 days therapy is required for treatment of meningitis.

CEFTRIAXONE

Ceftriaxone is longer acting than cefuroxime with a half-life of approximately 8 hours permitting once daily administration but initially it is given as 4 g/day in two divided doses for meningitis. It is the drug of choice in the treatment of meningitis due to *H. influenzae*. Hypoprothrombinemia, hemolysis and bleeding can occur as side effects.

CEFUROXIME

Cefuroxime is effective against β-lactamase expressing gram-negative bacteria including ampicillin resistant strains of *H. influenzae*. It attains only 10% concentration in CSF compared to its plasma level that is inadequate to be useful in meningitis. Therefore it is inferior to ceftriaxone in meningitis caused by *H. influenzae*.

Drug of Choice: Ceftriaxone

RATIONALE

The drug should reach effective therapeutic concentration in CSF to be effective in meningitis. The organism responsible should also be highly susceptible to the antibiotic used. Ceftriaxone and cefuroxime are both highly effective against *H. influenzae* but **ceftriaxone** reaches **higher** and **persistent concentration** in CSF. Therefore, it is more **effective**. Although **cefuroxime** suppresses the organism, its CSF concentration is just **adequate** and so it is **less effective**.

15. *Cefotaxime/Cefepime in meningitis due to resistant strains of N. meningitidis.*

BACKGROUND

Neisseria meningitidis causes meningococcal meningitis and most strains of *Neisseria* have developed resistance to penicillin. High fever, chills, confusion and delirium are the main symptoms. Neck stiffness, positive Kernig and Brudzinski are characteristic signs.

CEFEPIME

When compared to cefotaxime, cefepime has extended spectrum of activity. It has greater activity on *N. meningitidis* than cefotaxime. It has excellent penetration across BBB into CSF. Hence, cefepime is preferred to cefotaxime in *Neisseria meningitidis*.

CEFOTAXIME

Cefotaxime has good activity against many β-lactamase express-ing organisms. Since it has a short half-life of 1 hour it has to be administered frequently. Its metabolite desacetyl cefotaxime is less active on its own but acts synergistically with cefotaxime improving its efficacy.

Drug of Choice: Cefepime

RATIONALE

Since most of the strains of *Neisseria* have developed resistance to penicillins they are ineffective in meningitis due to *Neisseria* spe-cies. **Cefotaxime**, the third generation cephalosporin is **effective** against **resistant** strains of *N. meningitidis*. Its **metabolite** also **acts synergistically** with the parent compound. Fourth generation agent **cefepime** possess **superior efficacy** over *Neisseria* species and attains **very high concentration in CSF**. Hence, cefepime is preferred to cefotaxime.

16. *Ceftazidime/Cefepime in hospital acquired infections.*

BACKGROUND

Enterobacteriaceae and *Pseudomonas* cause nosocomial infections. Although third generation cephalosporins are less active against gram-positive cocci, a few agents of this group have selective action against *Pseudomonas aeruginosa*.

CEFEPIME

Fourth generation agents have extended spectrum of activity. Cefepime is a fourth generation cephalosporin. It is equieffective to ceftazidime against *P. aeruginosa* but is less effective against other species of *Pseudomonas*. It is very potent and highly resistant to β-lactamase. Hence, it is effective against hospital acquired or nosocomial infections.

CEFTAZIDIME

Ceftazidime is the only third generation cephalosporin that is effective against *Pseudomonas aeruginosa*. Although it is less effective against gram-positive and negative organisms it has excellent activity against *Pseudomonas* but its activity against *Enterobacteriaceae* is minimal. It is effective only through parenteral administration but its clinical efficacy is inferior to cefepime. Besides, it is effective only when coadministered with an aminoglycoside.

Drug of Choice: Cefepime

RATIONALE

Hospital acquired infections are commonly caused by *Enterobacteriaceae* and *Pseudomonas* species. Ceftazidime has inferior spectrum of activity than cefepime but it has excellent activity against *Pseudomonas*. Still its clinical efficacy is inferior to cefepime as it less effective against *Enterobacter* species. Cefepime has extended spectrum of action and specifically effective against *Pseudomonas* and *Enterobacter* species. It is highly resistant to many β-lactamase producing organisms. Cefepime is preferred due to its potency and extended spectrum of action.

17. *Imipenem/Meropenem in lower respiratory tract infection.*

BACKGROUND

Imipenem and meropenem belong to beta lactam antibiotic carbapenems. They are unsaturated carbon containing five member ring with fused β-lactam ring. They have broader spectrum of activity when compared to other β-lactam antibiotics. Imipenem and meropenem are both bactericidal inhibiting cell wall synthesis and effective against organisms causing lower respiratory tract infection.

MEROPENEM

Although the spectrum of activity of meropenem is similar to imipenem, it is more effective against imipenem resistant *P. aeruginosa*. Meropenem is not hydrolyzed by renal dipeptidase. Therefore, it does not require coadministration of cilastatin. The incidence of seizure is lesser with meropenem.

IMIPENEM

Imipenem is therapeutically effective only when combined with cilastatin which inhibits enzyme dehydropeptidase expressed in brush border of proximal convoluted tubule and hydrolyzing imipenem rapidly thereby reducing its serum concentration. Hence, cilastatin improves the action of imipenem. Nausea, vomiting, hypersensitivity and seizures are the side effects of imipenem.

Drug of Choice: Meropenem

RATIONALE

Carbapenems have greater spectrum of activity than many other beta lactam antibiotics as they are effective against many resistant organisms. They are bactericidal in activity and inhibit the cell wall synthesis. Imipenem and meropenem are both effective in lower respiratory tract infections but imipenem is effective only when **coadministered** with **cilastatin which inhibits** its **hydrolysis** by **renal dipeptidase**. The incidence of **seizures** in those with compromised renal function is **higher** with imipenem. Meropenem has **similar therapeutic efficacy** but **does not need** coadministration of **cilastatin**. Further, the **incidence** of **seizures** is minimal. Hence, meropenem is preferred.

18. *Imipenem/Aztreonam for organisms expressing class B β-lactamases.*

BACKGROUND

Gram-positive organisms express large quantity of β-lactamases. This information is encoded in plasmid and passed over to other bacteria. Gram-negative bacteria express very small amounts of β-lactamases but these enzymes are strategically located in gram-negative organisms. They are accumulated in periplasmic space of the bacteria between capsule and inner lipopolysaccharide layer. Four types of β-lactamases A, B, C and D are expressed by bacteria. Incorporation of 6-OH ethyl group improves the stability of carbapenems. They inhibit class A effectively and class D moderately but they inhibit the activity of class B and C enzymes very poorly. *Pseudomonas* and *Acinetobacter* species express class *B* β-lactamases which are zinc containing metallo β-lactamases.

AZTREONAM

Aztreonam has wide activity against many aerobic and anaerobic organisms including resistant *Streptococci, Staphylococci, Enterococci, Listeria* and against imipenem resistant *Pseudomonas* and *Acinetobacter*. Metallo β-lactamases expressed by class B β-lactamases do not inhibit aztreonam but inhibit all other β-lactam antibiotics. Therefore, aztreonam is effective against imipenem resistant organisms.

IMIPENEM

Imipenem has similar spectrum of activity. Many penicillinase or β-lactamases producing organisms are susceptible. Resistant *Streptococci, Staphylococci, Enterococci* and *Listeria* are sensitive. Most strains of *Pseudomonas* and *Acinetobacter* are sensitive to imipenem but organisms expressing class B β-lactamases resist its activity.

Drug of Choice: Aztreonam

RATIONALE

Although the amount of β-lactamases expressed by gram-negative organisms are lesser than gram-positive bacteria, they are strategically placed to inhibit the action of β-lactam antibiotics. Of the four types of β-lactamases class A and D are inhibited by carbapenems but **class B enzyme inhibits all β-lactam antibiotics except aztreonam**. *Pseudomonas* and *Acinetobacter* species express class B β-lactamases. Hence, aztreonam is effective even against imipenem resistant *Pseudomonas* and *Acinetobacter* species.

19. *Clavulanic acid/Sulbactam for coadministration with β-lactam antibiotics.*

BACKGROUND

β-lactamase inhibitors inhibit organisms expressing this plasmid coded enzyme. *Enterobacter, Acinetobacter* and *Citrobacter* species are not inhibited as they express type I chromosomal β-lactamases. Clavulanic acid and sulbactam are β-lactamase inhibitors. They do not have antibacterial activity. They require dose adjustment in renal insufficiency and can be given orally as well as parenterally.

CLAVULANIC ACID

Clavulanic acid is a 'suicide inhibitor' of β-lactamases as it binds irreversibly inhibiting this enzyme expressed by organisms. Hence, it is preferred for co-administration with β-lactam antibiotics. It is 20 times more active than sulbactam at inhibiting extended spectrum enzymes and 14 times more potent than sulbactam.

SULBACTAM

Sulbactam has structural similarity to clavulanic acid. Sulbactam may be given orally but its absorption is inconsistent. Its clinical efficacy is inferior to clavulanic acid.

Drug of Choice: Clavulanic Acid

RATIONALE

β-lactamase inhibitors are coadministered with beta lactam antibiotics. **Clavulanic acid** is a progressive **suicide inhibitor**. Initially it binds reversibly with β-lactamase **subsequently** it forms **covalent binding** resulting in permanent inhibition. Clavulanic acid is **20 times more active** and **14 times more potent** than sulbactam.[89] Hence, clavulanic acid is preferred to sulbactam.

20. *Aminoglycosides/Cephalosporins in meningitis.*

BACKGROUND

Causative organisms of meningitis include *S. pneumoniae, N. meningitidis, H. influenzae* and *P. aeruginosa*. Except *Streptococcus* all other organisms are gram-negative organisms and aminoglycoside antibiotics are effective against them. Third generation and fourth generation cephalosporins are also effective.

CEPHALOSPORINS

Cefotaxime and ceftriaxone are third generation cephalosporins and are indicated in the initial treatment of meningitis in children and adults. Meningitis caused by *S. pneumoniae, N. meningitidis* and *H. influenzae* is sensitive to cephalosporins. Ceftazidime, a third generation cephalosporin and cefepime, a fourth generation cephalosporin are effective against *P. aeruginosa*. Cefepime has also got greater activity against other organisms causing meningitis. Even resistant forms of *N. meningitidis* and *H. influenzae* are susceptible because cefepime is stable to hydrolysis by many plasmid mediated-β-lactamases. It penetrates BBB very freely and has excellent concentration in CSF. Cefepime is the drug of choice for meningitis due to these organisms. It is more suited compared to ceftazidime in *P. aeruginosa* meningitis. However, it is not so effective in meningitis due to other organisms.

AMINOGLYCOSIDES

Aminoglycoside antibiotics have rapid bactericidal activity. They are concentration dependent and peak concentration determines the activity. The rate of bactericidal activity is directly proportional to their concentration but, they attain only sub therapeutic concentration in CSF. They are highly polar compounds and do not penetrate BBB and achieve only 10% CSF concentration. Even in meningitis their concentration does not exceed 25%. Since higher dose potentiates their toxicity they are not recommended. Intrathecal administration improves CSF levels but the procedure is cumbersome. Hence, third and fourth generation cephalosporins are preferred.

Drug of Choice: Cephalosporins

RATIONALE

Aminoglycosides are highly polar in nature and do not penetrate BBB to achieve high concentration in CSF. Even in meningitis, their concentration is suboptimal and their toxicity limits any increase in dosage. The clinical activity of **aminoglycosides** is **concentration dependent**. Hence, they are not **useful** in the treatment of **meningitis**. Third generation **cephalosporins** like cefotaxime and ceftriaxone are **effective** in meningitis. They are the drugs of choice in meningitis due to *S. pneumoniae, N. meningitidis* and *H. influenzae* in immunocompetant children and adults. *P. aeruginosa* meningitis is sensitive to fourth generation cephalosporin cefepime.

21. *Levofloxacin/Ceftriaxone in typhoid fever caused by nalidixic acid resistant (NAR) S. typhi.*

BACKGROUND

Typhoid or enteric fever is caused by *Salmonella typhi* that infects and multiplies in intestinal mucosal epithelium. Infection spreads through macrophages in Payers patches and mesenteric lymph nodes, causing inflammation and ulceration during the third week. Improper treatment can result in intestinal hemorrhage and shock. Contamination, poor hygiene and reduced gastric acidity are some of the causes for typhoid infection. The incidence of *S. paratyphi* is on the rise in India. Levofloxacin and ceftriaxone are both being used in typhoid fever. In India, most strains of *S. typhi* are resistant to nalidixic acid and ciprofloxacin.

CEFTRIAXONE

Ceftriaxone is given in the dose of 1 to 2 g per day IV for 7 to 14 days. Ceftriaxone is highly protein bound and has long half-life with long duration of action. Most strains of *Salmonella typhi* are susceptible to ceftriaxone and it is effective in MDR typhoid including NAR (nalidixic acid resistant) and fluoroquinolone resistant strains. Hence, it is more suitable than levofloxacin in the treatment of NAR *S. typhi*. Ceftriaxone is started as empirical therapy for enteric fever. Following administration of Ceftriaxone fever subsides within the first week. It results only in 10% failure rate and less than 3% carrier rate.

LEVOFLOXACIN

Nalidixic acid is first generation and levofloxacin is second generation quinolone. Levofloxacin results in 95% cure rate, if organisms are susceptible. *Salmonella typhi* is generally highly susceptible to levofloxacin but organisms resistant to nalidixic acid (NAR *S. typhi*) do not respond to this fluoroquinolone. Its oral bioavailability is around 95% and has a long half-life permitting once daily dosage. It is administered in the dose of 500 mg once daily for 7 days in uncomplicated typhoid. In severe disease it is continued for 10 to 14 days.

Drug of Choice: Ceftriaxone

RATIONALE

In NAR *S. typhi* enteric fever **ceftriaxone** is the **drug of choice** as typhoid **organisms** are **highly susceptible**. It is given as intravenous infusion and **reduces** the **fever within a week**. The **relapse rate** is very **minimal**. It is effective even against fluoroquinolone resistant strains. Levofloxacin is very effective on susceptible organisms but not against NAR *S. typhi* strains. It has a longer half-life and can be given as once daily administration. Therefore, ceftriaxone is preferred in the treatment of enteric fever due to NAR *S. typhi*.

22. Ampicillin/Ciprofloxacin in typhoid carriers.

BACKGROUND

One to four percent of typhoid patients may become chronic asymp-tomatic carriers. Such patients excrete *S. typhi* in urine and faeces for about one year. Patients who excrete *S. typhi* in stools beyond three months qualify to be carriers. Carriers have to be treated for about 4 to 6 weeks with suitable agents. Relapse commonly occur in patients with cholelithiasis. The organisms accumulate in gall bladder creating problems in their clearance. Hence, a drug that reaches in high concentration in bile can reduce the failure rate.

CIPROFLOXACIN

Fluoroquinolones are effective provided that the strains of *S. typhi* are susceptible. Ciprofloxacin is very effective in treating chronic asymptomatic carriers as it is bactericidal against susceptible bacteria. It is well-absorbed and has good oral bioavailability. The concentration of ciprofloxacin in bile is higher than its serum concentration. Hence, its efficacy rate in eradicating carrier state is around 85%. The time kill curve of ciprofloxacin is significant and rapidly bactericidal. It is given in the dose of 400 mg twice a day for 4 to 6 weeks.

AMPICILLIN

Ampicillin is also an effective form of therapy in eradicating carrier state. The biliary concentration of ampicillin is also high, hence it is effective. Its efficacy is only around 60%, if organisms are suscep-tible. Most strains have developed resistance to ampicillin. So, it is only a second line drug in treating chronic carrier state of typhoid.

Drug of Choice: Ciprofloxacin

RATIONALE

The incidence rate of typhoid carrier state is around 1 to 4%. Since the organisms are present in gallbladder, a drug that attains high concentration in bile is preferred. **Ampicillin** and **ciprofloxacin** can **both attain high concentration in bile** but the **success rate** of **ciprofloxacin** is around **85%** while that of **ampicillin** is **highly variable** and ranges between **50** and **60%** depending upon the susceptibility of various strains of *S. typhi*. In India, **most strains** of *S. typhi* have **developed resistance** to **ampicillin**. Hence, ciprofloxacin is preferred to ampicillin for typhoid carriers.[90]

35

Aminoglycoside Antibiotics

1. *Gentamicin/Tobramycin in bacterial endocarditis, along with penicillin.*

BACKGROUND

Bacterial endocarditis, the bacterial infection of endothelial surface of heart is caused by gram-positive *S. aureus*, *Streptococci* and *Enterococci* species. *S. aureus* is more virulent and causes severe destructive lesion. *Streptococci* and *Enterococci* species are less virulent and cause subacute infection. Penicillin is bactericidal against rapidly multiplying gram-positive bacteria hence, effective against susceptible strains of *S. aureus* and *Streptococci* but it is only bacterostatic against *Enterococci* and is less effective. Aminoglycosides have lower activity against gram-positive organisms and their action is potentiated by penicillin that inhibits cell wall synthesis. Combination is synergistic and bactericidal, augmenting the effect of both drugs.

GENTAMICIN

Synergistic combination of gentamicin with penicillin for 2 weeks is effective in streptococcal endocarditis but longer therapy for 4 to 6 weeks is required in enterococcal endocarditis. They should not be combined in same syringe as penicillin inactivates gentamicin. It is predominantly vestibulotoxic and minimally cochleotoxic but its nephrotoxic potential is similar to tobramycin.

TOBRAMYCIN

Tobramycin shows poor activity against many strains of *Enterococci*. Hence, it is less suitable than gentamicin for *Enterococci endocarditis*.

Moreover, tobramycin affects both vestibular and cochlear function. Irreversible ototoxicity of aminoglycosides may occur even after single dose and deafness may occur several weeks after discontinuation of therapy. So, tobramycin should be used with caution as it affects both cochlear and vestibular function. Risk is high in those with pre-existing hearing impairment or genetic predisposition.

Drug of Choice: Gentamicin + Penicillin

RATIONALE

Gram-positive *S. aureus*, *Streptococci* and *Enterococci* species are the common causative organisms responsible for bacterial endocarditis. **Penicillin** is **bactericidal** against *S. aureus* and **Streptococci** but only bacterostatic against **Enterococci**. When **combined** with **Aminoglycosides** its action is augmented resulting in **bactericidal** action against **Enterococci**. Penicillin inactivates all aminoglycosides except amikacin when combined in the same syringe. **Gentamicin is more effective** against *Enterococci* when combined with penicillin. **Tobramycin is less effective, more toxic**, causes both auditory and cochlear toxicity hence not preferred.

2. *Amikacin/Netilmicin in serious hospital acquired infection, along with beta lactam antibiotics.*

BACKGROUND

Hospitalized patients are at a greater risk and prone for severe infections compared to normal healthy persons as their immunity is compromised. Most often they carry multidrug resistant (MDR) organisms and such nosocomial infections create problem in the selection of a suitable antibiotic. Prior antibiotic therapy during hospital stay also augments resistance. Resistant *Strepto-Staphylococci* and *Enterobacter* strains are involved. Other common organisms are *Klebsiella*, *Acinetobacter* and *Pseudomonas* species. Synergistic combination of aminoglycosides with β-lactam antibiotics is useful. Third or fourth generation cephalosporins are β-lactam antibiotics.

Amikacin and netilmicin are aminoglycosides for nosocomial infections because they are not inactivated by aminoglycoside-inactivating enzymes and are effective against organisms resistant to other aminoglycosides.

NETILMICIN

Netilmicin has the broad spectrum of activity and resistant to aminoglycosidase expressed by bacteria. It is more effective over gram-negative aerobic organisms. It is also effective against resistant forms of *Enterococci* and *Acinetococci*. Hence, it is most suitable for treating hospital acquired infections.

AMIKACIN

Resistance to aminoglycoside-inactivating enzymes is the main advantage of amikacin but it is less effective against many organisms when compared to netilmicin. The causative organisms *Enterococci* and *Acinetococci* are resistant to it. Hence, it is not very suitable for nosocomial infections.

Drug of Choice: Netilmicin

RATIONALE

The risk of nosocomial infections is high in hospitalized patients due to their compromised immune status. Prior treatment with antibiotics during hospitalization increases the risk of antibiotic resistance in such patients. Administration of aminoglycoside-cephalosporin combination is more effective as it is synergistic in action. Amikacin and netilmicin are not inhibited by enzyme aminoglycosidase expressed by bacteria and are effective in organisms resistant to other aminoglycosides, but **amikacin** is **less effective against aminoglycosides resistant *Enterococci* and *Acinetococci*,** the main causative organisms. **Netilmicin** is **more effective** even against aminoglycosides resistant causative organisms. Hence, netilmicin is more suitable to amikacin in the treatment of serious hospital acquired infections.

3. *Streptomycin/Doxycycline in plague.*

BACKGROUND

Plague is caused by gram-negative organism *Yersinia pestis* in rodent endemic area characterized by sudden high fever, tachycardia, myalgias and delirium. Hematogenous spread causes black plague with purpuric spots in skin.

STREPTOMYCIN

Streptomycin and gentamicin are indicated in some unusual infections like plague. Streptomycin is preferred due to vast experience related to its use in this condition. *Yersinia pestis* is an aerobic gram-negative bacterium highly susceptible to streptomycin as it diffuses through porin aqueous channels of the capsule in plague organism. It is transported from periplasmic space through cytoplasmic membrane and known as energy dependent phase-I. This phase is rate limiting and impairs the ability of streptomycin. When given IV at the dose of 1g every 12 hours for 10 days it effectively inhibits the organism.

DOXYCYCLINE

Although doxycycline is highly effective and most suitable for mass treatment in endemic areas, streptomycin is preferred as it acts faster. Doxycycline results in slow onset of action therefore it is a second line drug. It is also bacterostatic inhibiting protein synthesis and a broad spectrum antibiotic. Dose of doxycycline is 100 mg given either orally or intravenously for 10 days.

Drug of Choice: Streptomycin

RATIONALE

Yersinia pestis is gram-negative aerobic bacteria highly susceptible to both streptomycin and doxycycline. **Streptomycin** often acts **rapidly** but the onset of therapeutic benefit of **doxycycline** is **slow**. Vast experience related to the use of streptomycin in plague favours its use as the first line drug. Doxycycline is devoid of ototoxicity and nephrotoxicity usually seen with streptomycin and preferred for mass treatment.

4. *Gentamicin/Doxycycline in tularemia.*

BACKGROUND

Tularemia is caused by gram-negative *Francisella tularensis*. It is a zoonotic infection of rabbits and wild rodents. The organism is classified as high priority agent for potential bioterrorism because it is highly virulent and spreads easily. In humans it often manifests as local lesion with widespread organ involvement.

GENTAMICIN

Gentamicin is preferred as the drug of choice in tularemia. Its efficacy is comparable to streptomycin but it is less toxic. It is the most favored aminoglycoside due to its low cost and reliable activity. Gentamicin is given as a loading dose of 2 mg/kg intravenously, continued as 3–5 mg/kg/day and one third dose is given every 8 hours. Gentamicin should be given for a period of 7 to 14 days for complete cure. It offers therapeutic benefit with minimal relapse rate.

DOXYCYCLINE

Doxycycline is recommended as the second agent in this condition. It is effective but the failure rates may be higher. Its clinical effectiveness is masked by its relapse rate.

Drug of Choice: Gentamicin

RATIONALE

Tularemia, caused by gram-negative *Francisella tularensis* is susceptible to both aminoglycosides and broad spectrum antibiotics. Gentamicin and streptomycin are equieffective but **gentamicin** is **preferred** due to its **tolerability**, **low cost and reliability**. **Doxycycline** is **effective** but often **results in relapse**. Its **clinical efficacy** is **overshadowed** by its **failure rate**. Therefore, it is not preferred.

5. *Neomycin/Lactulose in hepatic encephalopathy.*

BACKGROUND

Hepatic encephalopathy occurs due to failure of hepatic detoxification of noxious substances originating from gut. Symptoms may be mild with cognitive and psychomotor deficits in initial stage. It progresses to stupor and coma in late stages due to increase in ammonia level.

LACTULOSE

Lactulose is a synthetic disaccharide of galactose and fructose, non-digestible sugar that is not metabolized by intestinal disaccharidases. It is hydrolyzed into short chain fatty acids that stimulate colonic activity and draws water into the lumen through osmosis stimulating peristalsis. Short chain fatty acids formed from lactulose favor formation of ammonium ion that is not absorbed into circulation preventing ammonia induced neurotoxicity. Additionally, lactulose inhibits the bowel flora that can synthesize ammonia. When given at the dose of 30 mL three to four times a day it reduces the frequency of recurrence.

NEOMYCIN

Neomycin is poorly absorbed and generally used only for topical application but is given orally for preoperative preparation of bowels. For hepatic encephalopathy, the recommended daily dose is 4 to 12 g in divided doses. Although it suppresses ammonia producing organisms in the bowel it causes malabsorption, ototoxicity, super-infection and nephrotoxicity. Since renal function is already compromised in acute hepatic encephalopathy and neomycin can potentiate the renal toxicity, it should not be used.

Drug of Choice: Lactulose

RATIONALE

Failure to remove noxious substances such as ammonia produced by intestine due to hepatic disease potentiates cerebral accumulation of ammonia resulting in hepatic encephalopathy. **Lactulose inhibits ammonia production** by inhibiting organisms involved in the synthesis of ammonia and **preventing** its **absorption** into circulation by converting ammonia into ammonium ion. **Neomycin inhibits synthesis** of ammonia in bowel but is highly toxic. It has to be given in **higher dosage** which can **potentiate** its **renal toxicity**. Since renal function is already compromised in such patients, neomycin is not preferred.

CHAPTER
36
Broad Spectrum Antibiotics

1. *Doxycycline/Demeclocycline in patients with renal dysfunction.*

BACKGROUND

Most tetracyclines are excreted through kidney and require a dosage modification in renal dysfunction. They aggravate azotemia in patients with kidney disease as they are basically catabolic. Few tetracyclines such as minocycline, doxycycline and tigecycline are safe in renal dysfunction.

DOXYCYCLINE

Doxycycline is a semisynthetic derivative of tetracyclines and excreted unchanged through bile and urine. Since it is excreted through bile it is partially reabsorbed in intestine, undergoes enterohepatic circulation. Hence, its action continues even after its discontinuation. It does not need dosage adjustment in renal dysfunction because it is not primarily excreted through renal route.

DEMECLOCYCLINE

Since demeclocycline has long half-life of 16 hours it need not be given frequently. Its plasma concentration is sustained for 48 hours due to high protein binding. It is primarily excreted through kidneys and not through bile. So, its toxicity is enhanced in renal failure which requires dose reduction. It is avoided in renal dysfunction as it causes nephrogenic diabetes insipidus.

Drug of Choice: Doxycycline

RATIONALE

Renal route of elimination forms the major pathway for most tetracyclines but few also undergo biliary excretion. Such tetracyclines are reabsorbed in intestine and undergo enterohepatic circulation. Drugs that are excreted through bile need dosage adjustment in liver disease or obstruction of common bile duct but not in renal failure. **Demeclocycline** is mainly **excreted** through **kidney**, so **requires dosage adjustment** but **doxycycline** is **excreted** through **both bile and kidney** and therefore **does not require alteration of dose** in patients with renal dysfunction.

2. *Demeclocycline/Minocycline suitable for oral administration.*

BACKGROUND

Tetracyclines are mainly absorbed from stomach and small intestine. Most tetracyclines are incompletely absorbed from GIT and absorption is improved, if administered on an empty stomach. Divalent cations like calcium and magnesium decrease their absorption. Iron, aluminum, milk, dairy products, antacid, dietary iron and zinc interfere with their absorption. Tetracyclines chelate these divalent cations and form complexes which have poor solubility and not absorbed.

MINOCYCLINE

The absorption of minocycline is very high and is almost 100%. Food does not interfere with its absorption. Its plasma concentration after oral or parenteral administration is similar. Its absorption is less influenced by milk or calcium containing food and the incidence of pseudomembranous colitis is minimal. Hence, it is preferred to demeclocycline for oral administration.

DEMECLOCYCLINE

Demeclocycline is incompletely absorbed even on empty stomach. Its rate of absorption is modest and ranges around 60% to 80%.

Higher concentrations occur in GIT as it is incompletely absorbed resulting in marked alteration of intestinal flora on prolonged therapy. It inhibits sensitive aerobic, anaerobic coliform and gram-positive organisms favoring growth of opportunistic organisms as resistance develops. This results in superinfections and pseudomembranous colitis, a life-threatening infection caused by *Clostridium difficile*.

Drug of Choice: Minocycline

RATIONALE

Many factors interfere with absorption of tetracyclines thereby influencing their bioavailability. Their absorption is reduced by milk, dairy products, divalent cations and iron. Tetracyclines chelate divalent cations and form insoluble complexes that cannot be absorbed. Incomplete absorption can potentiate the incidence of pseudomembranous colitis as it inhibits normal intestinal flora favoring overgrowth of tetracycline resistant organisms. Demeclocycline is incompletely absorbed. Hence it has lower bioavailability and can cause pseudomembranous colitis on long- term administration. **Minocycline** is **completely absorbed** with almost **100% absorption rate**. Hence, it has **higher bioavailability** and **lesser tendency** to cause **superinfections**. So, minocycline is preferred to demeclocycline.

3. *Doxycycline/Tigecycline in patients taking enzyme inducers.*

BACKGROUND

'Enzyme inducers' such as phenytoin, phenobarbitone and rifampin stimulate synthesis of microsomal enzymes of liver inducing the rate of biotransformation. They potentiate their self-metabolism as well as the metabolism of coadministered drugs, altering their duration and intensity of action. Enzyme induction either results in drug tolerance or potentiates drug toxicity. Doxycycline is a synthetic tetracycline and tigecycline is a glycylcycline.

TIGECYCLINE

Tigecycline is improperly absorbed through oral administration. Hence, it is administered only through parenteral route. It is widely distributed with good tissue concentrations. Tigecycline has long elimination half-life and prolonged duration of action. It does not undergo any interaction with enzyme inducers. So, it can be safely given in patients on therapy with enzyme inducers.

DOXYCYCLINE

Doxycycline is well-absorbed and has longer half-life, its action persisting even after its discontinuation. Doxycycline undergoes drug interaction and it should not be coadministered with enzyme inducers.

Drug of Choice: Tigecycline

RATIONALE

Phenobarbitone, phenytoin, rifampin and carbamazepine induce microsomal enzyme system and so are called 'enzyme inducers'. These drugs either stimulate their own metabolism or induce the metabolism of coadministered drugs. **Tigecycline**, a glycylcycline, is **minimally absorbed** through GIT and can be given **only** through **parenteral** route. It **does not interact with enzyme inducers** and can be safely coadministered with them. **Doxycycline** is **absorbed** nearly **completely** has a longer duration of action **but undergoes drug interaction** with enzyme inducers. Hence, it should be avoided in patients on therapy with enzyme inducers.

4. *Doxycycline/Minocycline in treating resistant S. aureus due to tet-K machanism.*

BACKGROUND

Tetracyclines are effective against aerobic and nonaerobic gram-positive and negative organisms. They are also effective against *Rickettsiae*, *Chlamydiae* and *Mycoplasma* but not against fungi. Most organisms have developed resistance to tetracyclines that is often inducible and mediated through 'plasmids'. Decreased influx or increased efflux results in lower intracellular concentration of tetracycline. Physiological role of efflux pumps is to eliminate endogenous noxious substances.

MINOCYCLINE

Minocycline is lipophilic and more active than tetracycline. *S. aureus* resistance occurs through plasmid mediated *tet-K* mechanism. Such *S. aureus* is resistant to doxycycline but susceptible to minocycline. Hence, resistance does not develop to minocycline through *tet-K* expressed by *S. aureus* and it is effective against methicillin resistant *Staphylococcus aureus* (MRSA). It is used in the treatment of mild to moderate MRSA infections.

DOXYCYCLINE

Staphylococcus aureus develops resistance through many mechanisms. One such mechanism is mediated through efflux pump. *Tet-K* is a Tetracycline efflux pump that decreases intracellular accumulation of antibiotic. This protein functions as an anti-port for net potassium uptake. An electrical potential-dependant K^+ leak mode facilitates potassium entry. Increased expression of the protein *tet-K* results in development of resistance to tetracycline. *Staphylococcus aureus* has developed resistance to all tetracyclines including doxycycline.

Drug of Choice: Minocycline

RATIONALE

Efflux pump plays a role in elimination of endogenous noxious substances from accumulating in the cell. *Tet-K* is a tetracycline efflux pump that prevents its entry into cell. Although **Staphylococcus aureus** develops resistance through increased **expression of tet-K** it is sensitive to **minocycline** as **development of resistance** to this antibiotic is **not** through **tet-K mediated efflux** pump.

5. *Tigecycline/Minocycline for treatment of resistant S. aureus infection due to tet-M mechanism.*

BACKGROUND

Organisms producing ribosomal protection protein prevent binding of tetracyclines by displacing them from their target. This process may be triggered by mutation and confers resistance to tetracyclines. Ribosomal protection is mediated through *tet-M* in *S. aureus*.

TIGECYCLINE

Tigecycline is a glycylamido derivative of minocycline. It inhibits *Staphylococci* expressing *tet-K* and *tet-M* proteins. Most efflux pumps have minimal affinity for tigecycline as its glycylamido moiety prevents its efflux thereby restoring the activity by stimulating its accumulation. Hence, *Staphylococcus aureus* expressing *tet-K* is not resistant to this drug. Binding of tigecycline to ribosomes is high and is not affected by *tet-M*. So, it is effective even against organisms showing ribosomal protection. Therefore, tigecycline is effective in the treatment of *S. aureus* expressing *tet-M*.

MINOCYCLINE

Tetracyclines develop resistance to *S. aureus* expressing *tet-M* gene that confers resistance to all drugs of tetracycline group. It is due to the similarity of target site of binding in all tetracyclines. So, *tet-M* expressing *S. aureus* develops cross resistance to all tetracyclines. Hence, minocycline is not useful in the treatment of *tet-M* expressing *S. aureus*.

Drug of Choice: Tigecycline

RATIONALE

One way of development of resistance by **Staphylococci** to tetracyclines is through ribosome protection mediated through **tet-M** protein located on bacterial chromosome. *Tet-M* gene *confers resistance to all tetracyclines*. Hence, *S. aureus* expressing tet-M is resistant to minocycline. The **glycylamido moiety** of **tigecycline** has **minimal affinity** for efflux pump and its ribosomal binding is high irrespective of the organism having high level of **tet-M**. Although tigecycline is a derivative of minocycline, it is *effective* in the *treatment* of *S. aureus* expressing both **tet-K** and **tet-M**.

6. *Doxycycline/Minocycline for moderate inflammatory acne.*

BACKGROUND

Acne is provoked by androgens in genetically predisposed individuals and is caused by overgrowth of acne bacillus *Propionibacterium acnes*. Retention of sebum and bacillus overgrowth in infundibular follicles triggers the events. Release of accumulated fatty acids provokes the inflammatory reaction. The incidence is higher and more severe in men until fourth decade. It does not often clear spontaneously but progresses to cystic inflammatory stage. For mild papular acne topical antibiotics are adequate and effective. Topical antibiotics are also preferred in those who do not tolerate oral antibiotics. Oral tetracyclines are the mainstay in the treatment of inflammatory acne. They inhibit overgrowth of *Propionibacterium* present in sebaceous follicles and are effective due to their anti-inflammatory and antibacterial action. Doxycycline and minocycline are both bacteriostatic agents and lipophilic in nature.

DOXYCYCLINE

The rate of oral absorption of doxycycline is high, around 95% and it is not reduced by milk, dairy products or calcium. It has prolonged action due to its long half-life and can be administered less frequently. It achieves similar plasma concentration through oral or parenteral administration. Doxycycline is given at 100 mg twice daily for 6 weeks. The dose is then reduced to 100 mg once daily for 3 to 4 months. It is usually well-tolerated but can result in photosensitivity reactions. It can cause esophagitis, GIT irritation, abdominal discomfort and pancreatitis.

MINOCYCLINE

The rate of minocycline absorption is absolute 100%. Milk, dairy products and calcium do not impair its absorption. Minocycline is often very effective even in unresponsive or resistant acne but it is expensive and frequently results in vestibular toxicity. Patients suffer from dizziness, ataxia, nausea and vomiting. The symptoms of vertigo start soon after the first dose. Hence, minocycline is preferably started as evening dose in the first few days. Prolonged therapy causes brownish discoloration of skin. It can also cause rashes, urticaria, dermatitis and drug eruptions complicating acne. Hence, doxycycline is preferred to minocycline in inflammatory acne.

Drug of Choice: Doxycycline

RATIONALE

Tetracyclines exert both antibacterial and anti-inflammatory action in inflammatory acne. They inhibit *Propionibacterium* that is present within sebaceous follicles decreasing the production of irritating fatty acids that trigger inflammation. **Doxycycline** is **effective**, **well-tolerated** even in prolonged use. **Minocycline** is very **effective** even in unresponsive or resistant acne but often causes vestibular toxicity immediately **after** the **initial dose**. Long term treatment causes brownish discoloration of skin, rashes, urticaria and dermatitis. Hence, it is not preferred in treatment of acne.

7. *Doxycycline/Chloramphenicol in Rocky Mountain spotted fever.*

BACKGROUND

This condition is caused by *R. rickettsiae* infection due to tick bite in endemic area. If left untreated it can progress into multiorgan failure. It is characterized by abrupt onset fever, chills, myalgias and irritability. Macular rash often progresses to maculopapules and petechiae. Diagnosis is confirmed by presence of *R. rickettsiae* in skin biopsy.

DOXYCYCLINE

Doxycycline at 100 mg twice daily orally for 4 to 10 days is preferred. It is often very effective and life saving in rickettsial infections. Clinical improvement is seen within 24 hours after initiating the treatment. When compared to chloramphenicol, it is well-tolerated, hence preferred.

CHLORAMPHENICOL

Chloramphenicol, a broad spectrum antibiotic is equally effective but can be administered only when its benefit outweighs the risks. It is more toxic than doxycycline and can cause aplastic anemia. It is reserved for treatment of Rocky Mountain spotted fever in pregnant women.

Drug of Choice: Doxycycline

RATIONALE

Rocky Mountain spotted fever is caused by *R. rickettsiae* infection. If left untreated it can progress to life-threatening multiorgan failure. **Doxycycline** is **life saving** and is given at the dose of 100 mg twice daily up to 10 days. **Chloramphenicol** is **equally effective** but **highly toxic**. It can result in **dose related bone marrow depression** causing aplastic anemia. It is not used routinely and is only a reserve drug. However, it is preferred to tetracyclines in pregnant women.

Macrolide and Miscellaneous Antibiotics

1. *Azithromycin/Linezolid in MDR resistant community acquired pneumonia.*

BACKGROUND

Diminished lower airway clearance increases the risk for pneumonia. Compromised phagocytic function or reduced immunoglobin G (IgG) synthesis form the main pathogenesis. Hence, pneumonia is most commonly seen at extremes of age. Chronic lung disease, smoking, malnutrition and immunosuppression are a few predisposing causes that are usually multifactorial in elders. Few causative organisms are *Streptococcus, Chlamydia* and *Mycoplasma. Streptococcus* is the more common causative organism for community acquired pneumonia. Hence, local prevalence of drug resistant *S. pneumoniae* causes problem in therapy.

LINEZOLID

Linezolid is an oxazolidinone that is selectively bactericidal against *Streptococcus*. Although it is very effective against community acquired pneumonia due to multidrug resistant (MDR) strains, it is a reserve drug and indiscriminate or overuse should be reduced to prevent development of resistant strains.

AZITHROMYCIN

Azithromycin attains extensive tissue concentration compared to its serum level. Its intracellular phagocytic concentration is very high. It is effective in mild to moderate pneumonia due to *Chlamydia* and

Mycoplasma but *Streptococcus* develops resistance to azithromycin through efflux pump mechanism. Since *Streptococcus* is the most common causative organism, azithromycin is less effective.

Drug of Choice: Linezolid

RATIONALE

Common causative organisms of community acquired pneumonia are species of *Streptococcus, Chlamydia* and *Mycoplasma*. Of these organisms, the most common causative organism is *Streptococcus pneumoniae*. Although azithromycin is very effective against *Chlamydia* and *Mycoplasma* it is more often ineffective against *Streptococcus pneumoniae* as many strains of this organism have developed resistance. Linezolid is effective even against macrolides-resistant strains of *S. pneumoniae*. Hence, it is very effective in MDR resistant community acquired pneumonia.

2. *Erythromycin estolate/Clarithromycin for treatment of pertussis.*

BACKGROUND

Pertussis is an acute infection caused by *Bordetella pertussis* which means 'violent cough'. It is predominantly seen in infants below two years of age while adults act as reservoir. Preventive immunization or antibodies due to active disease does not confer protection therefore empirical treatment should be started in suspected cases to prevent further progression.

ERYTHROMYCIN ESTOLATE

The absorption of erythromycin estolate is often adequate. It is more stable to inactivation by gastric acid than erythromycin base. It is the drug of choice for treatment of active pertussis as well as for post-exposure prophylaxis of family members. The dose of erythromycin estolate is 1 to 2 g in 3 divided doses per day for 14 days. It has to be administered early in the course of disease to shorten the duration of disease but has minimal efficacy if given during paroxysmal stage. Development of resistance by *Bordetella pertussis* to erythromycin is rare.

CLARITHROMYCIN

Clarithromycin undergoes high first pass metabolism so its bio-availability is only around 55%. It is less effective in pertussis and is only an alternative to erythromycin in the management of pertussis.

Drug of Choice: Erythromycin Estolate

RATIONALE

Development of **resistance** by *Bordetella pertussis* to **erythromycin estolate** is **rare** but therapy should be started early in the course of disease because its efficacy is minimal if started during late paroxysmal stage. It is given for both active disease as well as post-exposure prophylaxis of family members. **Clarithromycin** is **less effective**. Hence, it is only an **alternative** to erythromycin estolate.

3. *Erythromycin/Clarithromycin for middle ear infection due to organisms susceptible to macrolides antibiotics.*

BACKGROUND

Mild acute otitis media resolves on its own with minimal role for antibiotics. Anti-inflammatory agents are also added for initial management of severe pain. Antibiotics should be started immediately to prevent further secondary complications. *S. pneumoniae, H. influenzae* and *M. catarrhalis* are the common organisms. Most of these organisms are resistant to penicillin and amoxicillin but the latter drug is still highly effective in treatment of otitis media.

CLARITHROMYCIN

Clarithromycin achieves high concentration in many tissues and tissue concentration exceeds its plasma concentration. Its concentration in middle ear fluid is 50% higher than plasma level and it shows nonlinear pharmacokinetics with higher dosage. The half-life of clarithromycin is longer at higher dosages resulting in long duration of action. Clarithromycin is preferred due to its higher concentration and longer half-life.

ERYTHROMYCIN

Distribution of erythromycin in intracellular fluids is very high. It does not effectively cross blood-brain barrier (BBB) so its concentration in cerebrospinal fluid (CSF) and brain is inadequate. The concentration of erythromycin in middle ear fluid is very low and accounts to only half its plasma concentration. Hence, erythromycin is less suitable for treatment of middle ear infection.

Drug of Choice: Clarithromycin

RATIONALE

Most organisms causing otitis media have developed **resistance** to **amoxicillin** but **still** it is very effective and used as **first line agent**. **Erythromycin** reaches high intracellular concentration but its **middle ear concentration is 50% less than** its **plasma** concentration. **Clarithromycin attains 50% higher concentration than** its **plasma** level in middle ear fluid. Besides, its duration of action is prolonged at higher dose. Hence, it is preferred to erythromycin for middle ear infection.

4. *Erythromycin/Penicillin in the treatment of diphtheria.*

BACKGROUND

Diphtheria is caused by *Corynebacterium diphtheriae* that spreads through respiratory secretions. Gray membrane over tonsils and pharynx is the common feature of pharyngeal diphtheria. Bull neck diphtheria occurs due to edema of submandibular and paratracheal region. The exotoxin expressed by causative organism potentiates myocarditis and neuropathy. The antitoxin, a horse antiserum, reduces acute disease and further complications.

ERYTHROMYCIN

Erythromycin is given orally in the dose of 500 mg 4 times a day for 14 days. It is very effective in controlling the acute stage and also eradicates carrier state. Only erythromycin is approved by Food and Drug Administration (FDA) for this condition as other macrolides are less effective. Although antibacterial effect is inferior to penicillin, its relapse rate is lower. Since it is a bacteriostatic agent, it inhibits protein synthesis by binding to 50 ribosomal subunit (RSU) leading to rapid arrest in synthesis of exotoxin by the organism. Hence, erythromycin is preferred to penicillin for the treatment of diphtheria.

PENICILLIN

Procaine penicillin G is given IV at the dose of 6,00,000 units every 12 hours. It is switched over to oral penicillin V 125 to 250 mg 4 times a day for 14 days. It results in rapid resolution and lower rate of bacterial resistance. It eliminates the bacilli from pharynx and from other areas but relapse rate is high and more common with penicillin than with erythromycin. Since it inhibits cell wall synthesis it does not effectively reduce exotoxin production.

Drug of Choice: Erythromycin

RATIONALE

The causative organism is *Corynebacterium diphtheriae* and the exotoxin produced can cause myocarditis and neuropathy. Penicillin is very effective in the active stage of disease but it does not completely eradicate the carrier state resulting in higher relapse rate. Further, being a bactericidal agent it inhibits cell wall synthesis and does not inhibit exotoxin production rapidly. Although less effective than penicillin in suppressing active disease, erythromycin eradicates the carrier state absolutely, inhibits production of exotoxin by the organism more rapidly. Hence, it is preferred.

5. *Erythromycin/Azithromycin in legionellosis.*

BACKGROUND

Legionnaire's pneumonia is caused by *Legionella pneumophila*. It is an aerobic gram negative bacterium residing in aquatic bodies. Since the host defense is cell mediated immunity and triggered in legionella, it only occurs in immunodeficient individuals with suppressed cell mediated immunity. Less productive cough with severe pleuritic pain is the characteristic feature.

AZITHROMYCIN

Azithromycin is very effective in the treatment of Legionnaires pneumonia. Oral administration results in rapid absorption with excellent bioavailability. It attains higher concentration in lung, respiratory secretions and even in phagocytes. It accumulates in tissue fibroblasts and is released slowly from them. It exerts superior antibacterial effect as its intracellular concentration is high. It has better tolerability and is effective as a single daily dose. Comparatively hepatotoxicity and gastrointestinal (GI) distress are minimal with azithromycin. It does not cause cardiotoxicity such as QT prolongation like other macrolides. Azithromycin is relatively free of drug interactions. Hence, it is safe.

ERYTHROMYCIN

Erythromycin was once preferred for pneumonia due to various *Legionella* species but compared to azithromycin, it has inferior tissue concentration. Besides, it stimulates motilin receptors and peristalsis. It causes QT prolongation, hepatotoxicity and higher incidence of drug interaction.

Drug of Choice: Azithromycin

RATIONALE

Legionnaires pneumonia, caused by *Legionella pneumophila* is commonly seen in immunodeficient individuals with suppressed cell mediated immunity. **Azithromycin** is preferred to erythromycin due to its **better tolerability, greater therapeutic efficacy**, convenience of **single dosage** and **excellent oral bioavailability**. Erythromycin is not preferred due to its lesser therapeutic efficacy and greater side effects. **Erythromycin** causes **QT prolongation**, prone for drug interaction, hepatotoxicity and GI distress.

6. *Quinupristin-dalfopristin/Linezolid for vancomycin resistant strains of Enterococci.*

BACKGROUND

Enterococcal infections are caused by *E. faecalis* and *E. faecium*. They can cause urinary tract infection (UTI), septicemia, endocarditis or wound infections. *Enterococci* have developed resistance to penicillin, vancomycin and gentamicin. Most commonly *E. faecium* develops resistance to these antibiotics. Daptomycin and tigecycline are active in vitro against vancomycin resistant strains but they are not approved by FDA for treatment of vancomycin resistant *Enterococci*.

LINEZOLID

Linezolid is a synthetic oxazolidinone effective against both *E. faecalis* and *E. faecium*. Although it is only a bacteriostatic against *Enterococci* it is effective against vancomycin resistant strains. It is given orally, well absorbed with 100% bioavailability, well tolerated but can cause myelosuppression, optic neuritis and peripheral neuropathy.

QUINUPRISTIN-DALFOPRISTIN

Quinupristin is a streptogramin B and dalfopristin is streptogramin A. They are semisynthetic pristinamycins and combined in the ratio of 30:70. Each agent is bacteriostatic but combination causes synergistic bactericidal activity. It is administered IV in 5% dextrose solution over a period of one hour. It should never be administered with saline solution as it is incompatible with saline. Quinupristin-dalfopristin is effective only against vancomycin resistant *E. faecium*. It is not active against *Enterococcus faecalis* so not preferred in enterococcal infections. It causes infusion site pain, phlebitis, myalgias and arthralgias.

Drug of Choice: Linezolid

RATIONALE

E. faecalis and *E. faecium* can cause UTI, septicemia, endocarditis or wound infections. *Enterococci* have developed resistance to penicillin, vancomycin and gentamicin. **Quinupristin/dalfopristin** is **not effective** against *Enterococcus faecalis* so is less useful in enterococcal infections. **Linezolid** is **effective** against **MDR strains** of *Enterococci*. It has **100% oral bioavailability** and well tolerated but **long-term therapy** can **cause myelosuppression**, optic neuritis and peripheral neuropathy.

7. *(Polymyxin B + neomycin)/(Ofloxacin + ciprofloxacin) in otitis externa.*

BACKGROUND

Otitis externa is common in those who had recent water exposure (swimmer's ear). Mechanical trauma also results in otalgia, erythema and edema of external canal. Corticosteroids are added to antibiotic therapy in severe otitis externa. Gram negative rods *Pseudomonas*, *Proteus* or fungi *Aspergillus* are causative organisms. These organisms grow very well in an atmosphere of excessive moisture. *S. aureus*, *S. epidermidis* and *Corynebacterium* are also frequently involved. Usually auditory canal is self-cleansing structure due to its cerumen coat. Malignant or persistent external otitis is common in immunocompromised patients.

CIPROFLOXACIN + OFLOXACIN

Fluoroquinolones combination is very effective in the treatment of otitis externa. Topical application of combination is more effective against most causative organisms. They are antipseudomonal and act against *Pseudomonas* species. Topical application is well tolerated and devoid of severe untoward reactions.

POLYMYXIN B + NEOMYCIN

Polymyxins are cationic detergent and simple basic peptide. Polymyxin B is a mixture of polymyxin B_1 and polymyxin B_2. It is a surface active agent, interacts with polypeptide and bactericidal in nature. Its efficacy depends on the phospholipid content of cell wall of bacteria and its interaction with phospholipids is prevented by resistant bacteria. It is effective against strains of *Pseudomonas* but not against *Proteus* species. Hence, it is used as topical application against otitis externa due to *Pseudomonas*. Neomycin is effective against *Proteus* hence the combination is more effective but combined preparation can cause hypersensitivity reaction at the site of application. Generally the preparation is not absorbed when applied topically but if absorbed polymyxin present in the combination can result in nephrotoxicity.

Drug of Choice: Ofloxacin/Ciprofloxacin

RATIONALE

If the symptoms are severe in acute otitis externa corticosteroid-antibiotic ear drops are indicated. Polymyxin is bactericidal and inhibits the phospholipid of cell wall but it is effective only against *Pseudomonas* and less effective against *Proteus* and *Aspergillus*. Neomycin augments its effect as it is also effective against *Proteus* species. Systemic absorption can cause nephrotoxicity. Ciprofloxacin + Ofloxacin combination is more effective against most causative organisms. Fluoroquinolones are more effective against *Pseudomonas* species. The combination is well tolerated when applied topically. Even if absorbed systemically it is devoid of severe toxicity as very little is absorbed.

8. *Bacitracin/Mupirocin in nasal vestibulitis along with oral dicloxacillin.*

BACKGROUND

Folliculitis of nasal hairs causes inflammation of nasal vestibule and the most common causative organism is *Staphylococcus aureus*. Most strains of *S. aureus* are resistant to methicillin so known as Methicillin-resistant *Staphylococcus aureus* (MRSA). Dicloxacillin is given systemically and topical agents are added for local action.

MUPIROCIN

Mupirocin is derived from *Pseudomonas fluorescens*. It has a broader spectrum, inhibits *Pseudomonas* and has antifungal activity.[91] It is available as 2% ointment and can be applied as a cotton wick. It is very effective in eradicating *S. aureus* and abolishes carrier state. It can sensitize skin at the site of application and can cause skin irritation.

BACITRACIN

Bacitracin is a polypeptide antibiotic with bacitracin A as a major component. It is bactericidal and inhibits cell wall synthesis of susceptible organisms. Bacitracin inhibits many gram positive cocci and bacilli. *Pseudomonas, Enterobacteriaceae, Candida* and *Nocardia* are resistant but *Neisseria, H. influenzae* and *Treponema* species are susceptible. It is also available as topical application with polymyxin, neomycin and corticosteroids. Although it is effective in treating acute nasal vestibulitis, it does not eradicate carriers and topical application causes hypersensitivity reactions.

Drug of Choice: Mupirocin

RATIONALE

S. aureus induced nasal vestibulitis is chiefly treated by systemic antibiotics. Oral dicloxacillin is very effective. Topical antibiotics are given additionally. **Bacitracin** is a polypeptide and **bactericidal**. It is also available in combination with polymyxin and neomycin. It is effective in inhibiting *S. aureus* but **does not eradicate carrier** states. **Mupirocin** has a **broader spectrum**, effective against many organisms. It also has **antifungal** action. It is highly effective in **eradicating carrier** states.

38 Chemotherapy of Sexually Transmitted Diseases

1. *Benzathine penicillin G/Procaine penicillin G in syphilis.*

BACKGROUND

Treponema pallidum, a spirochete is the causative agent of syphilis and it is classified into primary, secondary and tertiary stages. Primary stage results in painless ulcers and secondary stage causes skin and mucosal lesions. Tertiary or late syphilis presents as neuro and cardiovascular syphilis. Till date penicillin is the drug of choice and organism has not developed resistance so far. *Spirochete* is extremely sensitive to penicillin even at lower concentrations. Penicillin is spirocheticidal and is effective in all types of syphilis. Jarisch-Herxheimer reactions occur due to rapid destruction of spirochetes and the endotoxin released from the killed spirochetes causes mucocutaneous lesions. It is caused by the first spirocheticidal dose and cannot be prevented by small doses.

BENZATHINE PENICILLIN G

Benzathine penicillin G 2.4 MU is given as deep intramuscular (IM) injection. It is effective as a single dose in primary and secondary syphilis. In tertiary syphilis, it is given weekly for a period of three weeks. Benzathine penicillin G is released slowly from the site of injection as it is long acting, maintaining low and persistent plasma concentration. *Spirochetes* multiply very slowly, so a low persistent concentration is very effective. Hence, cure rate of benzathine penicillin G in syphilis is 95%. It has an advantage of single dose that improves the compliance of patients. Its prolonged action is very effective in killing the slowly multiplying spirochetes.

PROCAINE PENICILLIN G

Procaine penicillin G is absorbed much more quickly than benzathine penicillin G. The dose is 2.4 million units daily for a period of ten days. It does not attain persistent concentration and has to be given daily. Hence, it is less effective and daily administration affects patient's compliance.

Drug of Choice: Benzathine Penicillin G

RATIONALE

Penicillin is the drug of choice in the treatment of syphilis and the organism has not developed resistance so far. Primary and secondary syphilis can be treated by a single dose of **benzathine penicillin G**. For tertiary syphilis it should be given at 3 doses, once every week. It **maintains steady low concentration for prolonged period**. Such prolonged plasma concentration kills **spirochetes** as they multiply very slowly. It has a cure rate of 95% and preferred. **Procaine penicillin G is short acting, does not maintain steady concentration** so is less effective.

2. *Ceftriaxone/Ofloxacin as single dose in uncomplicated urethral, cervical, rectal and pharyngeal gonorrhea.*

BACKGROUND

The causative organism of gonorrhea is gram negative *Neisseria gonorrhoeae*. Burning micturition, milky discharge that may turn into bloody mucus are the main features. If chronic, it causes inflammation of prostate, epididymis and periurethral glands. Rectal gonorrhea in homosexuals and pharyngeal gonorrhea are other types. Patient's adherence to therapy is vital to prevent development of resistant organisms. Hence, single dose regimens are preferred in therapy of gonococcal infections.

CEFTRIAXONE

Third generation cephalosporins are preferred as they are effective as a single dose. Parenteral ceftriaxone and oral cefixime are the preferred cephalosporins but cefixime is less effective and needs confirmatory 'test for cure' after a week. A single large intramuscular dose of 250 mg of ceftriaxone is very effective. Cephalosporin-resistant organisms necessitate use of higher doses. It has a longer half-life, prolonged action and half its dose is excreted in urine. It is effective even against penicillinase producing strains of *Gonococci*. Coadministration of doxycycline 100 mg orally twice daily for seven days is preferred as doxycycline is effective in treating the frequent co-infection by *Chlamydia trachomatis*.

OFLOXACIN

Most organisms are insensitive to penicillins, cephalosporins and fluoroquinolones. Single oral dose of 200 to 400 mg ofloxacin effectively suppresses susceptible strains. It has high bioavailability and attains high plasma concentration. Its concentration in urine, stool and prostate are higher than plasma so, it is effective. It results in 100% cure rate in susceptible strains but ineffective in resistant strains. Hence, it is no more the first line drug in the treatment of gonorrhea.

Drug of Choice: Ceftriaxone

RATIONALE

A single large dose of **ceftriaxone** is very **effective** in the treatment of gonococci infections in pharynx, urethra, cervix and rectum. It is effective **even against penicillinase producing** organisms. Doxycycline is coadministered to treat a possible co-infection by *Chlamydia* organisms. Although once susceptible, **most strains** of *Gonococci* have developed **resistance** to **ofloxacin**. Despite the fact that ofloxacin reaches high concentration in urethra, prostate and rectum, the sites of infection, it is no longer preferred as the first line drug due to the development of resistance.

3. *Doxycycline/Azithromycin in chlamydial infections.*

BACKGROUND

Chlamydia trachomatis causes urogenital infection in both sexes. They are urethritis, proctitis, cervicitis, salpingitis, bartholinitis and epididymitis. It is most often totally asymptomatic for many months in women. Co-infection of *Chlamydia* with *Gonococci* is a common occurrence.

AZITHROMYCIN

A single oral dose of azithromycin, 1 g is the drug of choice and equivalent to 7 days of oral therapy with doxycycline. *Chlamydia* is highly sensitive and has not developed resistance to azithromycin as it inhibits the organism even at a low plasma concentration of 2 µg/mL. It is well tolerated and achieves very high intracellular concentration in tissues. Therefore, it is preferred as it can be given as a single dose supervised therapy.

DOXYCYCLINE

Doxycycline is equally effective but it has to be given at 100 mg once daily for 7 days. In patients with poor compliance reinfection occurs. So far there is no evidence for development of resistance but improper or inadequate therapy can lead to resistance of organisms.

Drug of Choice: Azithromycin

RATIONALE

Azithromycin and doxycycline are equally effective in the treatment of *Chlamydia* infections but **azithromycin** is preferred to doxycycline because it can be given as a **single** supervised **dose**. This is more **convenient** and **prevents reinfection** and development of resistance by organisms. It attains very high intracellular concentration compared to its plasma level and is effective as a single dose. **Doxycycline** is not preferred as it has to be given for **seven days** and is **less convenient** to patient. Besides, in patients with poor compliance the **success** of therapy with doxycycline is **minimal**.

4. *Azithromycin/Ciprofloxacin in chancroid.*

BACKGROUND

The causative organism of chancroid is *Haemophilus ducreyi*. It is characterized by genital ulcers and inguinal lymphadenopathy. Multiple small or giant painful bleeding ulcers without inflammation are common. Infection evokes cell mediated immunity with macrophages and lymphocytic infiltration.

AZITHROMYCIN

Azithromycin is preferred as it is effective against the organism. It is given as a single convenient oral dose of 1 g in the treatment of chancroid. It attains higher concentration within macrophages and phagocytes. It is given as a single dose observed therapy and so is very effective in chancroid.

CIPROFLOXACIN

Haemophilus ducreyi is highly susceptible to ciprofloxacin and its concentration in macrophages is high. Hence, ciprofloxacin is equally effective in the treatment of chancroid but it is given in 500 mg dose twice a day for 3 days, less convenient than azithromycin.

Drug of Choice: Azithromycin

RATIONALE

Haemophilus ducreyi evokes delayed hypersensitivity reaction or cell mediated immunity resulting in phagocytic infiltration. Azithromycin and ciprofloxacin can both concentrate in phagocytes and so are equally effective but **azithromycin** is effective even as a **single oral dose** that is convenient to the patient. **Ciprofloxacin** should be given in **multiple doses** so, it is not preferred.

39

Chemotherapy of Malaria

1. *(Atovaquone+Proguanil)/Doxycycline as chemoprophylaxis during short travel.*

BACKGROUND

Travel for less than six weeks duration is considered as short-term travel and prophylaxis is necessary when persons travel from non-endemic to endemic areas. Therapy has to be started one to two days before travel, has to be taken daily during stay and continued for few days after leaving the area. For chloroquine sensitive areas, Centers for disease control and prevention (CDC) recommends chloroquine as chemoprophylaxis but in case of travel to chloroquine resistant areas other drugs are required.

DOXYCYCLINE

Doxycycline at the dose of 100 mg is started two days before journey to endemic areas. It should be continued for four weeks after the completion of journey. Although the required course is long it is still preferred as first line drug. It is recommended as drug of choice by National Institute of Malaria Research, India. It inhibits translation of proteins of parasites causing delayed onset of death. It is a slow acting blood schizonticide and suitable for prophylaxis but not for active disease. It causes abdominal pain, esophagitis, odynophagia, hypersensitivity and dizziness. Persons taking doxycycline should be advised to take lot of fluids and also not to lie down for at least one hour after taking the tablet to reduce the incidence of esophagitis and odynophagia. Doxycycline is unsafe during pregnancy and in children and should not be given to both.

ATOVAQUONE + PROGUANIL

P. falciparum has developed resistance to atovaquone and so it cannot be given alone but atovaquone results in higher cure rates when combined with proguanil. It is toxic to mitochondria of parasite and proguanil enhances its action. The combination is effective against asexual erythrocytic and hepatic parasites. Fixed dose combination contains atovaquone 250 mg and proguanil 100 mg. It is started 2 days before, taken daily and continued for 7 days after journey. The total duration of course is shorter than doxycycline. Fatty meal promotes absorption and it should be taken with food. Common side effects are nausea, vomiting, abdominal pain, headache and rashes. Since it is not safe in pregnancy it should not be used in pregnant women.

Drug of Choice: Doxycycline

RATIONALE

Chemoprophylaxis is required for those who travel to endemic areas. As per guidelines of national institute of malaria research, India, **doxycycline** is the **preferred** agent for chemoprophylaxis during short travel.[92] Doxycycline is a **slow acting** blood **schizonticide** and inhibits the translation of proteins. Persons on doxycycline should take lot of fluids and should not lie down for at least an hour to reduce the incidence of **esophagitis** and **odynophagia**. The combination of **atovaquone and proguanil** is only an **alternate** agent in spite of its short duration of course. CDC recommends this combination only for *P. falciparum* malaria. It is effective in chloroquine resistant *P. vivax* malaria but results in higher recrudescence rate. It is continued only for seven days while doxycycline has to be given for a period of four weeks after completion of the journey.

2. *Mefloquine/Chloroquine as chemoprophylaxis for long-term travel.*

BACKGROUND

Travel beyond six weeks is considered as long-term travel and requires a different drug for chemoprophylaxis. It is important to ensure safety and efficacy as it is given for long period. Hence, the drug should be effective and therapy should be convenient.

MEFLOQUINE

Mefloquine is effective only in areas where the *Plasmodium* is sensitive. It is given as 250 mg once weekly and therefore it is very convenient. It is started 2 weeks before journey, taken once on the same day of every week. It is continued up to 4 weeks after completion of journey. It is preferred for those who travel for weeks, months or years in endemic areas. It is best documented and well tolerated but it is contraindicated in persons with history of convulsions and cardiac problems. It is also absolutely contraindicated in persons with neuropsychiatric disorders as it can cause vivid dreams and neuropsychiatric symptoms in 10% of patients.

CHLOROQUINE

Chloroquine is safe at doses used for prophylaxis for long-term travel. It is given as 500 mg every week on the same day. It is started 2 weeks before and continued for 4 weeks after completion of journey. Malarial parasites across the World are resistant to chloroquine. The risk of ocular toxicity is high and periodic retinal examination has to be done. It is contraindicated in persons with glucose-6-phosphate dehydrogenase (G6PD) deficiency as it can induce hemolysis. On account of its high toxicity profile, it is not preferred.

Drug of Choice: Mefloquine

RATIONALE

Travel beyond six weeks is considered to be long-term travel. **Mefloquine** is more suited for long term travel as its **safety and efficacy** are well documented but is effective **only** on susceptible strains of ***Plasmodium*** and unsuitable for areas where the organisms have developed resistance. It is given as a convenient once a week dose starting two weeks before and continued for four weeks after journey. It can cause vivid dreams and neuropsychiatric problems in 10% of patients. **Chloroquine** is also started two weeks before and given for four weeks after journey but chloroquine resistance is a global phenomenon. Besides, it can cause **oculotoxicity** and requires periodic retinal examination. Therefore, it is not preferred.

3. *Primaquine/Pyrimethamine for radical cure.*

BACKGROUND

P. falciparum and *P. malariae* are seldom found in liver after completion of erythrocytic stage but *P. vivax* and *P. ovale* remain quiescent in liver in dormant form called 'hypnozoites' for a long period ranging from months to years. Relapse of malarial fever occurs whenever the hypnozoites become active. Hence, a drug that suppresses exoerythrocytic stage can result in radical care.

PRIMAQUINE

Primaquine has very high activity against the latent tissue forms or hypnozoites. It is the only antimalarial agent inhibiting latent stage and can prevent relapse and inhibit exoerythrocytic tissue stages of *P. vivax* and *P. ovale*. Bioavailability of primaquine is 100% and its elimination half-life is 7 hours. It is gametocidal against *P. falciparum*, reaches peak plasma concentration within 3 hours.

PYRIMETHAMINE

Pyrimethamine is a slow acting blood schizonticide of *P. falciparum*. It does not destroy hypnozoites or gametocytes of *P. vivax* and so does not prevent relapse. It increases number of mature gametocytes of *P. falciparum* in blood favoring transmission of *Plasmodium falciparum* infection.

Drug of Choice: Primaquine

RATIONALE

Hypnozoites are the dormant forms of *P. vivax* and *P. ovale*. These **hypnozoites** are **responsible** for **relapse** as the hypnozoites can **remain quiescent** for months to years. Of all the antimalarial agents only **primaquine** eradicates exoerythrocytic stage in liver. Hence, it is suitable for **radical cure**. **Pyrimethamine** is not effective against hypnozoites or gametocytes of *P. vivax*. It **increases** the number of circulating **gametocytes** of *P. falciparum* promoting transmission of infection.

4. *Quinine/Artesunate for severe malaria due to P. falciparum.*

BACKGROUND

Parenteral therapy with antimalarials should be started immediately in severe malaria. Follow-up oral therapy is required and initiated as soon as patient recovers sufficiently. Severe malaria is common in *P. falciparum* infection and it is a medical emergency. Severe and toxic symptoms occur within 12 to 24 hours leading to death. It presents as hyperthermia, coma, convulsions, hypoglycemia, pulmonary edema and shock. High creatinine > 3 mg/dL indicates renal failure and bilirubin >3 mg/dL implies jaundice.

ARTESUNATE

Aqueous solubility of artesunate, the artemisinin derivative, is high so it is given parenterally. It reduces the mortality rate up to 35% in *P. falciparum* infection. Artemether and arteether are oily preparations and absorbed erratically so they are not advisable for oral administration. They are effective when given through intramuscular route. Artesunate is given at 2.4 mg/kg IV every 12 hours on day 1 and continued once daily for 2 more days. It is very effective, safer and better tolerated than quinine so preferred in severe malaria. Parenteral administration is followed by a full course of ACT (artemisinin combined therapy) as oral therapy. Either artemether-lumefantrine or artesunate-sulfadoxine-pyrimethamine is given.

QUININE

Quinine is an alternative and given at 20 mg/kg in 5% dextrose or dextrose saline. It should never be administered as bolus dose but given over a period of 4 hours because rapid administration can lead to severe hypotension and shock. Acute over dosage can also result in cardiac arrhythmias, sinus arrest or atrioventricular (AV) block. Maintenance dose is 10 mg/kg, 8th hourly and infusion rate should not exceed 5 mg/kg/hour. Oral quinine 10 mg/kg three times daily with doxycycline 3 mg/kg/day is given for 7 days. In countries where quinine is not available, intravenous quinidine gluconate is an alternative. Quinine can cause 'black water fever' characterized by a triad of symptoms such as hemolysis, hemoglobinemia and hemoglobinuria. So it is not the first line drug.

Drug of Choice: Artesunate

RATIONALE

Severe malaria occurs due to *P. falciparum* infection causing toxic symptoms such as renal failure, jaundice, hyperthermia, hypoglycemia and convulsions. Parenteral therapy should be instituted immediately and should be followed up by oral therapy soon after the patient recovers. **Artesunate** is a water soluble hemisuccinate ester of dihydroartemisinin, the reduced form of artemisinin is most **ideal** for **parenteral** therapy. Once the patient recovers sufficiently, a full course of ACT should be given orally. Either artemether-lumefantrine or artesunate-sulfadoxine-pyrimethamine combination is given. **Quinine** is only an **alternative**, can cause hypotension, hypoglycemia or black water fever. Hence, it is not preferred.

5. *Chloroquine/Mefloquine for uncomplicated malaria due to P. vivax along with primaquine.*

BACKGROUND

Uncomplicated malaria is caused by *P. vivax* species and results in lower parasitemia. Prevalence of both *P. falciparum* and *P. vivax* is almost equal in Indian subcontinent. Erythrocytic replication cycle of *P. vivax* lasts for 48 hours. Hence, in uncomplicated malaria, tertian fever pattern is seen. Primaquine is added in therapy for 14 days to eradicate the exoerythrocytic stages but it is contraindicated in G6PD deficient individuals.

CHLOROQUINE

Chloroquine is the drug of choice for chloroquine sensitive, uncomplicated malaria. *P. ovale, P. malariae* and *P. knowlesi* are highly susceptible to chloroquine. It results in 100% success rate for sensitive strains of *P. vivax* along with primaquine. It is given at 1 g orally followed by 500 mg at 6, 24 and 48 hours. Nausea, vomiting, headache, dizziness, urticaria and pruritus are a few side effects.

MEFLOQUINE

Mefloquine is a reserve drug for the treatment of *P. vivax*. It is a very effective blood schizonticide. It is adequately absorbed after oral administration and undergoes enterohepatic circulation. It results in biphasic peak plasma concentration with prolonged half-life of 24 days. Although effective it is not preferred and reserved for resistant strains. It is given orally at the dose of 750 mg initially, followed by 500 mg, 6 to 12 hours after initial dose. It can result in neuropsychiatric reactions, encephalopathy and nightmares.

Drug of Choice: Chloroquine

RATIONALE

Chloroquine is the drug of choice for uncomplicated, chloroquine sensitive *P. vivax* malaria. It is highly **effective**, results in **excellent degree of suppression of erythrocytic** stage of *P. vivax* with **100% success rate**. **Primaquine** is given for two weeks for **radical cure** to **eradicate the hypnozoites** in liver. Mefloquine is the reserve drug for resistant strains and causes many unwanted side effects at therapeutic doses. It causes nightmares, neuropsychiatric problems so, not preferred.

6. *(Artemether-lumefantrine)/(Artesunate-sulfadoxine-pyrimethamine) for malaria due to mixed infections in North Eastern states.*

BACKGROUND

Mixed infection is caused by both *P. falciparum* and *P. vivax*. Chloroquine results in 100% success rate in *P. vivax* infection as it is very sensitive but most stains of *P. falciparum* in Indian subcontinent are resistant to chloroquine. While resistance is very high in North Eastern states, AP, MP, Chhattisgarh and Jharkhand, it is minimal in states like Tamil Nadu and Kerala. Since half-life of artemisinins is very short they are unsuitable for monotherapy and are always combined with other drugs known as artemisinin combined therapy (ACT). The success rate of ACT in mixed infection is around 98.8%. Primaquine is given for a period of 14 days in mixed infection for radical cure.

ARTEMETHER-LUMEFANTRINE

Artemisinin combined therapy (ACT) improves efficacy of therapy and reduce the emergence of resistance. Artemisinins are very effective against *P. falciparum* and *P. vivax*. They reduce parasite burden significantly and also reduce transmission of infection. They do not develop cross resistance with other antimalarial drugs. Mutant *pfcrt* (*Plasmodium falciparum* chloroquine resistance transporter) gene confers chloroquine resistance to *P. falciparum* but increases its susceptibility to artemisinins and lumefantrine. Lumefantrine is structurally similar to halofantrine and mefloquine. This combination is first line drug for mixed infections in North Eastern states. Artemether 20 mg and Lumefantrine 120 mg combination four tablets twice daily is given for 3 days.

ARTESUNATE-SULFADOXINE-PYRIMETHAMINE

Sulfadoxine-pyrimethamine combination inhibits folate synthesis. Pyrimethamine is a slow acting blood schizonticide with long half-life. It has higher potency than its active metabolite cycloguanil. It causes sequential blockade of folate synthesis of *Plasmodium*. North Eastern states have developed resistance to sulfadoxine-pyrimethamine combination. All other states are still sensitive to artesunate-sulfadoxine-pyrimethamine combination.

Drug of Choice: Artemether-Lumefantrine

RATIONALE

Mixed infection is caused by *P. falciparum* and *P. vivax*. Since *P. falciparum* is resistant to chloroquine in most parts of India, ACT is preferred. The success rate of ACT is 98.8%. Primaquine is added for 14 days to prevent further relapse. Sulfadoxine-pyrimethamine combination inhibits folate synthesis of *Plasmodium* through sequential blockade. **Artesunate-sulfadoxine-pyrimethamine** is very **effective** in **most states** of India **except** in **North Eastern states**. Artesunate acts by forming toxic heme adducts. Artemether-lumefantrine is a synergistic combination and *Plasmodium* causing mixed infection in North Eastern states is highly susceptible to this combination.

40 Amebiasis, Giardiasis and Other Protozoal Infections

1. *(5-Nitroimidazole + Luminal amebicide)/5-Nitroimidazole monotherapy in acute intestinal amebiasis.*

BACKGROUND

E. histolytica, E. dispar and *E. moshkovskii* are morphologically similar organisms. Although both *E. histolytica* and *E. dispar* colonize large intestine only *E. histolytica* is virulent. While *E. dispar* is asymptomatic, *E. histolytica* causes invasive disease in 10% of affected individuals. Trophozoite of *E. histolytica* invades lumen causing micro ulcerations of mucosa.

5-NITROIMIDAZOLE + LUMINAL AMEBICIDE

Luminal amebicides eradicate cysts colonized in the lumen of large intestine. Paromomycin 25 to 35 mg/kg thrice daily should be given with 5-nitroimidazole for 7 days. So far, resistance to 5-nitroimidazoles such as metronidazole, tinidazole and ornidazole by *E. histolytica* has not been reported. Metronidazole is a prodrug, becomes active due to reductive activation of nitro group that is toxic to the organism.

5-NITROIMIDAZOLE MONOTHERAPY

5-Nitroimidazoles are effective against *E. histolytica* as they are potent amebicides but they are well absorbed and so are less effective against cysts present in intestine. These cysts can develop into trophozoites and can cause reinfection in carriers. Unless the cysts are eradicated the chances of recurrence is very high.

Hence, a luminal amebicide should be added to the therapy of intestinal amebiasis. 5-Nitroimidazoles selectively inhibit microaerophilic or anaerobic organisms. Few of such organisms are *Giardia, Entamoeba* and *Trichomonas species*. Ferredoxins present in these organisms donate electron to 5-nitroimidazoles converting it to a highly reactive nitro radical anion that is toxic to amebic DNA but they can eradicate reinfection only when luminal amebicides are added.

Drug of Choice: 5-Nitroimidazole + Luminal Amebicide

RATIONALE

5-Nitroimidazoles are potent amebicides and so far resistance by *E. histolytica* to these agents has not been reported but these agents have **higher bioavailability** as they are **completely absorbed**. Although they are effective in destroying the trophozoite that invades intestinal lumen, they are **ineffective** in **eradicating cysts**. **Luminal amebicide** like **paromomycin** is **not absorbed**. Therefore, it is **effective** in **destroying cysts**. Hence, the combination of 5-nitroimidazole with luminal amebicide is more effective than monotherapy with 5-nitroimidazole.

2. *5-Nitroimidazole/Chloroquine in extraintestinal amebiasis along with luminal amebicide.*

BACKGROUND

Most common form of extra intestinal amebiasis is hepatic amebiasis and frequently manifests as single abscess in the right lobe. Asymptomatic intestinal colonization may precede liver abscess. Amebic trophozoites reach liver through portal circulation because they cannot be lysed by complement mediated immune mechanism. These trophozoits can lyse neutrophils, and monocytes. The liberated neutrophil toxins are toxic to the hepatocytes resulting in necrosis. A luminal amebicide is indicated in extra intestinal form even in asymptomatic people to eradicate the cysts.

5-NITROIMIDAZOLE

5-Nitroimidazole is the drug of choice in extraintestinal amebiasis. It attains a very high concentration in blood and tissues including liver. Being a tissue amebicide, it kills trophozoites concentrated in tissues. When given with luminal amebicide they prevent further recurrences.

CHLOROQUINE

Chloroquine is completely absorbed and highly concentrated in liver. Unlike 5-nitroimidazoles it does not accumulate in intestinal wall. Hence, it is not effective in intestinal amebiasis and in carriers. When compared to 5-nitroimidazoles its efficacy is lower and relapse rate is higher. Prolonged therapy often results in frequent side effects such as nausea, vomiting and headache. Chloroquine should be avoided as first line drug due to its higher relapse rate.

Drug of Choice: 5-Nitroimidazole

RATIONALE

Hepatic amebiasis is the most **common form** of extraintestinal amebiasis. **5-nitroimidazoles** reach very **high concentration in blood and tissues**. They are potent amebicides and are very effective in hepatic amebiasis. A **luminal** amebicide should be **coadministered** to prevent the recurrence. When compared to chloroquine, their efficacy is **superior** and **relapse rate is minimal** if given with luminal amebicide. Although chloroquine is a potent amebicide and highly concentrated in liver it is not preferred as it has to be given for prolonged period that may potentiate its side effects with higher relapse rate.

3. *Metronidazole/Tinidazole in trichomoniasis.*

BACKGROUND

Trichomonas vaginalis is a pathogen of genitourinary tract. Trichomoniasis is the most common infection among sexually transmitted diseases. It causes vaginitis in women and nongonococcal urethritis or prostatitis in men. To prevent reinfection concurrent treatment of sexual partners is necessary. Metronidazole and tinidazole reach high concentration in urine and semen. Hence, they both are very effective against *Trichomonas vaginalis*.

TINIDAZOLE

Tinidazole provides either equivalent or better therapeutic response than metronidazole in *T. vaginalis*. It is given at the dose of 2 g as it has a longer half-life (12 hours) and slower metabolism. It is better tolerated as a single large dose with minimal side effects. *Trichomonas vaginalis* has not developed resistance to tinidazole.

METRONIDAZOLE

Single dose of 2 g of metronidazole effectively controls the infection. If such high dose of metronidazole is not tolerated then it can be split into small twice daily dose of 375 mg and therapy is continued for 7 days. The cure rate for 5-nitroimidazoles in *Trichomonas vaginalis* is around 90%. Metronidazole has a half-life 8 hours, its distribution approximating total body water. It maintains linear relationship up to 2 g dose, beyond which it accumulates in body. The half-life of its hydroxy metabolite is longer around 12 hours. Fifty percent of its activity against *Trichomonas vaginalis* is due to its hydroxy metabolite but resistance of *Trichomonas vaginalis* to metronidazole has been reported. It often results in nausea, metallic taste, tinnitus, headache, dysuria, antabuse like action and pelvic pressure. Very rarely it results in Stevens-Johnson syndrome or toxic epidermal necrolysis.

Drug of Choice: Tinidazole

RATIONALE

As a pathogen of genitourinary tract *Trichomonas vaginalis* causes vaginitis, urethritis or prostatitis. Tinidazole is either equally effective or more effective in trichomoniasis. It is well tolerated with minimal side effects. It has a longer half-life with slower metabolism requiring single dose. These **organisms** have **not yet developed resistance** to **tinidazole**. Therefore it is preferred due to its **superior efficacy, simpler dosing** and **better tolerability**. Metronidazole and its metabolite are effective in suppressing *Trichomonas vaginalis* but the drug can accumulate on repeated dosage often resulting in side effects. Treatment failure is often reported and is due to development of resistance by organisms.

4. *Tinidazole/Nitazoxanide in giardiasis.*

BACKGROUND

Giardiasis is a protozoal infection of small intestine caused by *Giardia lamblia*. It is also known as giardia intestinalis or giardia duodenalis. It can occur as asymptomatic carrier state, acute or chronic diarrhea. Acute stage is often self-limiting but flagellated trophozoites and cysts are excreted. The infectious cyst form is transmitted from faeces, through oral route but the trophozoites are not infectious as they are destroyed by gastric acid.

TINIDAZOLE

Tinidazole is highly effective and is the first line drug in the treatment of giardiasis. It is well tolerated and can be administered as a single dose of 2 g. Simpler dosing and ease of single administration makes tinidazole the drug of choice.

NITAZOXANIDE

Nitazoxanide is approved for the treatment of acute giardiasis. Nitazoxanide has high efficacy around 85 to 90% but repeated doses are required. It is given for 3 days at the dose of 500 mg twice a day. It can result in GIT side effects like abdominal pain, diarrhea and vomiting. Since the symptoms of giardiasis overlap with its side effects it is not preferred.

Drug of Choice: Tinidazole

RATIONALE

Giardiasis is caused by *Giardia lamblia*. It can present as asymptomatic cyst carriers, acute diarrheal stage that is often self-limiting and chronic diarrhea. The advantage of **tinidazole** is its **simpler dosing** and **higher efficacy**. Just a single dose of 2 g is effective in acute giardiasis. Such a high dose is usually well tolerated so, it is preferred. **Nitazoxanide** has a **high cure rate** of around 85 to 90% but requires **frequent dosing** and causes side effects such as abdominal pain or diarrhea that overlap with symptoms of giardiasis.

5. *Pentamidine/Suramin in early stage of West African trypanoso-miasis.*

BACKGROUND

Trypanosomiasis is caused by *Trypanosoma brucei rhodesiense* and *Trypanosoma brucei gambiense.* The organisms are transmitted through tsetse fly bites. West African (Gambian) form is seen in forests of West and Central Africa. West African trypanosomiasis is caused by *Trypanosoma brucei gambiense.* The principal mammalian hosts are the humans and rarely domestic animals. The early form of disease is known as hemolymphatic stage. It is characterized by fever, headache, arthralgia, myalgia and lymphadenopathy.

PENTAMIDINE

Pentamidine is given at 4 mg/kg intramuscularly daily for 7 days. It is not effective in late stage of West African trypanosomiasis that involves central nervous system because it does not cross blood-brain barrier. It is a diamidine and accumulates in millimolar concentration in organisms that have high affinity selective uptake system that accumulates the drug. The positively charged diamidine binds to negatively charged cellular organelles. Trypanocidal effect is due to inhibition of DNA, enzymes and protein synthesis. It is 70% plasma protein bound and its plasma half-life is short but its elimination half-life lasts for weeks to months. In around 50% of patients, it is highly toxic and can result in life threatening hypoglycemia during any time of therapy. Hyperglycemia, nephrotoxicity and neutropenia are other side effects. Immediate hypersensitivity reaction causes vomiting, hypotension and tachycardia. Although frequent, this reaction is transient but does not necessitate cessation of therapy. It has high stability and can be administered easily, so, preferred.

SURAMIN

Suramin is a slow acting trypanocide against *Trypanosoma brucei gambiense*. It is not absorbed orally, causes inflammation and necrosis when given by subcutaneous or intramuscular route. So it is given as intravenous infusion. It is 99.7% bound to plasma proteins but less effective in early stage trypanosomiasis, and more toxic, so not preferred. Its untoward effects vary in intensity and more common in severely ill patients. It results in Mazzotti reaction characterized by rash, arthralgia, tachycardia and blindness if the patient is coinfected with onchocerciasis. Hence, it is only an alternative in the treatment of early stage African trypanosomiasis.

Drug of Choice: Pentamidine

RATIONALE

West African trypanosomiasis is caused by *Trypanosoma brucei gambiense*. It is characterized by hemolymphatic stage. **Pentamidine** is the drug of choice as it is an effective **trypanocide** and has **longer elimination half-life**. Frequent immediate hypersensitivity reaction is characterized by nausea, vomiting, hypotension and tachycardia but these reactions are transient and the drug need not be stopped. **Suramin** is **less effective** against early stage hence is only a **second line drug**.

6. *(Eflornithine + nifurtimox)/Melarsoprol for late stage West African trypanosomiasis.*

BACKGROUND

The onset of late stage West African trypanosomiasis called meningoencephalitic stage. Progress from early stage is slow and insidious. After many months the hemolymphatic stage progresses to meningoencephalitic stage. Symptoms such as somnolence, irritability, personality changes and motor in coordination are characteristic. It is called 'sleeping sickness' due to day time somnolence. The late stage neurologic abnormalities are associated with changes in cerebrospinal fluid (CSF).

EFLORNITHINE + NIFURTIMOX

Eflornithine is a suicidal inhibitor of ornithine decarboxylase, an enzyme which is the rate limiting enzyme of polyamines biosynthesis. It inhibits both trypanosomal and human ornithine decarboxylase irreversibly but human enzymes can be biosynthesized rapidly. So, it causes only selective toxicity. It penetrates BBB more effectively when that barrier has been disrupted by trypanosomes. Adverse effects are comparatively minimal. It mainly causes GIT irritation and myelosuppression. Coadministration of nifurtimox reduces frequency of dosing and duration of therapy. Dose of eflornithine is 400 mg/kg/day intravenously every 12 hours as 2-hour-long infusion for 7 days. Nifurtimox 15 mg/kg/day can be given orally in 3 divided doses.

MELARSOPROL

Melarsoprol is a prodrug and metabolized within 30 minutes to active melarsen oxide. Trypanocidal actions are due to glycolysis inhibition and glutathione substitution. The rate of treatment failures is higher with melarsoprol so, it is not preferred. It is very toxic and causes encephalopathy, hypertension and cardiac damage.

Drug of Choice: Eflornithine + Nifurtimox

RATIONALE

Late stage West African trypanosomiasis is characterized with CNS manifestations and it is called meningoencephalitic stage. **Eflornithine irreversibly inhibits** both mammalian and trypanosomal **ornithine hydroxylase** but mammalian enzyme is synthesized quickly and so is not affected much. In trypanosomiasis it penetrates BBB more effectively. **Coadministration** of **nifurtimox** reduces both frequency and duration of the course of treatment. **Melarsoprol** is an alternate drug because the rate of **treatment failures** is **high** and is **more toxic** causing encephalopathy.

7. *Suramin/Pentamidine in East African trypanosomiasis.*

BACKGROUND

East African (Rhodesian) Trypanosomiasis is caused by *Trypanosoma brucei rhodesiense*. The course of disease is more acute and symptoms occur within few days of insect bite. Hemolymphatic stage is characterized by severe fever along with rash but lymphadenopathy is not significant and less common than West African type. It progresses to meningoencephalitic stage with predominant somnolence.

SURAMIN

Suramin has high activity against *Trypanosoma brucei rhodesiense*. Except lysosomes all other membranes of intracellular organelles of trypanosomes are damaged. It inhibits dihydrofolate reductase, thymidine kinase and other glycolytic enzymes. It is the first line drug against East African trypanosomiasis. It is given only as supervised therapy as it can cause immediate hypersensitivity reactions. Incidence of hypersensitivity is rare (1 in 2,000) but it can be fatal so it requires test dose. Following test dose it is given by slow intravenous infusion on 1st, 3rd, 7th, 14th and 21st day. Nephrotoxicity, arthralgias and skin eruptions occur frequently.

PENTAMIDINE

Pentamidine has minimal efficacy against *Trypanosoma brucei rhodesiense*. Hence it is only an alternate drug in the treatment of East African trypanosomiasis. Life-threatening hypoglycemia can occur during any time of therapy.

Drug of Choice: Suramin

RATIONALE

East African trypanosomiasis caused by *Trypanosoma brucei rhodesiense* follows an acute pattern. There is no significant lymphadenopathy in the early hemolymphatic stage. Somnolence is predominant in late or meningoencephalitic stage. **Suramin** has

high efficacy against *Trypanosoma brucei rhodesiense*. Although it is the first line drug, it has to be given under observation as it **can result** in **fatal immediate hypersensitivity** reaction. **Pentamidine** is **less effective** and can cause life-threatening hypoglycemia any time during therapy.

8. *Nifurtimox/Benznidazole in Chagas disease.*

BACKGROUND

American Trypanosomiasis or Chagas disease is caused by *Trypanosoma cruzi*. It is mainly seen in South American countries mostly in rural areas. Acute stage is characterized by raised, tender skin nodules or chagoma, unilateral edema of eye and conjunctivitis. Symptomatic latent or intermediate stage can extend for long time. Cardiac and smooth muscle abnormalities are seen in chronic stage. Benzimidazole and nifurtimox are often ineffective in chronic stage because they need to be given for longer time resulting in side effects. Both drugs are activated by nitroreductase and generates nitroanion radicals that damage parasites. Both these drugs are very effective and reduce parasitemia to the extent of 80%.

BENZNIDAZOLE

Metacyclic trypomastigotes, the infective stage of the parasite, enter macrophages within human body through the protozoan parasite *Trypanosoma cruzi* and transform into 'amastigote form' which multiply by binary fission. Intracellular amastigotes become 'trypomastigotes', burst open the cell and enter the bloodstream. Benznidazole kills trypomastigotes and amastigotes. It has better therapeutic efficacy and higher safety profile. Hence, benznidazole is considered to be better than nifurtimox. It results in 90% cure rate in congenitally infected infants. It causes peripheral neuropathy and granulocytopenia.

NIFURTIMOX

Nifurtimox is a nitrofuran analog, cidal against trypomastigotes and amastigotes. It reduces parasitemia, duration of symptoms and mortality rate. It undergoes extensive first pass metabolism and has elimination half-life of 3 hours. It causes anorexia, vomiting, insomnia, headache, seizures and ataxia. Side effects are mostly reversible and reduce after dose reduction.

Drug of Choice: Benznidazole

RATIONALE

Nifurtimox and benznidazole are used in the treatment of Chagas disease. Both drugs have cidal activity against trypomastigotes and amastigotes but lack efficacy and often result in severe side effects. Yet, **benznidazole** is preferred to nifurtimox as it has better **therapeutic efficacy** and **higher safety profile**. **Nifurtimox** has **lesser efficacy** but has severe, reversible side effects. Hence, it is not preferred.

41

Chemotherapy of Tuberculosis and Leprosy

1. *Moxifloxacin/Levofloxacin as a suitable fluoroquinolone in tuberculosis.*

BACKGROUND

Fluoroquinolones are one of the most effective second line antituberculous drugs. They are added to therapy when first line drugs are ineffective or intolerant. Since monotherapy results in quick development of resistance they are added to first line drugs. Fluoroquinolones inhibit DNA synthesis by inhibiting DNA gyrase. *M. tuberculosis, M. leprae, M. marinum, M. kansasii* and *M. fortuitum* are susceptible. Levofloxacin and moxifloxacin are the most effective respiratory quinolones.

MOXIFLOXACIN

Moxifloxacin is well absorbed and reaches very high concentration in lungs. Its area under curve/minimum inhibitory concentration (AUC/MIC) ratio of microbial kill is higher than that of levofloxacin. Its kill rate is higher and faster than other fluoroquinolones in early phases of disease. Moxifloxacin also delays the emergence of resistance in *M. tuberculosis* bacilli. It is bactericidal at the dose of 400 mg daily and has similar efficacy to isonicotinic acid hydrazide (INH) but its safety profile at daily dose of more than 400 mg is not well established. Moxifloxacin reduces the duration of therapy and does not require dosage reduction in renal dysfunction. Currently a phase III trial is evaluating its efficacy as 4th drug in reducing antituberculous therapy to 4 months.

LEVOFLOXACIN

Levofloxacin is also well absorbed and well distributed in most tissues. *Mycobacteria* are less susceptible to levofloxacin when compared to moxifloxacin. Hence, its kill rate is inferior and development of resistance is quicker. Levofloxacin should not be given to persons with compromised renal function.

Drug of Choice: Moxifloxacin

RATIONALE

Respiratory fluoroquinolones such as levofloxacin and moxifloxacin are now being evaluated as one of the four first line drugs in pulmonary tuberculosis due to their superior efficacy against *Mycobacteria*. **Moxifloxacin** is **preferred** to levofloxacin as it is **more effective** with **greater kill ratio** and **delayed** development of **resistance**. As agents of wider use, development of resistance to fluoroquinolones is one of the major problems. Currently it is being evaluated as a replacement for ethambutol as fourth drug in reducing the course of therapy from 6 months to 4 months and it does not require dosing reduction in renal disease. **Levofloxacin** results in **lesser kill rate** and **organisms develop resistance** much **faster**. Hence, it is not preferred.

2. *Azithromycin/Clarithromycin in non-tuberculous pulmonary infection caused by Mycobacterium avium.*

BACKGROUND

Non-tuberculous pulmonary infection is caused by *M. avium* and *M. kansasii*. They are less pathogenic than *M. tuberculosis* but can cause dissemination. Triple drug therapy is given for the treatment of newly diagnosed *M. avium* and commonly includes macrolides with rifampin and ethambutol. Clarithromycin and azithromycin are the macrolides indicated for triple drug therapy as they both have enhanced activity against *Mycobacterium avium* intracelullarly.

AZITHROMYCIN

When compared to its serum level, intracellular and tissue concentration of azithromycin is high. The concentration of azithromycin within phagocytes and fibroblasts is very high. It has long elimination half-life (40–68 hours) and can be given as intermittent therapy. It undergoes minimal drug interaction, a factor suitable for combined therapy. Unlike clarithromycin it does not cause *torsades de pointes* and not cardio toxic and it belongs to pregnancy category B with no evidence of teratogenic risk. It does not require dose reduction in renal failure as it undergoes hepatic metabolism.

CLARITHROMYCIN

Clarithromycin also reaches higher intracellular and tissue concentration than plasma. Clarithromycin prolongs QT interval and undergoes drug interaction. Rifampin reduces its level while clarithromycin increases the plasma level of rifabutin. Since rifampin is one of the primary drugs in triple therapy, clarithromycin cannot be added. It belongs to pregnancy category C and should be avoided during pregnancy. It requires dosage reduction in renal disease as 30% of drug is excreted through kidney.

Drug of Choice: Azithromycin

RATIONALE

Macrolides are included in triple therapy in non-tuberculous pulmonary infection as they are very effective against *M. avium*. Azithromycin and clarithromycin are both equally effective against *M. avium* but clarithromycin interacts with rifampin, the primary drug in triple therapy. Besides, it results in cardiotoxicity and requires dose reduction in renal dysfunction. It belongs to pregnancy category C and should be avoided during pregnancy. Azithromycin has minimal drug interactions, does not require dosage modification in renal dysfunction and is neither cardio toxic nor teratogenic. Hence, it is more suitable macrolide in the treatment of pulmonary infection due to *M. avium*.

3. *Rifabutin/Rifampin in HIV associated TB.*

BACKGROUND

Rifampin, rifabutin and rifapentine are the three rifamycins used in therapy. Being macrocyclic compounds, rifabutin and rifapentine are rifampin derivatives. They are primary agents in treatment of TB and belong to first line group of drugs. Rifampin is first line essential drug and commonly included in all regimes. Rifabutin and rifapentine are first line supplemental drugs. They are highly effective with acceptable range of toxicity. Routine first line therapy is effective against HIV associated tuberculosis but incidence of adverse effects is severe as these patients are immunocompromised.

RIFABUTIN

Rifabutin inhibits *M. tuberculosis* bacilli at a lower minimum inhibitory concentration (MIC) than rifampin. It is lipophilic and its levels are higher in tissues than plasma. In comparison to plasma it attains 70% higher cerebrospinal fluid (CSF) concentration in HIV meningitis. HIV patients who develop monoresistance to rifamycin respond better to rifabutin. It is a substrate for CYP3A4 but is a weak inducer of the enzyme. Therefore, it does not reduce plasma levels of coadministered non-nucleoside reverse transcriptase inhibitors (NNRTI) and protease inhibitors. Unlike rifampin, it has a prolonged half-life of 32 to 67 hours and longer therapeutic effect. It has very high intracellular concentration, almost double the level of rifampin. Of the 14 mutant alleles of *rpoB* gene only 9 alleles confer resistance to rifabutin. So, bacilli do not develop resistance even when it is given as intermittent therapy. Hence, rifabutin is preferred to rifamycin in the treatment of HIV associated TB.

RIFAMPIN

Frequently drug interaction between rifampin and antiretroviral drugs has been documented. Development of monoresistance to rifampin also occurs frequently. Highly immunosuppressed patients (CD4+ < 100 μL) develop such resistance quickly. Resistance to rifampin is due to 14 mutant alleles of *rpoB* gene. Incidence is higher in those receiving once or twice weekly dose or intermittent therapy. It can be significantly reduced if rifampin is given either once daily or thrice weekly. Half-life of rifampin is only 5 hours so the bacilli develop resistance in intermittent therapy. Rifampin is not a substrate for CYP3A4 but causes pronounced enzyme induction reducing levels of coadministered anti-HIV agents. It reduces plasma level of many NNRTI and protease inhibitors, the primary drugs in HIV.

Drug of Choice: Rifabutin

RATIONALE

Rifampin is the first line essential drug while rifabutin and rifapentine are first line supplemental drugs. They are highly effective with acceptable range of toxicity. In HIV associated TB, **rifampin** is not suitable as patients quickly develop **monoresistance** because of its **shorter half-life**. It **augments** development of **resistance** when given less frequently. Besides, it is a **potent enzyme inducer** and **reduces** the **plasma level** of coadministered anti HIV drugs. **Rifabutin** has higher intracellular concentration and **prolonged** half-life so **does not develop resistance** even when given **intermittently**. It is a weak enzyme inducer and does not reduce the plasma level of coadministered anti HIV drugs. When compared to rifampin, the MIC required for inhibiting *Mycobacteria* are lower for rifabutin. Hence, rifabutin is preferred to rifampin in the treatment of HIV associated tuberculosis.

4. *Kanamycin/Amikacin in MDR tuberculosis.*

BACKGROUND

The aminoglycosides streptomycin, amikacin and kanamycin are used in multidrug resistant tuberculosis (MDR TB). Since organisms have developed resistance to streptomycin it is no longer advised. These drugs are second line antituberculous drugs and used as alternatives. Amikacin and kanamycin are preferred in 'extensively drug resistant MDR TB'. Organisms are generally resistant to INH, rifampin and fluoroquinolones in this type of TB.

Minimum inhibitory concentration of both drugs for *M. tuberculosis* is similar but the MIC required in *M. avium* for amikacin is lower than kanamycin.

AMIKACIN

Ninety percent of *M. tuberculosis* bacilli are suppressed by amikacin and it is not inactivated by aminoglycosidase enzyme produced by organisms. It is effective against extracellular organisms also. Small dose for shorter duration and avoidance of daily therapy reduces its adverse effects. It is very effective when given in thrice weekly regimen as it reduces the incidence of side effects.

KANAMYCIN

Kanamycin is the most toxic drug among aminoglycoside agents. Moreover it causes superinfection and has no therapeutic advantage to amikacin. Its susceptibility to organisms expressing aminoglycosidase enzyme leads to quick resistance. It is more ototoxic, nephrotoxic and causes malabsorption if given orally.

Drug of Choice: Amikacin

RATIONALE

Kanamycin and amikacin are **second line drugs** and are indicated in MDR tuberculosis. Ninety percent of *M. tuberculosis* bacilli are inhibited by **amikacin**. It is **very effective** on thrice weekly administration. It is **not inactivated by aminoglycosidase enzyme** expressed by organisms. Since it is **not administered frequently**, it causes **fewer side effects**. Although effective, **kanamycin is highly toxic** and has no therapeutic advantage to amikacin as it is susceptible to organisms expressing aminoglycosidase enzyme.

5. *Ethionamide/Cycloserine in 'totally drug resistant' type MDR TB in patients prone for psychosis.*

BACKGROUND

Multidrug resistant organisms can be either 'extensively drug resistant' or 'totally drug resistant'. 'Totally drug resistant' organisms are resistant to the primary drugs INH and rifampin. Resistance is also noted for ethambutol, pyrazinamide, streptomycin and para-amino salicylic acid (PAS). Although 'totally drug resistant' organisms are resistant to ethionamide and cycloserine, these drugs are still included in intensive phase of MDR tuberculosis. Intensive phase of 6 drugs for 9 months is continued with 4 drugs for 18 months. Ethionamide and cycloserine are included as agents for therapy in intensive phase.

ETHIONAMIDE

Ethionamide, a derivative of isonicotinic acid is bacteriostatic and very effective in MDR tuberculosis but causes frequent side effects. To minimize gastric irritation, it is advisable to take it along with food. It causes postural hypotension, drowsiness and asthenia. It frequently causes neurological symptoms such as mental depression, paresthesia, diplopia, dizziness and tremors. Coadministration of pyridoxine relieves the neurological symptoms of ethionamide. So, ethionamide can be administered with pyridoxine for patients prone for depression.

CYCLOSERINE

Cycloserine is a structural analog of D-alanine and has extensive oral absorption. It is called 'psych-serine' as it causes intense neuropsychiatric symptoms. Frequently it causes somnolence, headache, psychosis, seizures and suicidal tendencies. Symptoms occur in 50% of patients who receive a daily dose of 1 g and pyridoxine does not relieve or reduce the neuropsychiatric symptoms of cycloserine.

Drug of Choice: Ethionamide

RATIONALE

Cycloserine and ethionamide are given with other 4 drugs in intensive phase of therapy for totally drug resistant type MDR TB. **Cycloserine** or **'psych-serine'** should not be given in patients who are prone for psychosis because it results in **neuropsychiatric**

symptoms such as somnolence, psychosis, seizures and suicidal tendencies in 50% patients receiving the drug. Administration of pyridoxine does not relieve the symptoms. Although **ethionamide causes neuropsychiatric symptoms** that vary from drowsiness to mental depression, these symptoms are reversed by coadministration of pyridoxine. Hence, ethionamide can be safely given with pyridoxine in totally drug resistant type MDR TB in patients prone for psychosis.

6. *Prednisolone/Thalidomide in recurring erythema nodosum leprosum (ENL) in type 2 lepra reaction.*

BACKGROUND

Type 2 lepromatous reaction is common in patients with lepromatous leprosy. Erythema nodosum leprosum (ENL) usually occurs after chemotherapy is instituted. Painful papules that occur may resolve spontaneously within weeks to months but (ENL) may recur with profound symptoms such as neuritis, lymphadenitis, orchitis, uveitis or glomerulonephritis. Tumor necrosis factor (TNF) is generally elevated as it is involved in the pathogenesis of ENL. Inflammation may progress to ulceration creating cosmetic problems in areas like face.

THALIDOMIDE

For persisting and recurring ENL, thalidomide is the drug of choice. Thalidomide decreases synthesis of TNF and increases the level of immunoglobin M (IgM). It also slows down migration of polymorphonuclear cells to the site of inflammation. Daily dose of 100 to 300 mg is reduced to 50 to 200 mg once lepra reaction is controlled, but thalidomide is contraindicated during pregnancy as it can cause phocomelia.

PREDNISOLONE

Erythema nodosum leprosum with skin lesions is managed with prednisolone 40 to 60 mg/day for 1 to 2 weeks. Prednisolone is a potent anti-inflammatory agent and effectively inhibits inflammation

Although inflammation subsides lesions recur. Besides, prolonged therapy augments its side effects as it is an immunosuppressant, since immune status in lepromatous leprosy is already compromised. Hence, long-term therapy with steroids is not preferable in such patients.

Drug of Choice: Thalidomide

RATIONALE

Type 2 lepromatous reaction occurs commonly in patients with lepromatous leprosy. **Prednisolone** is very effective as it is a **potent anti-inflammatory** agent but it **does not reduce recurrence rates**. In case of recurrent ENL, prednisolone is not preferred as it has to be given for a long period, thereby inducing side effects. **Thalidomide** is very effective as it **inhibits TNF synthesis**, main **factor responsible for aggravation** of the condition. It also increases the level of IgM and slows down migration of polymorphonuclear cells to the site of inflammation but it is **contraindicated** during **pregnancy** as it can cause phocomelia.

Anthelmintic Drugs

1. *Albendazole/Mebendazole in roundworm, hookworm, whipworm and pinworm infestation.*

BACKGROUND

The most common intestinal helminth is the roundworm or *Ascaris lumbricoides*. Eggs ingested through contaminated food hatch larvae in small intestine that migrate to lung through blood and back to intestine to become adult worms. *Ancylostoma duodenale* and *Necatar americanus* are two species of hookworms. Infection commonly occurs in tropical and subtropical regions. Pinworm or *Enterobius vermicularis* has maximal prevalence in school children. Whipworm is *Trichuris trichiura*, infests children most frequently. These are soil-transmitted helminths (STH) and are also known as 'geohelminths'. Albendazole and mebendazole are benzimidazoles used in worm infestation. They bind to β-tubulin and inhibit polymerization of microtubules in worms. They are both versatile anthelmintics especially against intestinal nematodes. They kill both larval and adult stages of nematodes ovicidal, against *Ascaris* and *Trichuris*. They are slow in action and it may take many days for parasitic clearance from GIT. They are safely given in children above two years but not recommended in pregnancy.

ALBENDAZOLE

Albendazole is more effective than mebendazole against hookworm and *Trichuris*. It has variable bioavailability due to its improper absorption. Its absorption is enhanced up to 5 times by fatty food and bile salts. It is rapidly metabolized and its metabolite albendazole sulfoxide is also active. The advantage of albendazole is that it is effective as a single oral dose of 400 mg. against *Enterobius, Ascaris, Trichuris* and hookworm. It is well tolerated and just around 1% of patients experience minimal side effects. Epigastric pain, nausea, vomiting and diarrhea are frequent side effects and a rare side effect is dizziness.

MEBENDAZOLE

The bioavailability of mebendazole is around 22% as its aqueous solubility is very poor. Although extensively metabolized, none of its metabolites are active. For *Enterobius,* it is given as a single 100 mg dose but has to be repeated after two weeks. 100 mg twice daily for 3 days is given in *Ascaris, Trichuris* and hookworm infestation. It causes minimal side effects due to low bioavailability and can cause local GIT side effects. Rarely allergy, alopecia, hypospermia and blood dyscrasias can occur.

Drug of Choice: Albendazole

RATIONALE

Geohelminths or soil transmitted helminths are effectively killed by benzimidazoles mebendazole and **albendazole**. They cause slow death of worms by binding with β-tubulin and preventing polymerization of microtubules. Both are equally effective but the advantage of albendazole is **single dose therapy**. A single dose of 400 mg is effective against *Enterobius, Ascaris, Trichuris* and hookworm. **Mebendazole** has to be **given twice daily** for **three days** in *Ascaris, Trichuris* and hookworm infection while for *Enterobius,* it needs to be repeated after two weeks.

2. *Albendazole/Mebendazole in Echinococcus granulosus and Echinococcus multilocularis.*

BACKGROUND

Echinococcus granulosus causes cystic hydatid disease and alveolar hydatid disease is caused by *Echinococcus multilocularis. Echinococcus multilocularis* is more aggressive than

Echinococcus granulosus. Surgical resection is primary treatment in cystic hydatid disease and drugs are given in conjunction with surgery.

ALBENDAZOLE

Albendazole is very effective against helminths that reside in tissues due to its metabolite albendazole sulfoxide that exerts potent anthelmintic action. Albendazole sulfoxide is 70% bound to proteins with variable half-life of 4—15 hours. It is well distributed and its concentration in hydatid cyst is 20% higher than plasma. So it is the drug of choice in cystic and alveolar hydatid disease due to *Echinococcus.* As monotherapy it provides moderate cure rate but if given after surgery it is very effective as it reduces the risk of dissemination of organisms due to spillage of cyst fluid that occurs during surgery, puncture, aspiration or re-aspiration. Recommended dose is 400 mg twice a day for 1 to 6 months. It is the only active drug against alveolar hydatid disease but it exerts static and not cidal action against *Echinococcus multilocularis.* Hence, life-long therapy is required in treatment of *Echinococcus multilocularis.*

MEBENDAZOLE

Neither mebendazole nor its metabolites reach effective concentration in hydatid cyst. It undergoes extensive metabolism but the metabolites are not active and are excreted. Hence, mebendazole is not used in the treatment of *Echinococcus* infections.

Drug of Choice: Albendazole

RATIONALE

Echinococcus granulosus causes cystic hydatid disease and alveolar hydatid disease is caused by *Echinococcus multilocularis.* **Albendazole** and its **active metabolite albendazole sulfoxide** are **efficient** anthelmintic. Albendazole **sulfoxide** has a **long and variable half-life** of 4 to 15 hours. The **concentration** of albendazole sulfoxide in **hydatid cyst is 20% higher** than its plasma concentration. Hence, albendazole is useful adjunct to surgery in

E. granulosus and given for 6 months but life-long therapy is required in treatment of *Echinococcus multilocularis*. **Mebendazole** or its metabolites **do not** reach effective concentration in **hydatid cyst,** hence not useful in *Echinococcus granulosus* and *Echinococcus multilocularis*.

3. *Diethylcarbamazine citrate (DEC)/Ivermectin for filariasis due to W. bancrofti, B. malayi, B. timori and Loa loa.*

BACKGROUND

W. bancrofti is transmitted by *Culex, Aedes* and *Anopheles* mosquitoes. *W. bancrofti* is responsible for 90% of lymphatic filariasis. The remaining 10% of lymphatic filariasis is caused by *B. malayi*. Lymphatic obstruction with secondary bacterial infection causes cellulites and intense lymphedema leads to hydrocoele and elephantiasis. Tropical pulmonary eosinophilia occurs due to immune reaction to microfilariae. *L. loa* worms reside in subcutaneous tissue and cause 'calabar' swellings. Adult worm of *Loa loa* crosses across sclera causing 'eye worm'. Other complications include encephalopathy, nephropathy and cardiac problems. *B. malayi* and *B. timori* are transmitted by *Anopheles* and *Mansonia* mosquitoes. Larvae migrate through lymphatics to lymph nodes and mature into adult worms. Adult worms release microfilariae into circulation mainly at night. In Southern Pacific regions the microfilaria peak during night. Transmission of microfilariae to mosquitoes makes them more infective.

DIETHYLCARBAMAZINE CITRATE

DEC is first line drug for filariasis due to *W. bancrofti, B. malayi, B. timori* and *Loa loa*. It damages intracellular organelles promoting cellular death of microfilaria. It kills adult worms by inhibiting transport of macromolecules to plasma membrane. Microfilariae of *W. bancrofti, B. malayi, B. timori* and *Loa loa* are highly sensitive to DEC. They disappear rapidly from blood after institution of therapy. It does not reverse already existing lymphatic damage but prevents further damage. It is given as 6 mg/kg/day for 12 days.

IVERMECTIN

In *L. loa* infection with high microfilaremia pre-treatment with prednisolone is essential to minimize the reactions due to dying microfilaria that induce encephalitis. Ivermectin is the synthetic analog of insecticide avermectin. Its efficacy against lymphatic filariasis due to *W. bancrofti* is similar to DEC but the duration of therapy required is long and extends beyond 6 years. It causes encephalopathy if given in *Loa loa* infection with high microfilaremia.

Drug of Choice: Diethylcarbamazine Citrate

RATIONALE

Diethylcarbamazine citrate is **the drug of choice** in lymphatic filariasis due to *W. bancrofti, B. malayi* and *B. timori*. It is first line drug in the treatment of subcutaneous manifestation of *Loa loa*. **Microfilariae and not adult worms** are **more susceptible** to DEC. It is given as a 12 days course. In case of *L. loa* infection, pre-treatment with prednisolone is necessary before administering DEC or ivermectin to prevent complications such as encephalitis due to immune reaction to dying microfilariae. Although **ivermectin** is **equieffective** against *W. bancrofti, B. malayi, B. timori* and *Loa loa* infection, it results in **regression only** if **therapy** is **continued beyond 6 years**. Such prolonged therapy **increases** the incidence of its **adverse effects**. Hence, DEC is preferred to ivermectin in the treatment of *W. bancrofti, B. malayi, B. timori* and *Loa loa* infections.

4. *Diethylcarbamazine citrate (DEC)/Ivermectin for filariasis due Onchocerca volvulus.*

BACKGROUND

Onchocerca volvulus, the filarial nematode, causes onchocerciasis or river blindness. Larvae develop into adult worms in subcutaneous nodules and reside there for a period of seven months to three years, microfilariae released from adult female localises in skin. The lifespan of *Onchocerca volvulus* can extend around

18 years. It affects mainly the skin, eyes and causes subcutaneous nodules, pruritus, onchodermatitis, hyperkeratosis and eczema. Anterior uveitis, chorioretinitis, corneal scarring and opacities are a few ocular complications.

IVERMECTIN

Ivermectin, the semisynthetic macrocyclic lactone is the drug of choice. It is administered as a single dose and repeated once in 6 to 12 months. It induces tonic paralysis of muscles immobilizing these organisms. It reverses ocular inflammatory reactions and prevents further progression of disease. It further reduces microfilaria level in skin and causes relief from pruritus. Clearance of microfilaria occurs within a few days and persists for 6–12 months. It has only minimal effect on adult worms. Therefore, the therapy is not curative. It can result in 'Mazzotti-like reaction' due to dying microfilariae. These reactions are usually very mild and severe reactions respond to prednisolone. Ocular lesions in onchocerciasis are seldom exaggerated by ivermectin. Ivermectin causes minimal side effects compared to DEC, hence preferred.

DIETHYLCARBAMAZINE

DEC is contraindicated in filariasis due to *Onchocerca volvulus* infection because it can result in severe 'Mazzotti' reaction. These severe reactions are caused due to destruction of microfilariae. DEC can worsen the ocular lesions and can even result in meningo-encephalitis.

Drug of Choice: Ivermectin

RATIONALE

Onchocerciasis causes severe lesions of skin and eye. Ocular lesions are characterized by anterior uveitis, chorioretinitis, corneal scarring and corneal opacities. DEC is not preferred as it can exaggerate ocular lesions and can cause very severe 'Mazzotti reactions'. These reactions occur due to dead microfilariae. Severe reactions can cause high fever, tachycardia, hypotension, arthralgia, myalgia and facial edema. **Single dose** therapy of **ivermectin** is very **effective** in onchocerciasis. It causes tonic paralysis of microfilariae but does not kill adult worms. Hence, it has to be **repeated every 6 to 12 months**. When compared to DEC, it does not exaggerate ocular lesions and results in **minimal side effects**. Hence, ivermectin is preferred to DEC.

5. *Ivermectin/Thiabendazole in threadworm infestation.*

BACKGROUND

Strongyloides stercoralis or threadworm is less prevalent than *Nematodes infection*. It maintains a complete life cycle within human host and so is unique among helminths. Larvae enter into bloodstream, travel to lungs, reach alveoli, then travel back to intestine. They mature into adult worms, reside within intestine up to 5 years and lay eggs. Hyperinfection syndrome is due to release of huge volumes of larvae to lungs and tissues. In immunocompromised persons, this hyperinfection syndrome can result in death. Therefore, asymptomatic infection should also be treated to prevent hyperinfection syndrome.

IVERMECTIN

Ivermectin is drug of choice and given as a single dose. Second dose should be repeated after one week. By activating glutamate-mediated Cl^- channels, it causes paralysis of pharyngeal muscles of the worms, markedly inhibiting the feeding capacity of worms. It is better tolerated than thiabendazole with minimal side effects. Subcutaneous ivermectin is given in hyperinfection syndrome where GIT absorption is minimal.

THIABENDAZOLE

Since thiabendazole causes hypersensitivity, visual effects, liver and CNS toxicity, its clinical utility is highly compromised. Activities involving mental alertness should be avoided as it causes CNS toxicity. It also causes transient leucopenia and occasional Stevens-Johnson syndrome.

Drug of Choice: Ivermectin

RATIONALE

Strongyloides stercoralis completes its life cycle in human host. It has the potential to cause hyperinfection syndrome due to dissemination of huge amount of larvae to tissues and lungs. If not attended immediately, it may prove to be fatal in immunocompromised individuals. Due to the potential of *Strongyloides stercoralis* in causing hyperinfection syndrome, therapy should be instituted even in asymptomatic individuals. **Ivermectin** is **effective, better tolerated** than thiabendazole with **minimal side effects** and has an advantage of single dose that should be repeated after one week. **Thiabendazole** is **highly toxic** causing hypersensitivity and CNS side effects, so not preferred.

6. *Thiabendazole/Ivermectin in cutaneous larva migrans.*

BACKGROUND

Ancylostoma braziliense causes 'creeping eruption' or cutaneous larva migrans. Eggs of dog and cat hookworms are passed into feces and larvae hatch in soil. Skin contact with soil in such areas spreads the infection to humans. It causes intense pruritus and erythematous papules on hands and feet that migrate to other areas traveling many millimeters forming serpiginous tracts. The lesions turn into vesicles and prone for secondary bacterial infection. Mild lesions do not require therapy as the larva dies and gets absorbed.

IVERMECTIN

Ivermectin is highly effective against cutaneous larva migrans. Single oral dose of 200 µg/kg is the first-line treatment in larva migrans. Single dose therapy is successful as it has long half-life of 57 hours and low clearance. Besides, it has high tolerability with minimal side effects.

THIABENDAZOLE

Thiabendazole results in severe side effects, so seldom used orally but it can be given as topical cream for cutaneous larva migrans.

Marked relief of symptoms is noted in many patients treated by thiabendazole. Among benzimidazoles, it has high aqueous solubility and available as 15% cream. Cream base should be applied to the affected area thrice daily for 5 or more days. Since it is not given orally, it does not kill larvae, so has limited usefulness.

Drug of Choice: Ivermectin

RATIONALE

Topical application in cutaneous larva migrans can only have limited efficacy as the drug does not reach the site of action. **Thiabendazole** when applied topically as 15% cream base thrice daily for 5 or more days provides only **symptomatic** relief **but** it is not recommended for oral administration as it is **highly toxic** and has lower efficacy. **Ivermectin** is a very **effective** larvicidal when given as a single dose. It has a **prolonged half-life** with **slow clearance rate** that augments its duration of action. Hence, ivermectin is preferred to thiabendazole in the treatment of cutaneous larva migrans.

7. *Praziquantel/Niclosamide in cestode infestation.*

BACKGROUND

Four major tapeworms cause noninvasive human infestation. Beef tapeworm or *Taenia solium*, pork tapeworm or *Taenia saginata* are among them. Fish tapeworm or *Diphyllobothrium latum* is found in temperate climates. Dwarf tapeworm or *Hymenolepis nana* and *Taenia* species are widely distributed. Gravid segments of *T. saginata* passed in human feces are ingested by grazing cattle. Embryos release encyst as cysticerci in muscle and reinfect humans when they eat the infected beef. Similarly, *T. solium* is transmitted from pigs while eating undercooked pork. *D. latum* spreads through undercooked fish and *H. nana* spreads among humans.

PRAZIQUANTEL

Praziquantel increases intracellular calcium, resulting in spastic paralysis. Low doses of praziquantel are effective against *Taenia* species and *D. latum.* Single oral dose of 10 to 20 mg/kg is effective in *Taenia* species and *D. latum.* Slightly higher dose is required for treatment of *H. nana* as it is difficult to treat. Dose of 25 mg/kg is required for *H. nana* and it has to be repeated after 1 week. It causes pain, diarrhea, dizziness and occasionally pruritus and arthralgia.

NICLOSAMIDE

Niclosamide is the second-line drug for treatment of intestinal cestodes. It is cheaper and inhibits oxidative phosphorylation in mitochondria of worms. It is effective in injuring the worms but some segments may get digested in intestine. Digestion of dead segments is hazardous and risky in persons with *T. solium* infection because gravid worms that are partially damaged by the drug can release ova. Matured ova develop into larvae causing more severe visceral cysticercosis. Hence, saline purging is necessary when niclosamide is given for cestodes infestation and the scolex should be searched for in stools to rule out that residual worm is not left out. Two tablets of 500 mg are swallowed followed by two more tablets after one hour. Saline purging is given after 2 hours and for *H. nana,* procedure is repeated after five days. It is well tolerated but not preferred due to this cumbersome procedure because it requires additional purging.

Drug of Choice: Praziquantel

RATIONALE

Cestodes that cause noninvasive human infection are *T. solium, T. saginata, D. latum* and *H. nana.* **Praziquantel** expels the worms as it causes **spastic paralysis** and so **saline purging** is **not necessary** for patients taking praziquantel. **Niclosamide** is **cheaper** than praziquantel and **well tolerated**. It inhibits oxidative phosphorylation and interferes with generation of ATP. Therefore, it **only** injures the worms and causes **flaccid paralysis**. So, saline **purging is necessary** for complete expulsion of worms and scolex should be searched for in stools. If gravid segments of *T. solium* are digested, they can result in visceral cysticercosis. Though well tolerated, niclosamide is considered only as second line drug due to its possibility of causing visceral cysticercosis in *T. solium* infection as well as the necessity for purging and stool examination.

8. *Praziquantel/Albendazole in neurocysticercosis.*

BACKGROUND

Neurocysticercosis is an important cause for seizures and occurs due to cysts of *T. solium*. The organism results in subarachnoid, intracerebral and spinal cord lesions or intraventricular cysts leading to neurologic deficits, seizures and altered cognition. Intraventricular cysts can cause pappilledema. Cystic proliferation at base of brain results in racemose cysticercosis. Specialist opinion is needed to outweigh benefits and risks of rapid cyst clearance. The possible complications include vasculitis, arachnoiditis or cerebral edema because inflammatory response due to dead worms can aggravate CNS symptoms. Corticosteroids are administered along with anthelmintic drugs in neurocysticercosis.

ALBENDAZOLE

Albendazole is preferred as it is effective at a low dose of 400 mg/kg twice daily. Total therapy varies based on number, type and location of cysts and extends from 8 to 30 days. The efficacy of albendazole is high with 85% cure rate due to its active metabolite, albendazole sulfoxide that has wide distribution reaches higher concentration in cysts. Steroids that are given concurrently increase the plasma levels of albendazole sulfoxide. This explains the therapeutic superiority of albendazole in neurocysticercosis.

PRAZIQUANTEL

Praziquantel is also effective but has to be given in higher dose for longer period. It is given in the dose of 50 mg/kg/day in divided doses for a period of 30 days. Steroids reduce the bioavailability of praziquantel. It is contraindicated in ocular cysticercosis due to host inflammatory responses. These intense host responses can cause irreversible permanent damage to eyes. Tasks requiring mental alertness like driving are prohibited in those taking praziquantel.

Drug of Choice: Albendazole

RATIONALE

Neurologist should outweigh risks with benefits before instituting therapy for neurocysticercosis because rapid clearance of cysts can evoke severe inflammatory response resulting in vasculitis, arachnoiditis or cerebral edema. Corticosteroids should be given concurrently with anthelmintic drugs to reduce such inflammatory response. Albendazole is effective in clearance of cysts. The drug and its metabolite **albendazole sulfoxide** have anthelmintic activity. The **concentration** of albendazole sulfoxide in **cysts** is **higher** than its **plasma concentration. Corticosteroids increase plasma levels** of **albendazole sulfoxide** augmenting the therapeutic efficacy of albendazole. **Praziquantel** is effective only if given in **higher dose** and for **longer period** but its bioavailability is reduced by coadministered steroids. Hence, it is not preferred. Besides, it is contraindicated in ocular cysticercosis as it can cause irreversible damage to the eyes.

9. *Praziquantel/Artemether for treating adult worms in schistosomiasis.*

BACKGROUND

Schistosomiasis is caused by five species of trematode blood flukes, such as *S. mansoni, S. japonicum, S. mekongi, S. intercalatum* and *S. haematobium*. *S. haematobium* causes urinary schistosomiasis affecting venules of renal veins. Other species cause intestinal schistosomiasis affecting blood vessels of GIT. It spreads from water-containing cercariae that penetrate skin and mucous membranes. They enter portal circulation, mature, mate and migrate to various blood vessels.

PRAZIQUANTEL

Praziquantel is the drug of choice and causes spastic paralysis of worms. The paralyzed worms lose their grip, reach liver through mesenteric veins. It is a safer drug with proven efficacy so used for mass drug administration programs. It is given as 20 mg/kg at 4 to 6 hours interval for one day or as single 40 mg/kg/day. The cure rate is 70 to 95% or more than 85% with consistent reduction in egg counts. Single dose results in either complete cure or reduction in severity of infection. It is effective only against adult worms and not against juvenile worms. Therefore, praziquantel is not effective in early stage of schistosomiasis.

ARTEMETHER

Artemether is effective only against juvenile worms in early stage of schistosomiasis. It is not effective against adult worms, so cannot be used in late stage of infection. Dose of 6 mg/kg once in every 2 to 3 weeks reduces intensity of the condition. This dose is well tolerated and does not cause any significant side effects but indiscriminate use of artemether can induce drug-resistant malaria.

Drug of Choice: Praziquantel

RATIONALE

Praziquantel is effective against adult worms in schistosomiasis. It causes **spastic paralysis,** so the worms are dislodged from veins. It is **safe, well tolerated** with **proven efficacy** and preferred for mass drug administration programs. It is **simple** to **administer** and **relatively free of side effects**. Single dose reduces either the intensity of symptoms or causes complete cure. **Artemether** is effective **mainly against juvenile worms** and should be given only during the initial stage of disease, but indiscriminate use can result in drug-resistant *Plasmodium* species.

43

Antiviral Drugs

1. *Zanamivir/Oseltamivir for treatment of influenza-A swine flu (H1N1) in patients suffering from bronchial asthma.*

BACKGROUND

Orthomyxovirus or influenza virus is transmitted through respiratory route. Type-A virus is sub classified into hemagglutinin (H) and neuraminidase (N) subtypes. Seasonal influenza is of H3N2 type while swine flu is of H1N1 type. Swine flu originates from North American human and avian virus strains, North American swine or Eurasian swine virus strains. Pneumonitis, shock, myocarditis, renal failure and sepsis can occur. Oseltamivir and zanamivir are effective only if given within the first two days. They also reduce the pulmonary complications that occur due to influenza. The enzyme neuraminidase is vital for release of virus from infected cells. It cleaves sialic acid and destroys receptors recognized by viral hemagglutinin. Oseltamivir and zanamivir inhibit neuraminidase enzyme of influenza virus. They therefore inhibit viral release and its spread through respiratory tract. They are equally effective against both influenza A and B virus.

OSELTAMIVIR

Oseltamivir is available for oral administration as oseltamivir phosphate. It inhibits influenza-A strains resistant to amantadine, rimantadine and zanamivir. It is a prodrug, cleaved by esterases in GIT and liver to its active carboxylate derivative. Its bioavailability ranges around 80% and has half-life of 6 to 10 hours.

Nausea, abdominal pain and vomiting occur but are reduced if taken with food. Besides, the side effects resolve within 1 to 2 days on continuation of therapy.

ZANAMIVIR

Zanamivir is an analog of sialic acid, so has selective neuraminidase inhibiting activity. It has very low oral bioavailability and results in nausea and abdominal discomfort. Zanamivir is well tolerated and delivered through breath-activated inhaler device that deposits 80% of drug in oropharynx and 15% in lower respiratory tract. It can cause wheeze due to bronchospasm in patients without known airway resistance. Since acute deterioration of lung function leading to death can occur in asthmatic individuals, it is not suitable in patients with asthma or chronic obstructive pulmonary disease.

Drug of Choice: Oseltamivir

RATIONALE

Oseltamivir and zanamivir inhibit neuraminidase enzyme of influenza virus. **Zanamivir** is a **sialic acid analog**, hence has **selective neuraminidase inhibiting** activity. Oseltamivir is administered orally but zanamivir is **given through breath-actuated inhaler** device as it has very poor oral bioavailability. This results in high concentration of zanamivir either in lower **respiratory tract** or in **oropharynx**. Although such a high concentration in respiratory tract helps in its therapeutic efficacy it **deteriorates lung function** in persons with known **airway resistance**. Even in those with normal lung function it can cause bronchospasm resulting in wheeze. Hence, zanamivir is contraindicated in persons with bronchial asthma and chronic obstructive pulmonary disease (COPD).

2. *Oseltamivir/Rimantadine in influenza-A avian flu (H5N1).*

BACKGROUND

Avian flu strain H5N1 is highly contagious among birds but rarely spread from human to human. It is difficult to differentiate avian flu from regular influenza through symptoms. Fever, cough and dyspnea are common due to high level of circulating cytokines.

OSELTAMIVIR

Oseltamivir, the neuraminidase enzyme inhibitor is the first line drug. Dose is 75 mg twice daily orally for 5 days and should be started within the first two days. Higher dose for longer duration is required if the condition is progressive. Oseltamivir is effective even against rimantadine resistant strains. The GIT side effects are often mild and resolves as the drug is continued.

RIMANTADINE

Rimantadine inhibits replication of influenza virus more actively than amantadine. It inhibits two steps in viral replication, early viral uncoating and late viral assembly. It inhibits the ion channel M2 protein of influenza virus which is needed for uncoating. Avian H5N1 strains in most parts of the world are resistant to rimantadine.

Drug of Choice: Oseltamivir

RATIONALE

Influenza virus avian flu H5N1 strain is contagious among birds. Exposure to infected poultry can cause infection in human beings. The symptoms include cough, dyspnea and fever. **Rimantadine** inhibits **viral replication** but **most stains** around the world have become **resistant** to it. Hence, it is no more useful in avian flu. **Oseltamivir** is **effective even against rimantadine resistant strains** and so preferred. It causes mild GIT side effects that disappear as the drug is continued.

3. *Acyclovir/Valacyclovir in herpes zoster infection.*

BACKGROUND

Herpes zoster infection or shingles, the acute vesicular eruption is caused by varicella-zoster virus. Pain precedes 48 hours before eruption of vesicles and intensifies after its disappearance.

Deep seated colonies of vesicles occur most commonly on trunk and face. Persistent neuralgia, paralysis of nerves, scarring and encephalitis are common complications. If started within 72 hours both drugs reduce duration and severity of the condition. Early onset of therapy also reduces the risk of post herpetic neuralgia. These drugs inhibit viral thymidine kinase and DNA polymerase.

VALACYCLOVIR

Valacyclovir is more effective than acyclovir in varicella zoster infection. It results in better resolution of pain associated with herpes zoster. On oral administration it gets converted to acyclovir more quickly and completely. The intestinal and hepatic first pass metabolism is responsible for such rapid conversion. Hence, the bioavailability of valacyclovir is three to five times higher and it is effective at the dose of 1000 mg 3 times daily for 7 days. It can cause confusion, hallucination and nephrotoxicity.

ACYCLOVIR

Acyclovir has 200 times greater affinity for viral thymidine kinase than to human enzyme. Varicella zoster infection is less sensitive to acyclovir than herpes simplex virus. Hence, large doses of acyclovir are required for the treatment of varicella-zoster virus. Bioavailability of therapeutic dose is only 10 to 30% and decreases as the dose is increased. It is given for 7 days as 800 mg 5 times a day due to its poor bioavailability. It can cause nausea, headache, diarrhea, rashes but rarely neurotoxicity.

Drug of Choice: Valacyclovir

RATIONALE

Herpes zoster causes vesicular eruptions associated with severe pain that may intensify even after resolution of vesicles. Although acyclovir is more selective to viral enzymes, is well tolerated with minimal side effects, it is not preferred because of its low bioavailability and lesser sensitivity of the organisms. **Valacyclovir** gets **converted** to **acyclovir** and its **bioavailability** is **three to five times**

higher so it is administered only **three times** and **not five times**. Its **higher efficacy** and **more convenient three times administration** favors valacyclovir as the drug of choice, although it causes more severe side effects.

4. *Acyclovir/Ganciclovir in HSV infection.*

BACKGROUND

Herpes simplex type 1 (HSV-1) manifests as recurrent, self-limiting gingivostomatitis. HSV-2 causes similar lesions but these vesicles are typically located at genitalia such as labia, perianal skin, penile shaft and gluteal region. Complications are pyoderma, eczema herpeticum, proctitis, keratitis and encephalitis.

ACYCLOVIR

Acyclovir is very potent and selectively inhibits replication of HSV after phosphorylation into acyclovir triphosphate selectively within virus. It is highly effective against gingivostomatitis and genital HSV infections but only moderately effective against recurrent gingivostomatitis.

GANCICLOVIR

Similar to acyclovir, ganciclovir is effective against HSV infections. The inhibitory concentration for HSV is similar to both drugs but it is not preferred in HSV as it is more toxic. Since it can cause severe myelosuppression, reversible neutropenia and central nervous system (CNS) toxicity, it is reserved for treatment of cytomegalovirus infections.

Drug of Choice: Acyclovir

RATIONALE

Herpes simplex type 1 causes self-limiting mucocutaneous infection and HSV-2 causes genital lesions. Acyclovir is very effective in the treatment of HSV. It gets converted to its active phosphorylated derivative within viral cells. **Ganciclovir** is **equally effective** against

HSV but is more **toxic**. It can cause **myelosuppression** hence, avoided. **Acyclovir** has **good therapeutic efficacy** with minimal side effects hence, preferred.

5. *Foscarnet/Cidofovir for acyclovir resistant mucocutaneous lesions of HSV-1.*

BACKGROUND

Acyclovir inhibits HSV thymidine kinase and DNA polymerase. The HSV virus develops resistance to acyclovir through three mechanisms, reduced production of thymidine kinase, altered substrate specificity where the organisms phosphorylate viral thymidine instead of the drug and by alteration of viral DNA polymerase.

CIDOFOVIR

Cidofovir inhibits DNA synthesis of HSV by arresting its chain elongation. Topical cidofovir is effective in the treatment of acyclovir resistant mucocutaneous lesions. Cidofovir is active even against HSV strains that express lesser thymidine kinase because it is not phosphorylated by viral enzymes to become active but by host enzymes. Hence, it is active against resistant forms. It is also active against foscarnet resistant strains of HSV. Intravenous cidofovir has a very high intracellular half-life of more than 48 hours. So, it can be given once a week for first two weeks and then once every alternate week. It can cause nephrotoxicity which can be reduced through extensive hydration with saline.

FOSCARNET

Foscarnet interacts with herpes DNA polymerase inhibiting the synthesis of nucleic acids. Its affinity towards viral DNA polymerase is 100-fold higher than mammalian enzymes. It is very effective against acyclovir resistant HSV mucocutaneous lesions but few strains of HSV have developed resistance to foscarnet. It heals mucocutaneous lesions absolutely in 75% of patients. Since its oral bioavailability is very low it is given through intravenous infusion.

The main side effect is dose related nephrotoxicity and hypocalcemia. Other CNS related side effects are tremor, irritability, seizures and hallucinations. Topical application causes local irritation and ulceration.

Drug of Choice: Cidofovir

RATIONALE

Herpes simplex virus becomes resistant to acyclovir due to reduced production of thymidine kinase, altered substrate specificity of thymidine kinase or alteration of viral DNA polymerase. **Cidofovir** is effective against **acyclovir** and **foscarnet resistant** strains of **HSV**. Cidofovir **does not need viral thymidine kinase** for phosphorylation but becomes active due to host cell enzymes. The intracellular **half-life** is very high and extends to about **48 hours**. Hence, it can be administered less frequently. **Foscarnet** is effective against acyclovir resistant strains but some strains of HSV have developed **resistance** toward foscarnet. So, its **efficacy** is **inferior** to cidofovir. Since the side effects of foscarnet are very severe it is not preferred.

6. *Ganciclovir/Foscarnet in cytomegalovirus (CMV).*

BACKGROUND

Since CMV remains latent, the primary infection is most often asymptomatic. Three clinically recognizable types of CMV infection are prevalent commonly. It is usually seen in perinatal period, in immunocompromised and in immunocompetant persons. Congenital or perinatal CMV is the most common type and occurs in newly born infants. Although asymptomatic at birth, the infants develop neurologic defects in later part of life. Acquired CMV in immunocompetent persons causes severe complications. It also occurs in immunocompromised HIV patients and after transplantation.

GANCICLOVIR

Ganciclovir is the drug of choice as it is extremely effective against CMV. When compared to acyclovir, the MIC required for ganciclovir is 10 to 100 times lower. It is phosphorylated selectively within viral cells by thymidine kinase. Its concentration within CMV cells is 10 times higher than uninfected cells. Myelosuppression and reversible neutropenia are its side effects.

FOSCARNET

Foscarnet is also very effective against CMV resistant to ganciclovir and acyclovir. When given to HIV patients with CMV it inhibits development of Kaposi's sarcoma. It is given through IV route and has poor aqueous solubility so given in huge volumes. It is given at 60 mg/kg every 8 hours or 90 mg/kg every 12 hours for 14 to 21 days followed by daily maintenance dose for clinical stabilization. Foscarnet is highly toxic and such high doses result in severe side effects. Hence, it is not used routinely but reserved for ganciclovir resistant CMV. Nephrotoxicity, alterations of calcium, phosphate, low potassium and magnesium are a few side effects.

Drug of Choice: Ganciclovir

RATIONALE

Ganciclovir is the first line drug in CMV with a **lower MIC** when compared to acyclovir. It attains **10 times higher concentration within infected cells** compared to uninfected cells. Although few strains have developed resistance to ganciclovir it is still preferred due to its efficacy and **tolerable side effects**. Foscarnet is very effective even against ganciclovir resistant strains but is not used regularly due to its potential toxicity. It is only used as a reserve drug in ganciclovir resistant CMV.

CHAPTER

44

Antiretroviral Drugs

1. *3NRTI/2NRTI suitable for combination regime in ART along with 1NNRTI.*

BACKGROUND

Human immunodeficiency virus (HIV) is a retrovirus containing a small genome of RNA within the nucleocapsid. Three open reading frames, *gag, pol* and *env* are encoded by the viral genome. The *pol* encodes for three enzyme activities, integrase, reverse transcriptase and protease. Reverse transcriptase is a RNA dependent DNA polymerase with RNAase activity which converts viral RNA into proviral DNA that gets incorporated into host chromosome. Some virions remain dormant, survive for decades in host cells and cause reinfection. Suppressive combination antiretroviral therapy inhibits residual viremia and helps to prevent development of resistance to individual drugs. Once initiated antiretroviral therapy (ART) should not be stopped. 'Drug holidays' or 'structured treatment interruptions' will only potentiate its complications. Therapy should be interrupted only for valid reasons like adverse effects of drugs. Nucleoside reverse transcriptase inhibitors (NRTI) prevent infection of susceptible cells but do not eradicate virus from cells that already contain integrated proviral RNA. They enter cells, get phosphorylated and block replication of viral genome. They selectively inhibit viral reverse transcriptase but not the host cell DNA polymerase. They cause anemia, granulocytopenia, pancreatitis, myopathy and peripheral neuropathy and these toxicities increase many fold if they are given as monotherapy. Besides, HIV quickly develops resistance when they are given as single agent.

Hence, NRTIs should be given as combination therapy. NNRTI are non- nucleoside reverse transcriptase inhibitors, bind competitively to reverse transcriptase inducing conformational change to reduce enzyme activity.

TWO NUCLEOSIDE REVERSE TRANSCRIPTASE INHIBITORS (2NRTIs)

Three drugs with two different mechanisms instead of dual therapy should be started. Regimens containing 3 drugs with 2 potent active drugs are found to be very effective. So, 2NRTI with a single NNRTI are essential and preferred. Tenofovir + emtricitabine, abacavir + lamivudine are few such effective combinations that reduce the rate of progression of disease improving CD4+ counts.

THREE NUCLEOSIDE REVERSE TRANSCRIPTASE INHIBITORS (3NRTIs)

Addition of one more NRTI to the regimen does not offer any added advantage. The efficacy of 3NRTI is equivalent to 2NRTI and does not result in higher clinical benefit but increases the incidence of adverse effects due to an additional drug. Moreover, it creates inconvenience to patients causing problems of compliance making monitoring of anti retroviral therapy (ART) difficult and promoting resistance due to poor compliance. Hence, combination of three or four NRTI is reserved for drug-resistant virus.

Drug of Choice: 2NRTI

RATIONALE

Once initiated ART should not be stopped. The 'Drug holidays' or 'structured treatment interruptions' only potentiates the complications due to HIV. Hence, selection of proper drugs and suitable combinations are necessary. The efficacy of 3NRTI is equivalent to the efficacy of 2NRTI combination regimens. **Addition of one more NRTI** not only **potentiates** drug related **toxicities** but also **creates inconvenience** to patient leading to **poor compliance**. Since drug resistance develops due to poor compliance, more than required drugs should not be added to therapy. So, 2NRTI is adequate for combination regimes and 3 or more NRTI is not essential.

2. *(Tenofovir + emtricitabine)/(Zidovudine + lamivudine) as an effective NRTI combination.*

BACKGROUND

Success of combination therapy depends upon efficacy and safety profile of drugs used. Monitoring of CD4 cell count and HIV *viral load* gives a measure about drug's efficacy. Monitoring should be done 2 months after initiation of therapy and every 4 to 6 months thereafter. Regimen with good efficacy reduces *viral load* within 12 to 24 weeks. Nonadherence to therapy or development of resistance creates two problems. Either the viral load is not suppressed or rebound viremia occurs in such patients. Evaluation of toxicity in a patient on stable regimen should be done once in 3 to 4 months.

TENOFOVIR + EMTRICITABINE

Tenofovir disoproxil is the only nucleotide analog approved for treatment of HIV. It is a prodrug with good oral bioavailability, well tolerated, gets rapidly hydrolyzed to tenofovir. Phosphorylated tenofovir, the active metabolite gets incorporated into viral DNA, inhibits reverse transcriptase competitively and causes chain termination. It causes sustained reduction of viral RNA levels. Intracellular half-life of its triphosphate metabolite varies from 10 to 50 hours. Hence administration of tenofovir once daily is clinically effective in reducing *viral load*. It can cause flatulence but otherwise results in only few significant side effects but can rarely cause renal failure. Emtricitabine is related to lamivudine and inhibits HIV reverse transcriptase enzyme. It is one of the least toxic NRTI but causes hyper pigmentation on exposed areas. Co-formulation of tenofovir and emtricitabine can be given once daily and this combination is preferred due to its dosing convenience, efficacy and safety profile.

ZIDOVUDINE + LAMIVUDINE

Zidovudine causes blood dyscrasias due to bone marrow suppression. It also results in pancreatitis and lactic acidosis. A rare, fatal hepatic steatosis occurs due to its interaction with host DNA polymerase-γ, a mitochondrial enzyme. Lamivudine is less toxic due to its low affinity to host DNA polymerase. Combination of zidovudine and lamivudine is given twice daily and does not constitute a complete treatment due to its minimal efficacy. It is reserved as second or third line regimen due to its toxicity and frequent dosing schedule.

Drug of Choice: Tenofovir + Emtricitabine

RATIONALE

Drugs are combined to improve the efficacy of therapy and to reduce drug related toxicities. Combination of tenofovir and emtricitabine is very effective resulting in sustained reduction of viral RNA levels. **Tenofovir and emtricitabine** are both **less toxic** and cause minimal side effects such as flatulence or hyper pigmentation. Besides they have a convenient **once daily** dosage schedule. It is a preferred regimen due to its efficacy, dosing convenience and better safety profile. Combination of **zidovudine and lamivudine** is considered to be a second line regimen as they have **lesser efficacy** and can cause **blood dyscrasias, pancreatitis** and rarely hepatic steatosis that can be fatal. They are administered twice daily, less convenient to patients interfering with compliance.

3. *Didanosine/Ritonavir suitable for combination with tenofovir.*

BACKGROUND

Tenofovir is the only nucleotide reverse transcriptase inhibitor used in therapy. It has poor oral bioavailability hence it is available as a prodrug tenofovir disoproxil. Combination of tenofovir with abacavir or zidovudine or lamivudine is ineffective against organisms that are resistant to zidovudine or lamivudine.

RITONAVIR

Ritonavir is an HIV protease inhibitor and is effective against both HIV-1 and HIV-2. It is a potent inhibitor of CYP3A4 but also moderate inducer of CYP3A4. As an enzyme inhibitor, it increases plasma concentration of coadministered drugs. Hence, it is combined with other drugs as a pharmacokinetic inducer at low doses. High dose should be avoided as it drastically increases concentration of coadministered drugs. Besides, it also potentiates gastrointestinal (GIT) toxicity of ritonavir as this side effect is dose related. A low dose of 100 mg ritonavir increases the plasma level of tenofovir by 34%.

DIDANOSINE

Nucleoside reverse transcriptase inhibitor didanosine has long-term efficacy so combined with other NRTI, NNRTI or PI. It is acid labile and needs to be given 30 minutes before or 2 hours after food. This complicates the dosing schedule as most anti-HIV drugs are given after food. The toxicity of didanosine is very high ranging from peripheral neuropathy to pancreatitis. Purine nucleoside phosphorylase (PNP) is responsible for clearance of didanosine and converts it to hypoxanthine that further gets converted to uric acid. Tenofovir inhibits PNP and increases plasma concentration of didanosine. The level of didanosine increases around 44 to 60% potentiating its toxicity. Hence, combination of tenofovir and didanosine is also associated with high failure rates.

Drug of Choice: Ritonavir

RATIONALE

Didanosine is one of the most **toxic** drugs resulting in serious side effects such as acute pancreatitis, irreversible neuropathy and hypertriglyceridemia. **Tenofovir** inhibits purine nucleoside phosphorylase that is responsible for the clearance of didanosine thereby **increasing its level** to around **44 to 60%** and **potentiating** its **toxicity**. The combination is also less effective probably due to noncompliance on account of its side effects. **Ritonavir**, an HIV protease inhibitor is a potent enzyme inhibitor. It **inhibits CYP3A4** and **increases** the plasma **concentration** of **tenofovir, augmenting** its **clinical efficacy**. Hence, low dose ritonavir is suitable for combination with tenofovir. Ideally didanosine should not be combined with tenofovir. If combined, the dose of didanosine should be reduced from 400 mg to 250 mg.

4. *Indinavir/Darunavir for those living in warm climates with ritonavir.*

BACKGROUND

Indinavir, darunavir and ritonavir are HIV protease inhibitors. As CYP3A4 inhibitor, low dose ritonavir is used as pharmacokinetic inducer but seldom used as individual agent due to its dose related GIT toxicity. Except nelfinavir, it inhibits metabolism of all other HIV protease inhibitors enhancing their pharmacokinetic profile and reducing their dose as well as frequency.

DARUNAVIR

Ritonavir promotes oral absorption of darunavir and increases its bioavailability. It enhances the plasma concentration of darunavir by inhibiting its metabolism. Darunavir mainly undergoes metabolism in liver and only 8% of drug is excreted in urine. It is usually well tolerated and only 3% of patients discontinue the drug due to side effects. It does not cause crystalluria or nephrolithiasis hence preferred to indinavir.

INDINAVIR

High fat meal interferes with indinavir bioavailability reducing its absorption by 75%. Ritonavir decreases influence of food on indinavir absorption and bioavailability. By inhibiting CYP3A4, ritonavir enhances the plasma concentration of indinavir. Due to the poor solubility, at higher alkaline pH, indinavir precipitates in urine. High plasma concentration of indinavir results in its increased level in urine. Such high concentration in urine causes renal colic, crystalluria and nephrolithiasis. The incidence of crystalluria is 40% and nephrolithiasis occurs in 15% of patients. Hence, patients on indinavir therapy should take at least 2 liters of water daily because adequate hydration helps in preventing renal complications. Indinavir is given as a high dose more frequently and this increases its plasma level creating difficulty for patients in warm climates due to highly concentrated urine. Higher pH further reduces the solubility and so antacids should not be coadministered.

Drug of Choice: Darunavir

RATIONALE

As **pharmacokinetic inducer** at low dose 100 mg of **ritonavir enhances** plasma **concentration** of **coadministered** drugs. It increases bioavailability of indinavir by promoting its absorption and increases its plasma concentration through inhibition of its metabolism. The **solubility** of **indinavir** is **low** in **alkaline pH**. It is given at the dose of 800 mg thrice daily orally. Such high dose given more frequently increases its plasma concentration. High plasma level **increases** its urinary concentration promoting **urolithiasis** and **nephrolithiasis**. To **avoid** this problem the patient should take **adequate fluids** but this creates **inconvenience** to patients living in **warm areas** as chances of **concentrated urine** are very high in such patients. **Darunavir** is very effective when coadministered with ritonavir. It is mainly **metabolized** in liver and only 8% is excreted in urine. It **does not cause crystalluria** and **nephrolithiasis** and so preferred.

5. *Lamivudine/Stavudine suitable for combination with zidovudine.*

BACKGROUND

Antiretroviral therapy contains two NRTIs combined with other groups with different mechanism. Zidovudine the NRTI is included in most regimens. It is one of the oldest drugs but still used widely. It has good tolerability, high efficacy and well known toxicity profile.

LAMIVUDINE

Lamivudine is one of the least toxic antiretroviral drugs used for therapy. Resistance to lamivudine occurs due to amino acid substitutions at M184V or M184I. M184V and M184I mutations decrease the viral replication capacity. These mutations reduce the susceptibility of organisms to lamivudine by 1000 folds and also confer cross resistance to emtricitabine and abacavir but M184V mutation restores susceptibility of zidovudine resistant organisms. Hence, coadministration of both drugs contributes to sustained fall in *viral load*.

STAVUDINE

Stavudine, an NRTI, is phosphorylated by thymidine kinase to monophosphate which does not accumulate intracellularly unlike zidovudine. Synthesis of stavudine monophosphate is the rate limiting step for its clinical efficacy. Since both drugs compete for thymidine kinase and zidovudine has higher affinity, concomitant administration of these drugs is not advisable as they result in significantly inferior outcome of the therapy. Being a promotor of mitochondrial toxicity, stavudine is highly toxic resulting in agranulocytosis, pancreatitis and fatal hepatic steatosis.

Drug of Choice: Lamivudine

RATIONALE

Zidovudine is one of the oldest drugs with vast experience and it is still used due to its good tolerability, high efficacy and well known toxicity profile. Coadministration of lamivudine with zidovudine has certain advantages. **Lamivudine** resistant strains through M184V mutations **restore susceptibility** of **zidovudine resistant** strains resulting in **effective reduction of *viral load*.** Hence, coadministration of zidovudine with lamivudine is beneficial. **Stavudine competes with zidovudine for thymidine kinase** for synthesis of stavudine monophosphate, the rate limiting step that determines its clinical efficacy. Since the enzyme has more affinity to zidovudine than to stavudine it **inhibits clinical outcome potentiating the toxicity** of stavudine. Hence, stavudine should not be combined with zidovudine.

7. *Nelfinavir/Lopinavir as 'dual protease inhibitor' in HIV associated with TB in addition to ritonavir.*

BACKGROUND

Tuberculosis (TB) is one of the most common opportunistic infections in HIV patients. All HIV infected TB patients should be given ART irrespective of CD4+ count to prevent TB associated immune reconstitution inflammatory response. Although severe, these reactions are usually self-limiting. Preferred regime is zidovudine + lamivudine + lopinavir-ritonavir. Rifampin should not be given with protease inhibitors (PI) as it is an enzyme inducer and decreases the plasma concentration of PI. Rifabutin should be substituted instead of rifampin in patients treated with PI.

LOPINAVIR

Coadministration of lopinavir and ritonavir are given in ratio of 4:1. This oral dose results in high plasma concentration of lopinavir in the ratio of 20:1. Difference between oral dose and plasma level is due to inhibition of CYP3A4 by ritonavir. Hence, lopinavir is preferred for 'dual PI combination' with ritonavir. Lopinavir 400 mg-ritonavir 100 mg twice daily suppresses viral load. The dose can be doubled gradually over 2 weeks to lopinavir 800 mg and ritonavir 200 mg and is well tolerated but should be given only under close supervision. The risk for possible hepatotoxicity requires clinical and laboratory monitoring.

NELFINAVIR

Only PI that does not require pharmacokinetic enhancement by ritonavir is nelfinavir. A high fatty meal increases the concentration of nelfinavir by three to four fold. It is metabolized by both CYP3A4 and CYP2D6 and causes autoinduction. When compared to ritonavir the capacity to inhibit CYP3A4 is lower. Ritonavir does not modify plasma concentration of nelfinavir's active metabolite M8 hydroxy-t-butyl amide because the major metabolite is formed by CYP2D6. Ritonavir inhibits only CYP3A4 and not CYP2D6 enzyme. Hence, ritonavir does not interfere with plasma level of active metabolite M8. Hence, coadministration of ritonavir with nelfinavir is not advantageous. Besides, nelfinavir is associated with watery diarrhea and glucose intolerance.

Drug of Choice: Lopinavir

RATIONALE

It is mandatory for all HIV infected TB patients to be treated with ART irrespective of CD4 count. Protease inhibitors are part of combination therapy in such patients. Ritonavir increases the level of lopinavir by inhibiting CYP3A4 involved in its metabolism. **Oral administration** of **ritonavir-lopinavir** in the ratio of **1:4** results in **plasma concentration ratio** of **1:20**. Hence, lopinavir is **more suitable** for **coadministration** with ritonavir as 'dual protease inhibitor' but since the risk of hepatotoxicity is high with this combination, therapy should be given under close observation. **Nelfinavir** is the **only protease inhibitor** that is **not influenced** by **ritonavir**. It is **metabolized** by **both CYP3A4 and CYP2D6** and **does not undergo pharmacokinetic enhancement** by ritonavir. Hence, ritonavir offers no additional advantage to nelfinavir. Nelfinavir is associated with watery diarrhea, glucose intolerance and abnormalities in lipid profile. Ritonavir-lopinavir is also associated with diarrhea but the incidence is less common than nelfinavir.

CHAPTER
45

Antifungal Agents

1. *Conventional amphotericin-B (C-AMB)/Liposomal amphotericin-B (L-AMB) for initial therapy of cryptococcal meningitis.*

BACKGROUND

Amphotericin is a systemic antifungal drug used for deep and invasive fungal infections caused by species of *Cryptococcus*, *Histoplasma*, *Aspergillus* and *Blastomyces*. Presently four formulations such as conventional, colloidal dispersion, liposomal and lipid complex of amphotericin B are available for therapy.

LIPOSOMAL AMPHOTERICIN-B (L-AMB)

L-AMB is approved and found to be equieffective to C-AMB in cryptococcosis. It is a small unilamellar vesicle formulation of amphotericin B and available as lyophilized powder that is reconstituted with water before use. When administered IV it attains similar plasma levels to C-AMB with greater clinical efficacy. Since higher doses are tolerated, it can be given at doses much higher than C-AMB. Such doses achieve high tissue concentration mainly in spleen and liver. Infusion-related reactions, hypokalemia, nephrotoxicity are lower than C-AMB. Infusion-related pain in abdomen and other areas can occur after few doses. Azotemia and nephrotoxicity are less common than C-AMB.

CONVENTIONAL AMPHOTERICIN-B (C-AMB)

Conventional amphotericin B (C-AMB) is insoluble in water and combined with bile salt deoxycholate and given as lyophilized powder.

Filters in IV set block entry of particles with diameter more than 0.22 µm. Since C-AMB is a colloid with high particle size it is blocked by filters in IV infusion reducing its plasma concentration and efficacy. Electrolytes added to infusion can cause aggregation of colloids. Besides, infusion mediated effects such as fever, chills, hypotension or hypoxia is high and the incidence of azotemia, nephrotoxicity is also high. Hence, it is less preferred to L-AMB in cryptococcal meningitis.

Drug of Choice: Liposomal Amphotericin-B (L-AMB)

RATIONALE

L-AMB is **equieffective** to C-AMB in cryptococcosis. It is a small unilamellar vesicle formulation of amphotericin B and available as lyophilized powder that is reconstituted with water before use and intravenous administration results in **higher plasma levels** when compared to C-AMB. It is **well tolerated** with minimal incidence of infusion related reactions, azotemia and nephrotoxicity. **C-AMB** is a colloid preparation with **bigger particle size** and can **get blocked by filters** in IV infusion set **reducing its plasma concentration** and the efficacy. Hence, L-AMB is preferred to C-AMB although it causes higher rate of infusion mediated side effects, azotemia and nephrotoxicity.

2. *Liposomal amphotericin B (L-AMB)/Flucytosine for initial manage- ment of cryptococcal meningitis.*

BACKGROUND

Cryptococcosis is caused by yeast *Cryptococcus neoformans*. Lung infection remains localized and heals in immunocompetent patients but in immunocompromised patients it disseminates quite often. Dissemination can occur in any organ but meningitis is more com- mon. Azoles are not preferred in initial therapy due to lower efficacy.

LIPOSOMAL AMPHOTERICIN B (L-AMB)

Lyophilized powder releases amphotericin that is 90% bound to proteins. Liposomal amphotericin B at 3 to 4 mg/kg is very effective in cryptococcal meningitis. In 70% patients it improves clinical symptoms and causes cerebrospinal fluid (CSF) sterilization. It binds with ergosterol, the sterol moiety of fungal cell membrane forming pores, increasing cellular permeability and causing leakage of small cellular molecules. It can cause moderate infusion related chills, tachypnea and azotemia.

FLUCYTOSINE

Flucytosine is a fluorinated pyrimidine that impairs DNA synthesis. It either gets incorporated into RNA inhibiting thymidylate synthetase. UPRTase or uracil phosphoribosyltransferase converts flucytosine to its active metabolite. It is clinically active against *Cryptococcus neoformans* so useful in cryptococcosis. Monotherapy with flucytosine is not superior to monotherapy with amphotericin B as drug resistance is the main cause for therapeutic failure. Secondary resistance is due to loss of permease activity or reduced activity of UPRTase can also occur. Combination of amphotericin B and flucytosine improves survival rate but causes toxicity as flucytosine causes bone marrow depression. Other side effects are rash vomiting, diarrhea and severe enterocolitis.

Drug of Choice: Liposomal Amphotericin B (L-AMB)

RATIONALE

In immunodeficient individuals cryptococcal infection can disseminate into meningitis. Liposomal amphotericin-B **(L-AMB)** is very **effective** at the dose of 3 to 4 mg/kg. Infusion related reactions are minimal in liposomal preparation. It binds to ergosterol, damages cellular membranes causing leakage of cellular contents. **Monotherapy** with **flucytosine** is **inferior** to monotherapy with amphotericin B and its therapeutic failure is due to **drug resistance**. Secondary resistance occurs due to loss of permease activity or reduced activity of UPRTase. Besides it causes **bone marrow depression**. **Coadministration** of amphotericin B and flucytosine **improves survival rate** but also **potentiates toxicity**. Hence, flucytosine is neither preferred for monotherapy or as adjunct for amphotericin B.

3. *Fluconazole/Itraconazole in mucosal (oropharyngeal and vulvo-vaginal) candidiasis.*

BACKGROUND

Candida albicans is a normal flora but an opportunistic pathogen. Oropharyngeal and vulvovaginal candidiasis are two manifestations of mucosal form of candidiasis. Esophageal candidiasis is the most frequent form of oropharyngeal candidiasis. Vulvovaginal candidiasis occurs in two thirds of women during their life time. Few risk factors are pregnancy, uncontrolled diabetes mellitus and chronic steroid use. It causes severe pruritus, vaginal discharge, pain and dyspareunia. Invasive candidiasis is common among those treated with broad spectrum antibiotics, prolonged neutropenia, renal disease and recent abdominal surgery. Mucocutaneous disease occurs due to cellular immunodeficiency. If condition is less severe and patients are able to swallow then oral therapy is given. When compared to imidazoles, triazoles do not affect host cells, so they are preferred. They have a lower affinity to host cell sterol in contrast to imidazole antifungals.

FLUCONAZOLE

Fluconazole is a triazole, very effective against *Candida* species and against all forms of mucosal candidiasis including urinary tract candidiasis. It interferes with synthesis of ergosterol in cell membrane inhibiting the growth. Fluconazole tablets at the dose of 200 mg on day 1 and subsequently 100 mg for 10 to 14 days is very effective. It is completely absorbed from GIT with 90% bioavailability and is not altered by food or gastric acidity. Both oral and parenteral administration attains similar concentration. Distribution of fluconazole into body fluids and tissues is consistently high as the drug diffuses freely into body fluids higher concentrations are seen in saliva. Prolonged elimination half-life of 25 to 30 hours makes it suitable for once daily dosing and a single 150 mg oral dose is highly effective in vulvovaginal candidiasis. It has to be repeated every week to prevent recurrence. Ninety percent of its elimination is through renal route so it is also effective in urinary tract candidiasis. Daily dose of 100 to 200 mg reduces candiduria in candidiasis of urinary tract. It inhibits both CYP3A4 and CYP2C9 hence prone for more drug interactions but it is preferred due to its safety, cost and extensive usage.

ITRACONAZOLE

Itraconazole is also a triazole with similar advantages. Absorption is improved if oral solution of itraconazole is given on empty stomach but its tissue concentration is very high especially in skin and nails. Hence, it is more suitable for treatment of dermatomycosis and onychomycosis. It is effective in esophageal and vulvovaginal but not in urinary tract candidiasis. It is both substrate and inhibitor of CYP3A4 so prone for lesser drug interactions. Itraconazole and its active metabolite attain equal concentration and 99% protein bound. Its plasma concentration reaches steady-state concentration after 4 days. The time required for its active metabolite to reach steady-state level is 7 days. Neither the drug nor its active metabolite is present in urine so, it is ineffective in the treatment of urinary tract candidiasis. Itraconazole is equieffective to fluconazole in esophageal candidiasis. 70% of fluconazole resistant strains are susceptible to itraconazole. So, itraconazole is reserved as second line drug for fluconazole resistant candidiasis. 100 mg (10 mL) solution once daily should be swished aggressively before swallowing for topical action. Itraconazole results in more GIT side effects such as diarrhea, anorexia and GIT cramps. Hepatotoxicity is high, so it is reserved for persons who do not respond to fluconazole.

Drug of Choice: Fluconazole

RATIONALE

Being an opportunistic pathogen *Candida albicans* often results in disseminated infections in immunodeficiency states. Broad spectrum antibiotic therapy, prolonged neutropenia, renal diseases and recent abdominal surgery can all promote invasive candidiasis. Most common oropharyngeal candidiasis is esophageal candidiasis. Vulvovaginal candidiasis is frequent occurrence during pregnancy and in those with uncontrolled diabetes mellitus or in persons taking corticosteroids. Being triazoles, both fluconazole and itraconazole do not affect host cell sterol synthesis and are more selective in candidiasis. **Fluconazole** is **effective** against **all forms** of **mucosal candidiasis**, is **completely absorbed** irrespective of the presence of food. It is **well distributed** in tissues and body fluids such as **saliva** with prolonged excretion half-life. **Single oral** dose of fluconazole is highly effective in **vulvovaginal** candidiasis but it has to be **repeated** weekly to prevent **recurrence** in **vaginal candidiasis**. **Itraconazole** is **equally effective, less prone for drug interactions** but **causes more GIT side effects** when given as **oral** solution **in esophageal candidiasis**. **Fluconazole** is **first line** drug on account of its well known **efficacy and safety**.[93] Non-responsive candidiasis encountered in HIV patients respond well to itraconazole although its efficacy in other forms of mucosal candidiasis is not equivalent to fluconazole. Hence, itraconazole is reserved for those patients who do not respond to fluconazole.

4. *Itraconazole/Ketoconazole in non-meningococcal localized histoplasmosis.*

BACKGROUND

Histoplasmosis is caused by the organism *Histoplasma capsulatum*. Organism is engulfed by phagocytes in lungs and undergoes proliferation. These organisms spread from lungs to other areas through lymphohematogenous route and one such form is acute pulmonary histoplasmosis. Clinically it can manifest as mild flu-like state or as severe pneumonia, in HIV patients, progressive disseminated histoplasmosis can occur. Chronic pulmonary histoplasmosis occurs in persons with chronic lung disease. Granulomatous mediastinitis is the common complication.

ITRACONAZOLE

Itraconazole is a triazole which inhibits the ergosterol synthesis of these organisms, when compared to ketoconazole it has a broader spectrum of antifungal activity and is the drug of choice in non-meningeal localized histoplasmosis. Duration of therapy ranges from weeks to months depending upon severity. Generally 200 to 400 mg daily in divided doses is very effective. Oral solution has better bioavailability than capsules and capsule formulation requires acidic gastric pH for better absorption, so should be given in empty stomach.

KETOCONAZOLE

Ketoconazole is a broad spectrum antifungal imidazole effective in deep mycosis caused by *Candida, Coccidioides, Cryptococcus, Histoplasma* and *Aspergillus*. Being an imidazole it is not selective and interferes with host sterol synthesis. The only advantage of ketoconazole against itraconazole is its low cost. It causes gynecomastia, oligozoospermia, alopecia and loss of libido. Hence, it has been totally replaced by itraconazole as it is more effective and less toxic.

Drug of Choice: Itraconazole

RATIONALE

Itraconazole is used in non-meningeal localized form of histoplasmosis. The duration of therapy varies according to severity of condition. It has **good bioavailability** when given as oral solution. **Ketoconazole** is an imidazole, **interferes** with **host cell sterol synthesis**. Although it is **cheaper** than itraconazole it **more toxic** and causes gynecomastia, oligozoospermia, loss of libido and hair. Hence, itraconazole is preferred to ketoconazole.

5. *Voriconazole/Posaconazole in life-threatening invasive aspergillosis.*

BACKGROUND

Aspergillosis is most commonly caused by *Aspergillus fumigatus* involving lungs, sinuses and brain. The organism causes life threatening invasive form in immunodeficient individuals with prolonged neutropenia or chronic granulomatous disease and in those who have undergone recent hematopoietic stem cell transplantation.

These patients are exposed to steroid therapy and have leucopenia with a higher risk for CMV infection. From its source, the infection disseminates through circulation to CNS, skin and other areas. Early diagnosis is possible through estimation of 'galactomannan' levels in serum.

VORICONAZOLE

Voriconazole, a triazole has wider spectrum but poor aqueous solubility. It has 96% oral bioavailability, 56% protein binding and half-life extends to 6 hours. It is metabolized by CYPs 2C19, 2C9 and 3A4 hence, prone for many drug interactions. Generally well tolerated but can cause hepatotoxicity and *torsades de pointes*. Rapid IV administration of voriconazole 6 mg/kg twice is given on first day and subsequently reduced to 4 mg/kg every 12 hours till patient stabilizes. It should not be given IV in patients with impaired renal function due to accumulation of SBECD, a sulfobutyl ether β-cyclodextrin, a compound present in its IV formulation. Oral voriconazole is given as step down regimen following intravenous administration.

POSACONAZOLE

Posaconazole has prolonged terminal phase half-life of 25 to 31 hours. It has increased activity against *Aspergillus fumigatus* with higher clinical efficacy. It is given orally at the dose of 300 mg twice daily on day one and 300 mg once daily thereafter. If given four times daily it takes 7 to 10 days to attain steady-state concentration due to which its peak clinical action is delayed when given through oral route. Besides, posaconazole is not available as intravenous formulation. So, it has questionable clinical utility in emergencies like life-threatening aspergillosis. Hence, it is approved only for salvage therapy in mucormycosis due to its efficacy.

Drug of Choice: Voriconazole

RATIONALE

In immunocompromised persons, aspergillosis disseminates to form life-threatening infection and intravenous formulations are required for quick clinical benefit in such emergency situations. Although **posaconazole** is very effective with **higher efficacy** against *Aspergillus fumigatus* it is **not preferred** in life-threatening invasive aspergillosis as it is **not available** as **intravenous** formulation. When administered through oral route it takes 7 to 10 days to achieve steady-state concentration as it has wide volume of distribution. Hence, it is only approved as **last resort drug** for **salvage therapy** in **mucormycosis**. **Voriconazole IV** is the drug of choice and effectively tides over the situation. It is then given orally as a step down regime. Voriconazole is generally **well tolerated** but can cause **hepatotoxicity** and *torsades de pointes*.

6. *Caspofungin/Micafungin in azoles resistant disseminated Candida albicans infection.*

BACKGROUND

Disseminated candidiasis can vary from mild fever to severe septic shock. Skin lesions occur commonly but liver, spleen, kidney, eyes and heart can be involved. Diagnosis is difficult as blood culture for organism is positive only in 50% of cases. Management of disseminated candidiasis is individualized for each patient. For those with previous azoles exposure in recent past, fluconazole is ineffective.

MICAFUNGIN

Micafungin is equally effective as caspofungin in resistant candidiasis. Micafungin is given at 100 mg intravenously daily for two weeks. Increase in dose and frequency does not offer any significant clinical improvement. Abnormal liver function with increased levels of serum alkaline phosphatase can occur. It can cause allergy, rash, nausea, constipation, hypokalemia and rarely leucopenia but the intensity of these side effects is minimal. So, it is preferred.

CASPOFUNGIN

Caspofungin is a semisynthetic lipopeptide with good aqueous solubility. It has high efficacy against *Candida* species and

Aspergillus species. It is used as salvage therapy in invasive aspergillosis for those intolerant to first line drugs. Since it has poor oral bioavailability it is given as IV formulation. It has extensive 95% protein binding and half-life of about 10 hours. It is unable to cross BBB and has minimal CSF concentration. Caspofungin also causes similar side effects with higher intensity. Azoles resistant *Candida* species is highly susceptible to caspofungin IV, loading dose is 70 mg once daily and then 50 mg daily for 2 weeks.

Drug of Choice: Micafungin

RATIONALE

Management of disseminated candidiasis is individualized for each patient. Diagnosis is often difficult as blood culture is positive in only 50% of patients. Caspofungin and micafungin have high cure rates in azoles resistant invasive candidiasis[94] as the organisms are highly susceptible but the **intensity** and **frequency** of **side effects** are **more severe** with **caspofungin**. Hence, micafungin is preferred to caspofungin.

7. *Liposomal amphotericin B (L-AMB)/Fluconazole for treatment of febrile neutropenia in patients not responding to antibiotics.*

BACKGROUND

In febrile neutropenia 'absolute neutrophils count' or (ANC) is less than 500/µL. Antifungal agents should be withheld till patients are categorized under high risk group.[95] Such patients remain febrile even after 5 to 7 days treatment with broad spectrum antibiotics. Patients with profound neutropenia and comorbidities require intravenous empiric therapy and kept under close observation. Low risk patients have febrile neutropenia of less than 7 days duration but no comorbidity. They require oral therapy but need close monitoring at least once in 3 days. Each patient needs to be assessed for risk of complication due to severe infection. Appropriate risk assessment determines type (oral/IV) and duration of empiric therapy. Empiric antifungal treatment is not advised routinely but only in select cases. Despite overall risk, empiric therapy with antifungals is a valid and safe approach.[96]

FLUCONAZOLE

Fluconazole is effective in patients who have not been exposed to long-term azoles. Loading dose of 800 mg IV followed by maintenance dose of 400 mg is effective. Dose exceeding 400 mg causes dose related nausea, headache, skin rash and alopecia. Unlike L-AMB it does not cause neutropenia even as a rare side effect.[97] It is generally avoided in severe aspergillosis as posaconazole is more effective but posaconazole is not approved for initial therapy and reserved for salvage therapy. It is equieffective to L-AMB and causes minimal adverse effects so preferred.

LIPOSOMAL AMPHOTERICIN B (L-AMB)

L-AMB is often given as empirical therapy in high risk patients. It is given IV in patients with fever and profound neutropenia. It is active against species of *Coccidioides*, *Sporothrix*, *Histoplasma* and *Blastomyces* but few strains of *Candida* species and *Aspergillus* species have developed resistance.[98] An IV dose of 3–5 mg/kg is effective in high risk febrile neutropenia. It can cause infusion-related reactions such as fever, chills and hypotension. Renal tubular acidosis, hypokalemia and hypomagnesemia are less frequent. Although rare L-AMB itself can cause neutropenia, so has to be used cautiously.

Drug of Choice: Fluconazole

RATIONALE

In febrile neutropenia, antifungal agents are given after broad spectrum antibiotics have failed. **L-AMB has wide spectrum** of antifungal activity **but few strains** of *Candida* and *Aspergillus* have **developed resistance**. It causes severe infusion-related side effects and rare incidence of neutropenia. Hence, it has to be monitored carefully. **Fluconazole** is effective in patients not exposed to azoles earlier. When compared to L-AMB, it is **equally effective** and is much **safer**. So, fluconazole is preferred to L-AMB.

8. *Terbinafine/Itraconazole in onychomycosis (Tinea unguium).*

BACKGROUND

Onychomycosis is nail infection caused by *Trichophyton* species. More commonly it is caused by *T. rubrum*, less frequently by *T. interdigitale*. Nail becomes thickened, discolored and brittle as infection progresses. It is difficult to treat onychomycosis and prolonged therapy is required and recurrences are frequent. Fingernails respond better than toe nails and systemic therapy is more effective but topical application has limited value. Clinical improvement occurs in 75% of patients.[99] Cure rate for toenails is only 50% but cure rate is generally very high for fingernails and they can be cured completely. Since risk of hepatotoxicity for ketoconazole is high, it is not recommended. In case of griseofulvin, it has to be given for long time but still the cure rate is only 30 to 40%.

TERBINAFINE

Terbinafine accumulates in skin and nails and persists there for long period. It inhibits squalene epoxidase required for conversion of squalene to its epoxide which is necessary for biosynthesis of ergosterol of fungal cell membrane. It is both fungistatic and fungicidal so minimal inhibitory concentration is very low. It is fungistatic due to ergosterol depletion and fungicidal due to accumulation of squalene. It is the most active currently available antidermatophyte agent with 76% cure rate.[100] Terbinafine is given orally in the dose of 250 mg daily for 6 weeks.

ITRACONAZOLE

Itraconazole is mainly fungistatic but can achieve fungicidal concentration. Itraconazole is also highly concentrated in nails and skin for long period. When compared to terbinafine the MIC required for itraconazole is 10 times higher. It has moderate efficacy with cure rate around 63% only. Itraconazole at the dose of 400 mg daily orally for seven days is given monthly for a period of two months then reduced as 200 mg daily for two months for effective response. Drug interactions with coadministered drugs and risk of hepatotoxicity are high.

Drug of Choice: Terbinafine

RATIONALE

Onychomycosis is best treated with drugs that concentrate highly in nails for long period. Terbinafine and itraconazole can both accumulate in nails. **Terbinafine** is **fungistatic** and **fungicidal**, fungistatic as it inhibits ergosterol synthesis, fungicidal as it accumulates squalene. The **cure rate** for terbinafine is **76%** and the **MIC** required is **very low**. **Itraconazole** is generally **fungistatic**, requires **high MIC** and **cure rate is inferior** to terbinafine. Besides, drug interactions and risk of hepatotoxicity are high with Itraconazole. Hence, terbinafine is preferred to itraconazole.

9. *Tolnaftate/Terbinafine in Tinea cruris, Tinea corporis, Tinea pedis and Tinea manus.*

BACKGROUND

T. corporis is body ringworm. *T. cruris* occurs in groin and gluteal regions. *T. pedis* affects soles (athlete's foot) and *T. manus* involves palms. Body ringworm affects exposed area of body such as face and arms. These lesions have sharp margins, clear center with an active scaly periphery.

TERBINAFINE

Terbinafine is effective against dermatophytes and available for topical application. It is fungicidal and results in fast response and high clinical cure when applied once daily. Terbinafine causes most rapid response even when applied for a shorter duration.

TOLNAFTATE

Tolnaftate is equally effective and clinical response occurs within 48 to 72 hours. It has to be applied twice daily with cure rate around 80% in *T. pedis*. Although symptomatic improvement occurs quickly, relapse is common. Hence, it should be continued for long time till the infected tissue sheds off. It can cause irritation and allergic reaction at the site of application, so not preferred.

Drug of Choice: Terbinafine

RATIONALE

Tinea infections have characteristic lesions with sharp margins, clear centers with active spreading scaly peripheries. **Terbinafine** is **very effective** when applied topically **once daily** over the lesions. It is **fungicidal** and results in rapid clinical improvement even when applied for shorter duration. **Tolnaftate** is **equally effective** with **significant clinical response** occurring within 72 hours but has to be applied **twice daily**. If it is not applied until the shedding of infected tissue, it can result in **relapse**. It also causes allergic reactions and irritation at the site of application. Hence, terbinafine is preferred to tolnaftate for Tinea infections.

CHAPTER
46

Anticancer Drugs

1. *Non-cell-cycle specific agents/Cell-cycle specific agents for rapidly growing tumors.*

BACKGROUND

One complete cell cycle consists of four growth phases and one quiescent phase. These phases are required for synthesis of nucleic acid and cell division. All cells, cancer and normal, display similar pattern of progression in cell cycle. In quiescent phase (G_0) cells remain dormant for long periods of time. G_1 phase is the phase prior to synthesis of nucleic acid DNA. S phase is the DNA synthetic phase which involves synthesis of nucleic acid. G_3 indicates interval following DNA synthesis and is the premitotic phase. M or mitotic phase involves mitosis or cell division and formation of daughter cells. The two daughter cells formed enter into G_1 phase and cell cycle is continued. Cyclin dependent kinases are required for cell progression at each transition point.

CELL-CYCLE SPECIFIC AGENTS

Lymphomas and leukemias are rapidly growing tumors with rapid proliferation of cells. Rapidly dividing cells are highly vulnerable for destruction in mitotic phase. So, an anticancer agent that acts on mitotic phase is more effective on these cells. Drugs such as taxanes and vinca alkaloids block formation of functional mitotic spindle. Similarly, drugs that inhibit S phase or DNA synthetic phase are also effective. Purine, pyrimidine and folate anti metabolites and hydroxyurea inhibit S phase. Normal cells of bone marrow, GIT and hair follicles are highly susceptible to these drugs. They are toxic to these cells as they undergo rapid proliferation.

NON-CELL-CYCLE SPECIFIC AGENTS

Some tumors follow slow growth pattern as they do not multiply rapidly. Such tumors express only small population of cells at any given time. Carcinomas of colon and non-small cell cancer of lung belong to this category. These tumors do not respond or poorly respond to cell-cycle specific drugs. They are amenable only to cytotoxic drugs such as alkylating agents that damage DNA. They also respond to fluoropyrimidines that accumulate within cells. Alkylating agents, nitrosoureas, procarbazine and platinum derivatives are nonspecific to cell cycle. These drugs crosslink, damage or intercalate with DNA so effective on slow tumors.

Drug of Choice: Cell-Cycle Specific Agents

RATIONALE

Although cancer cells divide rapidly, most tumors vary in their growth pattern. While some tumors are rapidly proliferating with higher growth rate, others are slow growing with smaller growth fraction at a particular time. **Cell-cycle specific agents** are very effective against **rapidly proliferating** cells. Hence, they are very useful in treating **rapidly growing cancers**. **Taxanes** and **vinca alkaloids** act in mitotic phase. Cells of leukemias and lymphoma are highly vulnerable in mitotic phase. Hence, such cancers respond better to these agents. Similarly, S phase specific drugs such as anti metabolites are also effective against rapidly growing cancers. However, they also exert toxicity on normal, rapidly proliferating cells of bone marrow, GIT and hair follicles. Slow growing tumors respond better to non cell-cycle specific agents as these drugs affect DNA by intercalating, cross linking or damaging DNA.

2. *Cyclophosphamide/Ifosfamide as anticancer agent in Hodgkin's lymphoma.*

BACKGROUND

Cyclophosphamide and ifosfamide, the alkylating agents form highly reactive carbonium ion intermediates. These are second-line drugs used in combination therapy for Hodgkin's lymphoma. The active carbonium ion intermediates of these agents link covalently to nucleophilic moieties alkylating the key target N_7 of guanine forming a strong covalent linkage. This causes mispairing and instead of guanine pairing with cytosine it pairs with thymine. Less frequently N_1 and N_3 of adenine and O_6 of guanine can also be alkylated by these agents. These alkylating agents act slowly and cause cytotoxicity by interfering with DNA integrity.

CYCLOPHOSPHAMIDE

Cyclophosphamide is used with other drugs in Hodgkin's and non-Hodgkin's lymphoma. It is also indicated in cancers of breast, ovary and in childhood solid tumors. It is metabolized to aldophosphamide that forms phosphoramide mustard and acrolein. Phosphoramide has antitumor action while acrolein causes hemorrhagic cystitis. Therefore 6-mercaptoethane sulfonate (MESNA) an organosulfur compound, containing SH group that detoxifies acrolein is coadministered to prevent hemorrhagic cystitis. The intensity of myelosuppression, mucosal damage is lower with cyclophosphamide. It is less leukemogenic and unlike ifosfamide causes minimal renal and CNS toxicity.

IFOSFAMIDE

Ifosfamide is an analog of cyclophosphamide but causes more toxicity. Intensity of hemorrhagic cystitis is similar to cyclophosphamide so MESNA is given. It is metabolized to chloracetaldehyde that crosses BBB resulting in severe CNS toxicity. Seizures, ataxia, altered mental status are the CNS manifestations of ifosfamide. It causes irreversible renal damage and acute myelosuppression so, not preferred.

Drug of Choice: Cyclophosphamide

RATIONALE

The therapeutic **efficacy** of cyclophosphamide and ifosfamide are **similar**. They are second-line drugs used in combination regimes in Hodgkin's lymphoma. Incidence of **hemorrhagic cystitis** is **similar** for both drugs hence **coadministration** of **MESNA** is **required**. **Ifosfamide** is highly **neurotoxic** due to its **metabolite chloracetaldehyde**. At higher dosage it causes irreversible renal damage and acute myelosuppression. **Cyclophosphamide** is **less leukemogenic** and **does not cause CNS toxicity** or renal damage with similar intensity. Hence, cyclophosphamide is preferred to ifosfamide for combination regimes.

3. *Neoadjunctive chemotherapy/Adjunctive chemotherapy in stage I and stage II non-small cell carcinoma of lung (NSCLC).*

BACKGROUND

Surgical resection is main line of treatment in stage I and stage II in NSCLC. Without surgical resection cure rate in non-small cell carcinoma is questionable. Limited resection results in three fold recurrence compared to lobectomy. Chemotherapy is not curative but increases overall survival and performance rate.

ADJUNCTIVE CHEMOTHERAPY

Adjunctive chemotherapy means chemotherapy after surgery or radiotherapy. It is found to be effective in delaying recurrences in stage IB and II patients. Combination regimens confer overall survival benefit in such patients. It improves the survival period and quality of life from 5 to 11 months but survival benefit is not reported in patients with poor performance status.

NEOADJUNCTIVE CHEMOTHERAPY

Neoadjunctive chemotherapy means starting drugs before surgery or radiation. Trials indicate that such a therapy does not offer any superior advantage in NSCLC. Neoadjunctive therapy does not increase the survival period of patients. It is seldom indicated for stage I and stage II patients with NSCLC. It is indicated in select patients with stage IIIA and IIIB with NSCLC as these patients are not suitable for surgery due to severity of condition but neoadjunctive chemotherapy along with radiation can improve survival time. In few other cancers it is very essential to start neoadjuvant chemotherapy. In prostate cancer it is effective in high-risk patients and in breast cancer it is vital before surgery. In these conditions, neoadjunctive chemotherapy shrinks tumor size and prolongs survival rate by preventing disease progression.

Drug of Choice: Adjunctive Chemotherapy

RATIONALE

Neoadjunctive chemotherapy is given prior to surgery or radiotherapy. Adjunctive chemotherapy is given after surgery or radiotherapy. In NSCLC, **neoadjunctive chemotherapy does not benefit patients in stage I and II**. It is **only indicated** for patients with **advanced** condition with **stage IIIA or IIIB** who are **unsuitable for surgery**. In such patients it can be given prior to radiotherapy but **neoadjunctive chemotherapy** is **most essential in breast cancer** as it **shrinks tumor size** hampering progression of disease and **improving survival rate** of patients. In **prostate cancer**, it is **effective** in high-risk groups. **Adjunctive** chemotherapy is given for **stage I and II in NSCLC after surgery or radiotherapy**. It improves survival rate and quality of life from 5 to 11 months.

4. *Cisplatin/Carboplatin as adjunctive chemotherapy in non-small cell carcinoma of lung (NSCLC).*

BACKGROUND

The platinum coordination complexes such as cisplatin, carboplatin and oxaliplatin are included in combination regimen for therapy of NSCLC. They improve the survival period in 5% of patients up to five years. These drugs alkylate DNA and have broad antineoplastic activity and used in cancers of ovary, lung, bladder, colon, esophagus, head and neck. Cisplatin and carboplatin are indicated in NSCLC and oxaliplatin is given for colon cancer. Water displaces chloride group of cisplatin and cyclohexane moiety of carboplatin converting them into positively charged active compounds that crosslink with DNA.

CARBOPLATIN

Carboplatin is equieffective to cisplatin, the first platinum coordination complex, in the treatment of NSCLC. Major portion of carboplatin is in unbound form in plasma as it is less reactive. It is well-tolerated and causes less nausea, neurotoxicity, ototoxicity. It also causes intense thrombocytopenia therefore its dose limiting toxicity is myelosuppression. Hypersensitivity to carboplatin can be overcome by giving it in graded doses. Unlike cisplatin, it does not cause refractory nausea, ototoxicity or electrolyte changes. Hence, carboplatin is preferred to cisplatin for combination regimen in NSCLC.

CISPLATIN

Cisplatin is 90% plasma protein bound and remaining 10% is excreted quickly. It accumulates in kidney, liver, testes and intestine and does not effectively cross BBB and so its CSF concentration is very poor. Since it is slowly excreted and excretion is delayed over a period of 5 days it causes nephrotoxicity which can be reduced by amifostine, a thiophosphate. Immediate anaphylaxis can occur after administration of the drug. Its leukemogenic action can cause acute myeloid leukemia up to 4 years or even later. It causes refractory nausea, ototoxicity and severe electrolyte disturbances. It causes unilateral or bilateral tinnitus of intense severity and high frequency hearing loss. Rarely, it causes hyperuricemia, hemolytic anemia and cardiac problems.

Drug of Choice: Carboplatin

RATIONALE

Combination regimens including platinum coordination complexes such as cisplatin and carboplatin improve survival rate of patients with NSCLC up to 5 years. The clinical efficacy of carboplatin in NSCLC is similar to cisplatin. It is **better tolerated** and **does not cause nephrotoxicity**, high frequency hearing loss and refractory nausea but the incidence of **myelosuppression** may be **high. Hypersensitivity** reactions can be overcome by starting therapy with graded doses. **Cisplatin** is **nephrotoxic, ototoxic,** causes intense nausea, anaphylaxis and severe electrolyte disturbances. Hence, it is less preferred to carboplatin for combination regimens in NSCLC.

5. *Pemetrexed/Vinorelbine for non-small cell carcinoma of lung (NSCLC) in combination with cisplatin.*

BACKGROUND

NSCLC is epithelial lung cancer that accounts for 85% of all lung cancers. It is relatively insensitive to chemotherapy compared to small cell cancer. Most common types are squamous cell carcinoma, adenocarcinoma and large cell cancer. Adenocarcinoma accounts for 40% of NSCLC and occurs more commonly in young women and commonly found in outer part of lung. The next frequent type is squamous cell carcinoma with incidence around 25 to 30%. Squamous cell carcinoma occurs in central part of lung. Large cell or undifferentiated cell cancer occurs in 10 to 15% of patients with NSCLC. It can occur at any part of lung and tends to grow very quickly so, difficult to treat. Subtype of large cell cancer is called large cell neuroendocrine cancer. Of all chemotherapeutic agents, platinum coordination complexes are very effective. It is cytotoxic cell-cycle non specific agent so effective in slow growing NSCLC.

VINORELBINE

Vinorelbine a vinca alkaloid inhibits the formation of mitotic spindle. It is cell-cycle specific agent and inhibits mitosis at M phase. Vinorelbine combination with platinum coordination complexes is more effective if started early as it prevents progression of disease. It is given in the dose of 25 mg/m^2 either weekly or three out of every four weeks. In patients with poor performance status it can be given as single agent. When compared to other vinca alkaloids, the incidence of neurotoxicity is minimal but it can cause severe granulocytopenia and modest thrombocytopenia.

PEMETREXED

Pemetrexed is an antimetabolite and folic acid analog that inhibits dihydrofolate reductase. It readily enters tumor cells through folate carrier and also inhibits thymidylate synthase. Pemetrexed thus prevents one carbon transfer reactions necessary for synthesis of DNA. Unpredictable severe myelosuppression limits the use of pemetrexed. It also causes alopecia and 40% of patients suffer from erythematous and pruritic rash.

Drug of Choice: Vinorelbine

RATIONALE

Eighty five percent of lung cancers are of non-small cell lung carcinoma. It presents in four forms, adenomatous, squamous and 2 types of large cell carcinoma. Combination of **vinorelbine** and **platinum coordination complexes** is clinically **more active** and **well-tolerated**. In patients unable to tolerate cisplatin or carboplatin it is effective if given as monotherapy. Vinorelbine is **least neurotoxic** among vinca alkaloids but can cause granulocytopenia. **Pemetrexed** is a folate analog and acts by inhibiting DHFRase and thymidylate synthase. It is very effective but it causes **unpredictable** severe **myelodepression that limits its use**. Hence, vinorelbine is preferred on account of its efficacy and safety.

6. *Methotrexate/Etoposide in acute lymphoblastic leukemia (ALL).*

BACKGROUND

Eighty percent of all childhood leukemias are mainly acute lymphoblastic leukemia and peak incidence occurs in children in the age group between 3 and 7 years of age. Although seen only in 20% of adults, myeloblastic leukemia is the predominant type in adults and adequate chemotherapy causes complete remission in 90% of individuals.

METHOTREXATE

Methotrexate, the folate analog is a critical drug in the treatment of ALL in children. It is of limited use in adults suffering from acute myeloblastic leukemia. High dose methotrexate induces prolonged remission with rare recurrence. It reaches high steady state concentration and therefore associated with lower relapse rate. Leucovorin is coadministered to prevent the toxic effects of methotrexate. Although myelosuppression induced by methotrexate is reversible within two weeks high dose causes nephrotoxicity, alopecia and allergic interstitial pneumonitis.

ETOPOSIDE

Epipodophyllotoxin etoposide has significant therapeutic activity in pediatric leukemia. Etoposide inhibits topoisomerase II complex preventing re-sealing of DNA break. It causes leucopenia, nausea, stomatitis, hepatitis or reversible nausea. It is leukemogenic and causes acute nonlymphocytic leukemia within one to three years with variable cytological appearance. It may be either monocytic or monomyelocytic type and occurs among children treated with etoposide for acute lymphoblastic leukemia. It should not be included as therapy for ALL due to its leukemogenic action.

Drug of Choice: Methotrexate

RATIONALE

The incidence of acute lymphoblastic leukemia is 80% among childhood leukemias and children between three and seven years of age are affected. **Methotrexate**, the folic acid analog at higher dose results in **higher remission** and **lower recurrence rate**. **Leucovorin**, a fully reduced folate coenzyme is **coadministered** with methotrexate to **prevent** its **toxicity**. Methotrexate can cause **myelosuppression** that is **reversible** within two weeks after stopping therapy but high dose can result in nephrotoxicity, interstitial pneumonitis and alopecia. **Etoposide** has therapeutic activity against childhood leukemia but if given in acute lymphoblastic leukemia it **causes** an **unusual** type of leukemia, the **nonlymphocytic leukemia** that occurs within a period of one to three years after stopping therapy. The cytological appearance is variable and presents as either monocytic or monomyelocytic type. It should never be given in ALL due to its leukemogenic action occurring at a very short time interval.

7. *Chlorambucil/Fludarabine in chronic lymphocytic leukemia (CLL).*

BACKGROUND

Chronic lymphocytic leukemia mainly involves B lymphocytes where small lymphocytes with longer survival period accumulate gradually. Ninety percent of CLL occurs after 50 years of age and these cells are immunodeficient. Eighty percent of patients present with lymphocytosis and 50% with enlargement of liver or spleen. CLL generally follows slow course but sometimes may follow aggressive course. Prolymphocytic leukemia, a variant of CLL progresses much more rapidly.

FLUDARABINE

Fludarabine is a cytotoxic agent and effective against CLL and low-grade lymphoma. It is purine antagonist and inhibits DNA polymerase, DNA primase and DNA ligase. It is equally effective through oral and intravenous routes and effective both as monotherapy as well as combination therapy in CLL. As single agent the response rate in previously untreated patients is 80%. Combination of fludarabine with alkylating agents is synergistic because it prevents repair of DNA damage induced by alkylating agents. Myelosuppression, nausea and vomiting are few common adverse effects. An infrequent complication is 'tumor lysis syndrome' due to rapid destruction of cells where release of intracellular ions and metabolic by-products from destroyed cells can occur. Hyperuricemia, hyperkalemia, hypocalcemia and hypophosphatemia develop rapidly.

CHLORAMBUCIL

Chlorambucil is an alkylating agent and is clinically effective against CLL. It exerts cytotoxic action on bone marrow, lymphoid organs and epithelial tissues. It is administered orally and is generally well tolerated at small doses. It is given once a day for a period of 3 to

6 weeks and induces a fall in peripheral leucocyte count. Being an alkylating agent, it acts slowly and results in gradual clinical improvement. It causes myelosuppression that is reversible, pulmonary fibrosis and hepatotoxicity. It is leukemogenic and increases incidence of acute myelocytic leukemia.

Drug of Choice: Fludarabine

RATIONALE

CLL generally follows a slow course, but can also be aggressive. **Chlorambucil** is very **effective** against CLL and causes gradual clinical improvement **but** it is **leukemogenic** and increases the incidence of acute myelocytic leukemia in patients. Hence, it is **not preferred**. Although **fludarabine** is effective as **monotherapy** in CLL, **combination** therapy with **alkylating agents** is **more effective** because this **synergistic** combination prevents repair of DNA damage caused by alkylating agents. It is well-tolerated but **rarely** can cause **'tumor lysis syndrome'**. Fludarabine is preferred to chlorambucil due to its therapeutic superiority as well as tolerability. Besides, unlike chlorambucil, it is not leukemogenic.

8. *Temozolomide/Carmustine as monotherapy in malignant glioma in addition to radiation therapy.*

BACKGROUND

Around 50% of intracranial tumors belong to the category of gliomas and the remaining tumors may be adenomas, meningiomas or neurofibromas. Therapy depends on site and type of tumors and is also based on patient's condition. Radiation therapy increases median survival rates in malignant gliomas but long-term neurocognitive deficits may complicate radiation therapy. Chemotherapy in combination with radiotherapy provides additional benefit.

TEMOZOLOMIDE

Temozolomide is a standard agent used in combination with radiation therapy in malignant glioma. It is commonly used in glioma through both oral and intravenous route. It undergoes nonenzymatic activation to a triazine methyl-triazeno-imidazole-carboxamide (MTIC) that has significant clinical activity against glioma. It causes mild myelosuppression which is reversible within one to two weeks. Nausea and vomiting persist up to 12 hours after discontinuation in 90% patients.

CARMUSTINE

Nitrosoureas carmustine and lomustine are highly lipophilic agents. Hence they cross BBB, attain high concentration in CSF and are effective in brain tumors. These agents are bifunctional alkylating agents having two 2-chloroethyl active groups. Carmustine breaks down to a highly reactive intermediate 2-chloroethyldiazonium ion and alkylates DNA at guanine O_6 instead of guanine N_7. It also alkylates cytidine as well as adenine bases forming inter and intrastrand crosslink with DNA. Hence, carmustine is effective in inhibiting 30% of malignant glioma. Being lipophilic, it is unstable in aqueous solution and disappears from plasma quickly. Even a single dose of carmustine results in profound and delayed myelosuppression.

Drug of Choice: Temozolomide

RATIONALE

Fifty percent of intracranial tumors are malignant gliomas. Radiation therapy is the primary treatment for gliomas but combined chemotherapy provides additional advantage. **Carmustine** is a nitrosourea and **bifunctional** alkylating agent. It is highly lipophilic and enters CSF within 90 minutes of administration. It alkylates guanine O_6 instead of guanine N_7 but it causes severe, progressive and **delayed myelosuppression** hence is being **replaced by temozolomide** in the treatment of glioma. Temozolomide gets converted to its triazine intermediate methyl-triazeno-imidazole-carboxamide (MTIC) that exerts antineoplastic activity against glioma. It causes only **mild reversible myelosuppression**. Hence, temozolomide is preferred in glioma as single chemotherapeutic agent in addition to radiation therapy.

9. *Dacarbazine/Procarbazine in Hodgkin's lymphoma.*

BACKGROUND

Hodgkin's lymphoma is characterized by 'Reed-Sternberg' cells derived from B lymphocytes. It has 'bi-modal' age distribution and occurs either in twenties or after 50 years of age. It starts within single lymph node and spreads to neighboring nodes in an orderly fashion. Dissemination to other areas through circulation occurs only at late stages. Chemotherapy is the mainstay of treatment in Hodgkin's lymphoma. Prognosis is excellent for stage IA and IIA with 90% survival rate up to 10 years.

DACARBAZINE

Dacarbazine, the triazine derivative acts after its conversion to its active metabolite, methyl-triazeno-imidazole-carboxamide (MTIC) which is clinically active. Its primary clinical indication is combination therapy in Hodgkin's lymphoma ABVD or doxorubicin (adriamycin), bleomycin, vinblastine and dacarbazine. It induces nausea and vomiting that continues for around 12 hours after stopping therapy. Mild reversible myelosuppression is common while hepatotoxicity and alopecia are rare.

PROCARBAZINE

Procarbazine is a methyl hydrazine derivative rarely used now-a-days in Hodgkin's disease and is activated by CYP mediated hepatic metabolic pathway to active metabolites causing chromosomal damage and resulting in anticancer action. Since it is slow acting, DNA repair enzymes can reverse the damage induced by the drug leading to quick development of resistance and contributes to therapeutic failure. Common toxicities are nausea, vomiting, reversible leucopenia and thrombocytopenia. It is highly mutagenic, carcinogenic and causes antabuse like reaction. It is associated with higher toxicity and lack of definitive survival advantage. Hence, it is seldom used as combination therapy in Hodgkin's lymphoma.

Drug of Choice: Dacarbazine

RATIONALE

Hodgkin's lymphoma presents as 'bi-modal' fashion with peak occurrence in two age groups either at twenties or after 50 years. It often presents as painless lymph node that enlarges and spreads to nearby lymph nodes. 'Reed-Sternberg' cells are derived from B lymphocytes and are the characteristic feature in Hodgkin's lymphoma. Chemotherapy is the main line of management in Hodgkin's lymphoma. ABVD combination regimen includes **dacarbazine** as the primary drug. Its **metabolite** methyl-triazeno-imidazole-carboxamide (MTIC) is **clinically active**. It causes mild reversible myelosuppression. **Procarbazine** is **seldom used** now-a-days due to its **high toxicity** and **lack of definitive survival advantage**. **Resistance** to procarbazine **develops quickly** and this adds to its therapeutic failure. Besides it is **highly mutagenic** and **carcinogenic**. It causes antabuse-like reaction in those consuming alcohol.

10. *Doxorubicin/Idarubicin in acute myeloid leukemia (AML).*

BACKGROUND

Anthracycline antibiotics are derived from fungus *Streptomyces peucetius*. Structurally they contain tetracyclic ring attached to sugar daunosamine. They intercalate with DNA inhibiting transcription and replication. They form complexes with topoisomerase II and prevent re-ligation of DNA strand reducing DNA repair and replication leading to apoptosis of cancer cells. Quinone and hydroquinone moieties in their structure either gain or lose electrons thereby generating free radicals.

IDARUBICIN

Idarubicin is an analog of doxorubicin with half-life of 15 hours and it is given as slow intravenous infusion extending for 10 to 15 minutes. The active metabolite idarubicinol has significant clinical anticancer activity. It enhances long-term efficacy of coadministered drugs in combination regimen. It is combined with cytosine arabinoside for the treatment of AML. It is the least cardiotoxic drug among anthracyclines.[101] Hence, it is preferred.

DOXORUBICIN

Doxorubicin follows multiphasic pattern of clearance with terminal half-life of 30 hours. It is used in induction and consolidation therapy for AML with cytosine arabinoside. Doxorubicin causes 'adriamycin flare', an erythema at infusion site and the most important long-term toxicity of doxorubicin is cardiomyopathy. It can manifest as acute toxicity with ST or T wave abnormalities and arrhythmias. The chronic, cumulative, dose mediated toxicity is congestive cardiac failure.

Drug of Choice: Idarubicin

RATIONALE

Anthracyclines are naturally occurring anticancer agents and are derived from *Streptomyces peucetius*. They intercalate with DNA inhibiting transcription and replication as they form complex with topoisomerase II and prevents religation of DNA strand. Although **doxorubicin** is effective when given along with cytosine arabinoside it is **highly toxic**. It causes 'adriamycin flare' as well as acute and chronic cardiac toxicity. **Idarubicin**, an analog of doxorubicin enhances **long-term efficacy** of coadministered drugs. Its active metabolite idarubicinol accumulates in plasma and exerts significant anticancer activity. It is **least cardiotoxic**, improves efficacy of combination regimen,[102] so preferred.

11. *Oxaliplatin/Irinotecan for colon cancer along with 5-Fluorouracil + leucovorin.*

BACKGROUND

Colorectal carcinoma is second leading cause of death in the world. It is mostly of adenocarcinomatous type and arises from adenomatous or serrated polyps which may be of tubular, villous and tubulovillous type. Serrated polyps can be hyperplastic, traditional serrated and sessile serrated. A positive family history is reported in 20% of patients suffering from colon cancer.

OXALIPLATIN

Oxalate ligand of oxaliplatin, the platinum coordination complex, is displaced by water and this hydration results in positively charged highly reactive molecule leading to alkylation of guanine N_7. It has brief half-life and is rapidly taken up by tissues but forms DNA adducts slowly. DNA repair in cancer cells is mediated by mismatch repair pathway or MMR. Absence or inactivation by mismatch repair (MMR) pathway increases DNA damage. However, early recognition of DNA adducts is essential for such DNA repair of cancer cells. Since oxaliplatin adducts are bulkier, they are neither recognized nor repaired by MMR system. Hence, it has greater cytotoxicity and better clinical efficacy in colon cancer. It suppresses thymidylate synthetase, the target enzyme of 5-fluorouracil. This combination is synergistic and has greater therapeutic efficacy in colon cancer. FOLFOX is combination of 5-fluorouracil, leucovorin and oxaliplatin. This regimen is found to be effective in 73% of patients with colon cancer. It causes dose limiting reversible neurotoxicity in mouth, throat and lower extremities. It can result in delayed onset leukemia and pulmonary fibrosis even after many months of stopping therapy.

IRINOTECAN

The camptothecin analog irinotecan inhibits function of topoisomerase I. It is converted by carboxylesterases to its active metabolite SN-38. It follows linear pharmacokinetics, results in higher plasma concentration. It also induces *c-fos* and *c-jun* early response genes causing DNA fragmentation. It is S-phase specific and causes irreversible double strand DNA break. Being cell-cycle specific it needs prolonged exposure with cancer cells for cytotoxicity. Prolonged therapy causes lesser toxicity and greater antitumor activity in many patients but in about 35%, irinotecan can cause life-threatening diarrhea. In colon cancer it is given along with 5-fluorouracil + leucovorin as FOLFIRI regimen. Irinotecan is not recommended due to its toxicity that limits its clinical efficacy. Hence, FOLFOX is better than FOLFIRI regimen for colon cancer.

Drug of Choice: Oxaliplatin

RATIONALE

Colon cancer is the second leading cause of death and is mostly of adenomatous type. Family history is present in 20% of patients. FOLFOX and FOLFIRI regimens are both considered to be the first line regimens in colon cancer. FOLFOX contains 5-fluorouracil + leucovorin + oxaliplatin. FOLFIRI regimen is the combination of 5-fluorouracil, leucovorin and irinotecan. **Oxaliplatin** induced DNA damage cannot be repaired by MMR gene and so it exerts **greater clinical activity**. When given with 5-fluorouracil it results in synergistic action by inhibiting thymidylate synthetase, the target enzyme of 5-fluorouracil. Prolonged administration of **low dose irinotecan** results in **lower toxicity** and **greater antitumor activity** in many patients but it can cause **life-threatening diarrhea** in 35% of patients and therefore should be avoided. Hence, oxaliplatin is preferred to irinotecan for combination therapy in colon cancer.

12. *Cetuximab/Panitumumab for metastatic colon cancer.*

BACKGROUND

Epidermal growth factor receptor (EGFR) belongs to ErbB family of receptors. It is known as ErbB1 or HER1 and necessary for growth and differentiation. Ligand binding results in dimerization of EGFR receptor stimulating tyrosine kinase, causing autophosphorylation of tyrosine residues and triggering signaling pathways. Cetuximab and panitumumab are monoclonal antibodies and bind to EGFR.

CETUXIMAB

Cetuximab is a recombinant chimeric antibody and binds to EGFR. It prevents receptor dimerization inhibiting cell growth and differentiation. In addition it also mediates antibody dependent cellular cytotoxicity. It follows non-linear pharmacokinetics, reaches steady-state concentration after 3 weeks. Once EGFR receptor pools are saturated it follows only zero order kinetics. It is approved as single agent for EGFR positive metastatic colon cancer. It is reserved for patients resistant or unable to tolerate FOLFIRI or FOLFOX and improves the survival rate in such patients. Hence it is preferred. Acneform rash, pruritus, nail changes, headache and diarrhea are some of the side effects.

PANITUMUMAB

Panitumumab is a humanized monoclonal antibody that inhibits EGFR but unlike cetuximab it does not promote antibody mediated cytotoxicity. The pharmacokinetics and adverse effects of panitumumab are similar to cetuximab. In patients with metastatic colon cancer, it results in progression free survival period but its clinical efficacy is inferior to cetuximab as it does have an additional mechanism.

Drug of Choice: Cetuximab

RATIONALE

Cetuximab is a chimeric monoclonal antibody while panitumumab is a humanized monoclonal antibody. The pharmacokinetics and adverse effects are similar for both drugs. Cetuximab acts through **two mechanisms**, preventing receptor dimerization, inhibiting cell growth and differentiation. In addition it also mediates antibody dependent cellular cytotoxicity. **Panitumumab** acts by inhibiting EGFR mediated cell growth and differentiation but it **does not** have any **additional mechanism**. Hence, cetuximab is clinically more effective than panitumumab in metastatic colon cancer.

13. *Trastuzumab/Lapatinib in HER2/neu positive breast cancer.*

BACKGROUND

HER2 is a protein called human epidermal growth factor receptor-2 protein that promotes growth and differentiation of cancer cells in HER2 positive breast cancers. Genetic amplification in cancer cells causes excess expression of this protein. HER2 positive breast cancers are generally very aggressive than HER2 negative cancers. These cancers are less likely to be susceptible to hormonal therapy. Recurrence rate is high while response rate is low if treated with standard drugs. Therapy that specifically targets HER2 proteins is very effective in such cancers. The incidence of HER2 positive breast cancer is around 30%. Younger women tend to be more HER2 positive than older women.

LAPATINIB

Lapatinib is a tyrosine kinase inhibitor used in HER2 positive breast cancers. Being a small molecule, lapatinib inhibits tyrosine kinase activity of HER2 receptor. It is clinically superior and effective even in those unresponsive to trastuzumab. It binds and inhibits both ErbB1 and ErbB2 while trastuzumab binds to only ErbB2. Trastuzumab binds to external site while lapatinib binds to internal site of receptor. It inhibits truncated form of HER2 which lacks binding site for trastuzumab. Patients not responding to trastuzumab respond better to lapatinib. Trastuzumab is clinically inferior and lacks the multiple mechanisms of lapatinib. Due to its smaller size lapatinib crosses BBB and reduces the incidence of brain metastasis. Acneform rash, mild diarrhea, cramps and increased esophageal reflux can occur.

TRASTUZUMAB

Trastuzumab is a humanized monoclonal antibody that binds to HER2/neu and is indicated for metastatic breast cancers expressing HER2/neu protein. It is combined with paclitaxel for metastatic or unresponsive breast cancers. It causes infusion mediated effects such as fever, chills but can also cause cardiac failure. Unless cardiac failure is recognized early it can be either disabling or fatal.

Drug of Choice: Lapatinib

RATIONALE

HER2 positive breast cancers are generally very aggressive than HER2 negative cancers and are less likely to be susceptible to hormonal therapy. If given standard therapy the response rate is lower but recurrence rate is higher. Therapy that specifically targets HER2 proteins is very effective in such cancers. Trastuzumab is a humanized monoclonal antibody that binds to HER2/neu. **Lapatinib** binds and **inhibits both ErbB1 and ErbB2** while trastuzumab binds to only ErbB2. The binding of trastuzumab is to external site of receptor but lapatinib binds internally and unlike trastuzumab it inhibits truncated form of HER2 also. Being a **smaller** molecule it crosses BBB and **prevents brain metastasis**. **Trastuzumab** can cause **cardiac failure** that can be fatal if not attended to quickly but lapatinib causes manageable and mild side effects. Hence, lapatinib is preferred to trastuzumab in HER2 positive breast cancer.

14. *Bevacizumab/Sunitinib in clear-cell renal-cell carcinoma.*

BACKGROUND

Clear-cell renal-cell carcinoma arises from epithelial cells of proximal convoluted tubule within renal cortex. It has high propensity for vascular invasion than lymphatic spread. It extends into renal sinus and spreads through renal veins. Clear-cell renal-cell cancer is highly vascular so resistant to routine anticancer drugs and responds promptly to anti-angiogenic drugs. Stimulation of vascular endothelial growth factor (VEGF) prevents cancer cell apoptosis. VEGF inhibitors target pro-angiogenic function of VEGF inhibiting neovascularization. Targeting VEGF in renal cell carcinoma has strong biologic rationale.

SUNITINIB

Sunitinib inhibits binding of ATP to tyrosine kinase site of VEGF-2. It also inhibits protein kinases PDGFR-α, PDGFR-β, RET, CSF-1R and c-KIT. It causes 30% increase in survival rate and inhibits rapid progression of disease. It can be given orally once daily for 4 weeks with drug free interval of two weeks. It can cause bleeding, hypertension, proteinuria, fatigue and hypothyroidism.

BEVACIZUMAB

Bevacizumab is a humanized monoclonal antibody that inhibits angiogenesis. It inhibits VEGF and delays progression of the disease by three months. It is approved for monotherapy in clear-cell renal-cell tumor. Instead of monotherapy if combined with interferon its efficacy is improved. It causes vessel injury, bleeding, poor wound healing, stroke or myocardial infarction.

Drug of Choice: Sunitinib

RATIONALE

Clear-cell renal-cell cancer is highly vascular so resistant to conventional anticancer drugs but responds promptly to antiangiogenic drugs as they specifically inhibit neovascularization. **Sunitinib** is the most effective **antiangiogenic** drug and compared to any other drug in this group, it **prolongs** the **survival period** and **inhibits progression** of disease. Although **bevacizumab** is approved for monotherapy, it is more effective if combined with interferon. The **toxic profile** of bevacizumab is **very high** making it the **lesser preferred** drug compared to sunitinib. Since sunitinib has better efficacy and improves longevity it is preferred.

15. *Thalidomide/Lenalidomide as angiogenesis inhibitor in relapsed/ refractory multiple myeloma (MM).*

BACKGROUND

Vascular endothelial growth factor or VEGF is a potent angiogenic factor. It is an essential growth factor for vascular endothelial cells and is up regulated in many tumors. VEGF is also expressed in non-endothelial cells like macrophages, platelets and mesangial cells. It is also known as vascular permeability factor as it increases angiogenesis in tumors. Thalidomide and lenalidomide have multiple mechanisms of action. They have direct antiproliferative effect promoting apoptosis of tumor cells. They inhibit tumor growth by inhibiting cellular interaction with adhesion molecules. They are antiangiogenic by inhibiting interleukin-6 and tumor necrosis factor-α (TNF-α). They act as immunomodulators by enhancing natural killer and T-cell mediated cytotoxicity.

LENALIDOMIDE

Lenalidomide is effective in both newly diagnosed or refractory or relapsing MM. It causes less severe adverse effects with minimal sedation, neuropathy or constipation. It is safer than thalidomide as it is not teratogenic and may be given during pregnancy.

THALIDOMIDE

Thalidomide is a racemic mixture of S (–) and R (+) enantiomers. Teratogenic property of thalidomide is due to its R (+) enantiomer. S (–) enantiomer is responsible for the sedative activity of thalidomide. It is eliminated by spontaneous clearing through hydrolysis of S (–) form that undergoes elimination more rapidly than R (+) form. It is equally effective against newly diagnosed as well as refractory or relapsed MM. it is well-tolerated but causes sedation and constipation as common side effects. Dose and time dependent peripheral neuropathy occurs mainly in elderly patients. Neuropathy may involve pyramidal tract or may present as carpel tunnel syndrome. It is contraindicated during pregnancy as it is teratogenic and causes phocomelia.

Drug of Choice: Lenalidomide

RATIONALE

In addition to their antiangiogenic action, thalidomide and lenalidomide act through multiple mechanisms. They are immunomodulators, antiproliferators and inhibit cellular interaction with adhesion molecules. Both are effective in newly diagnosed multiple myeloma as well as in relapse. They are also effective in multiple myeloma resistant to other regimens. Although **well-tolerated, thalidomide** can cause common side effects such as sedation, constipation and severe side effects like peripheral **neuropathy**. The severity of peripheral neuropathy depends on duration of treatment and doses used. It **may involve pyramidal tract** or may present as **carpal tunnel syndrome**. Long standing sensory loss may not improve even after discontinuation of drug. It is **teratogenic** and should not be used in pregnant women. **Lenalidomide** is **equally effective** and causes **similar side effects** with minimal intensity. It is **not teratogenic**. Hence, lenalidomide is preferred to thalidomide.

16. *Everolimus/Temsirolimus in renal cell carcinoma.*

BACKGROUND

Everolimus and temsirolimus are mammalian target of rapamycin (mTOR) inhibitors and useful in renal and hepatocellular carcinoma. They inhibit mTORC1 of PI3 kinase pathway and have immunosuppressive action. They are also angiogenesis inhibitors and inhibit cell-cycle progression promoting apoptosis.[103]

EVEROLIMUS

Advantages of everolimus are its quick onset of action and long duration of action. Everolimus requires very short time to attain steady state concentration. Although half-life of everolimus is short, its action is not short lived. If given once weekly it inhibits white cells mTORC1 for about 7 days till the administration of next dose. Everolimus is effective in patients who do not respond to other angiogenesis inhibitors. While temsirolimus is administered intravenously, everolimus can be given orally. It shares similar toxic profile with similar intensity. When compared to temsirolimus the overall survival period is increased because it inhibits further progression of the disease increasing the progression free survival period and improving quality of life.

TEMSIROLIMUS

Temsirolimus prolongs survival period and delays progression of disease. It is metabolized to its active metabolite sirolimus that has longer half-life and equal efficacy in inhibiting mTOR. Half-life of temsirolimus is 30 hours and that of sirolimus is 50 hours. Greater efficacy of sirolimus contributes to improved therapeutic benefit.

Drug of Choice: Everolimus

RATIONALE

Everolimus and temsirolimus are antiangiogenic in nature and inhibit cell-cycle progression promoting apoptosis. They both share similar mechanism of action and toxicity profile. **Everolimus** can be given **orally** but **temsirolimus** requires **intravenous** administration. Given once weekly **everolimus** inhibits mTORC1 till next dose is due, for about 7 days **increasing overall survival period** and **increases progression free survival period**.[104] Temsirolimus and its metabolite sirolimus contribute to improved therapeutic benefit. Experience with both drugs proves superiority of everolimus to temsirolimus.

17. *Folic acid/Folinic acid for reducing 'high dose methotrexate' toxicity.*

BACKGROUND

Folate is a cofactor for single carbon transfer reactions required for purine synthesis and folic acid should be reduced to folinic acid or tetrahydrofolate for these reactions. One such important one carbon transfer reactions is conversion of dUMP to dTMP where one mole of tetrahydrofolate (TH4) is utilized for each mole of dTMP produced. Therefore, a continued DNA synthesis in rapidly multiplying tissues requires plenty of dTMP. During this reaction TH4 and reduced folate cofactor are oxidized to dihydrofolate that should again be reduced to tetrahydrofolic acid for continued synthesis of DNA. The enzyme DHFRase is responsible for continuous synthesis of TH4. Methotrexate inhibits the enzyme dihydrofolate reductase (DHFRase) inhibiting the synthesis of tetrahydrofolate and interfering with single carbon reactions. Since methotrexate is not selective it is also toxic to rapidly multiplying cells. Bone marrow, GIT, skin, hair follicles contains cells that divide rapidly. Hence, methotrexate causes bone marrow suppression, GIT toxicity and alopecia. It also potentiates organ toxicity, cellular injury through synthesis of free radicals. Many standard regimens of adult or pediatric cancer include 'high dose' methotrexate.

FOLINIC ACID

Leucovorin or citrovorum factor or folinic acid is given with methotrexate. It is a more stable, more potent form of folic acid, preventing methotrexate induced myelosuppression, alopecia and GIT toxicity. It is a folate enzyme that is fully reduced and replenishes tetrahydrofolate cofactors. Leucovorin should be administered within 24 to 36 hours of methotrexate therapy and is available as calcium or sodium salt for therapy.

FOLIC ACID

Folic acid supplements reduce efficacy of methotrexate, so not preferred. Methotrexate antagonizes reduction of folic acid to folinic acid. So folic acid supplementation will counter the therapeutic benefit of methotrexate but in contrast, folic acid can be supplemented with low dose methotrexate in rheumatoid arthritis. Folic acid improves the 'methotrexate survival' rate in this condition. It indicates the rate at which patients continue to use methotrexate. Hence, folic acid can be supplemented with low dose but not with high dose methotrexate.

Drug of Choice: Folinic Acid

RATIONALE

Clinical toxicities of methotrexate, the folic acid antagonist are due to depletion of folate cofactors. It is given as a high dose methotrexate therapy in cancer and as a low dose in rheumatoid arthritis. Methotrexate is not selective to cancer cells and affects both normal and cancer cells. As anticancer agent it causes bone marrow depression, alopecia and GIT toxicity. **Leucovorin** or citrovorum factor or **folinic acid** prevents toxicities induced by high dose methotrexate. It is a reduced folate cofactor and **replenishes folinic acid** and is available as sodium and calcium salts. **Folic acid** supplements only reduce the efficacy of methotrexate. Although **supplementation** of folic acid **increases 'methotrexate survival'** rate in **rheumatoid arthritis**, in **cancer** patients its **therapeutic benefit is reduced**.

Hence, folinic acid and not folic acid is preferred with high dose methotrexate in cancer.

18. *Tamoxifen citrate/Toremifene in ER positive breast cancer of postmenopausal women.*

BACKGROUND

Selective estrogen receptor modulators or SERM are used in ER+ breast cancer. These drugs act either as agonist or antagonist after binding to ER receptor. The estrogenic or antiestrogenic action is organ specific and variable for each drug. SERM are effective only in the presence of either estrogen or progesterone receptors. They induce long remissions and prevent further progression in hormone positive cancers. In ER and PR negative cancers they have questionable therapeutic benefit. The two estrogen receptors ERα and ERβ have diverse tissue distributions. These receptors undergo homo or hetero dimerization after binding with estrogen stimulating a cascade of events and inducing estrogen response element and transcription. Binding of SERMs with ER inhibits dimerization of ER thereby suppressing estrogen action.

TOREMIFENE

Toremifene is a derivative of tamoxifen with similar pharmacodynamic profile. Its therapeutic efficacy is similar to tamoxifen but has minimum toxicity profile. It has lesser estrogen agonistic activity and so is devoid of many side effects of tamoxifen. Its capacity to induce hepatocellular carcinoma in animals has not been reported so far in human beings. It has equal efficacy, higher long-term tolerability and better safety profile. Hence, it is preferred to tamoxifen in ER+ breast cancer of postmenopausal women.

TAMOXIFEN CITRATE

Tamoxifen is an SERM and exerts antiestrogenic action in ER+ breast cancer. It is used as an adjuvant in both premenopausal and post- menopausal women. In pre and postmenopausal metastatic ER+ breast cancer it is used as an initiating agent. It is used as an adjuvant in early disease for prevention in high-risk patients and also in metastasis but it has estrogen agonistic activity on endometrium, bone and clotting mechanism. It causes endometrial proliferation, increased bone density and thromboembolism. Increased endometrial proliferation increases the risk of endometrial carcinoma. Higher incidence of hepatocellular cancer in animals has been reported for tamoxifen.

Drug of Choice: Toremifene

RATIONALE

Selective estrogen receptor modulators (SERMs) are effective in ER+ and PR+ breast cancer. They bind to estrogen receptors and prevent their dimerization. Tamoxifen is useful as prophylactic in high-risk women, as an adjuvant in early cancer and in metastatic or advanced cancer in both pre and postmenopausal women. Toremifene is effective only in postmenopausal women. Although tamoxifen exerts antiestrogenic or antiproliferative action in breast cancer, it is agonistic promoting estrogenic action in uterus, bone and clotting pathway. Hence, it increases incidence of **thromboembolic manifestation, endometrial cancer**, increased mineral density of bone and vaginal bleeding. **Animal studies** indicate its capacity to induce **hepatocellular carcinoma. Toremifene** has lesser estrogen agonistic activity and so does not cause these adverse effects mediated by tamoxifen. It is **not a hepatocarcinogen** in animals. The **clinical efficacy** of toremifene in breast cancer is **comparable** to tamoxifen. It has higher **long-term tolerability** and **better safety profile** and so is preferred in ER+ breast cancer in postmenopausal women.[105]

Immunomodulators

1. *Azathioprine/Cyclosporine as immunosuppressant in patients undergoing renal transplantation.*

BACKGROUND

Immunosuppressives suppress immune response and are used in many conditions such as organ transplantation and autoimmune disorders. Prolonged administration of immunosuppressants is required in both these conditions. They result in nonspecific suppression of entire immune system for long periods increasing chances of severe infection due to low immune status. Calcineurin inhibitors inhibit T cell-receptor activated cell signaling pathways.

AZATHIOPRINE

Azathioprine is a purine antimetabolite and is converted into 6-mercaptopurine. It causes bone marrow depression and most commonly leucopenia. Therefore, its dose should be standardized to prevent organ rejection and toxicities. Increased susceptibility to infections, hepatotoxicity and alopecia are other side effects. Since it is not a potential nephrotoxic agent, it is preferred for renal transplantation.

CYCLOSPORINE

T-cell mediates immune response in transplant rejection and autoimmune conditions. Cyclosporine inhibits calcineurin by binding to immunophilin cyclophilin and specifically inhibits T-cell mediated responses triggered by antigens. Nephrotoxicity is the main side effect so first dose should be delayed until after transplantation and should not be given till renal function improves after organ transplantation. Yet nephrotoxicity occurs in majority of patients requiring cessation of therapy.[106] Renal toxicity is induced by both cyclosporine as well as renal transplantation and it is often difficult to differentiate one from the other. A low dose of cyclosporine can cause rejection and high dose causes nephrotoxicity. Fifty percent of patients receiving cyclosporine after renal transplant suffer from hypertension. Hence, cyclosporine should be avoided for patients undergoing renal transplantation.

Drug of Choice: Azathioprine

RATIONALE

Prolonged administration of immunosuppressants is required to suppress immune responses in organ transplantation and in autoimmune disorders. **Cyclosporine** inhibits T cell response in these two conditions. It causes **nephrotoxicity** hence the first dose is delayed until transplantation is completed. While low dose is insufficient and causes transplant rejection, higher doses result in nephrotoxicity. Following transplantation, **cyclosporine should not be given till renal performance is improved**. Most often symptoms of organ rejection after renal transplant overlap with nephrotoxic effect of cyclosporine. Half the patients receiving cyclosporine for renal transplant, suffer from hypertension. Hence, it should be avoided in patients undergoing renal transplant. **Azathioprine** improves **survival rate** and **reduces rejection** following renal transplant. It has superior efficacy when combined with steroids. It results in bone marrow depression but **does not cause nephrotoxicity**. Hence, azathioprine is preferred to cyclosporine as immunosuppressant in patients undergoing renal transplant.

2. *Tacrolimus/Sirolimus as immunosuppressant in liver and lung transplantation.*

BACKGROUND

Immunosuppressants have resulted in lower rejection rates of organ transplantation. They improve short-term outcome in recipient and allograft survival. Long-term improvement is yet to be achieved in allograft survival. Calcineurin inhibitors suppress T-cell activation but not B-cells activation. Hence, they do not adequately control acute and chronic B cell mediated rejection.

TACROLIMUS

Tacrolimus, the calcineurin inhibitor, *per se* does not act as an immunosuppressive agent. It combines with intracellular protein FKBP-12 to inhibit T-cell activation. Being calcineurin inhibitor, its immunosuppressive pathway is similar to cyclosporine. It causes nephrotoxicity, hypertension, hyperkalemia, seizures and tremor. It inhibits pancreatic beta cells causing impaired glucose tolerance and hyperglycemia. It also increases risk of opportunistic infections and secondary tumors.

SIROLIMUS

Sirolimus, the macrocyclic lactone inhibits T-lymphocyte function. It also inhibits B cell proliferation and T cell dependent or independent antibody production. When compared to tacrolimus, it does not increase overall survival period of allograft. It does not cause nephrotoxicity as it is not nephrotoxic *per se* but results in GIT toxicity. Sirolimus delays wound healing probably due to its antiproliferative action causing dehiscence of bronchial anastamosis in lung transplant patients. It can result in thrombosis of hepatic artery after liver transplant. Hence, sirolimus should be avoided in liver and lung transplantation.

Drug of Choice: Tacrolimus

RATIONALE

Calcineurin inhibitors act mainly by inhibiting T-cell activation. Generally, they do not interfere with B-cell function. In contrast to tacrolimus, sirolimus inhibits both T and B cells. But this does not improve its clinical efficacy. Although **sirolimus** does **not cause nephrotoxicity**, it **augments** risk of **neoplasms** such as **lymphomas**.

Since it has antiproliferative action and **delays wound healing**. In liver transplant patients, it potentiates risk of **hepatic artery thrombosis** and causes **dehiscence** of **bronchial anastamosis** due to impaired wound healing. **Tacrolimus** is the **most favored** calcineurin inhibitor for **liver and lung transplantation but** should be **avoided in renal transplant due to its nephrotoxicity**.

Endocrine Drugs

Section Outline

48 Introduction and Hypothalamic-Pituitary Axis

1. *Cabergoline/Bromocriptine in hyperprolactinemia.*

BACKGROUND

Regulation of prolactin secretion at hypothalamic level is predominantly inhibitory and this feature makes prolactin unique among other anterior pituitary hormones. Secretion of prolactin is regulated by dopamine released from tuberoinfundibular region which binds to D_2 receptor on lactotropes, inhibiting the secretion of prolactin. Oligoamenorrhea, amenorrhea or infertility occurs in women with hyperprolactinemia due to hypogonadotropic hypogonadism, secondary to hyperprolactinemia. Lactation or galactorrhea even in non-nursing women is a frequent occurrence. Bromocriptine and cabergoline are dopamine agonists and reduce prolactin secretion.

CABERGOLINE

Ergot derivative cabergoline has long half-life of 65 hours so can be given less frequently. The potency of cabergoline is four times high due to its affinity and selectivity. Unlike bromocriptine, it does not interact with D_1 receptors and binds only to D_2 receptors. Although it is a selective and potent agonist at D_2, its adverse effects are milder and cause minimal nausea but can cause dizziness due to hypotension. It reduces the size of prolactin adenoma and does not result in recurrence on withdrawal. It induces complete remission in hyperprolactinemia and so preferred.

BROMOCRIPTINE

The semisynthetic ergot derivative bromocriptine binds to D_2 receptors and inhibits both spontaneous as well as thyrotropin-releasing hormone (TRH) mediated secretion. It has minimal bioavailability due to very high hepatic first-pass metabolism. Its elimination half-life is also relatively short, so it has to be given frequently. It is also available as sustained release oral formulation to avoid frequent administration. On continuous administration it reduces prolactin to near normal levels but its level starts to increase on cessation of therapy resulting in recurrence. Hence, the cure rate in person with prolactin secreting adenomas is very low. As dopamine agonist it causes severe nausea and vomiting particularly during initial period but once daily vaginal administration can overcome such severe GIT symptoms. It can also cause postural hypotension, headache, vasospasm of digits and nasal congestion that can be diminished by low dose at bedtime and adding morning dose after one week.

Drug of Choice: Cabergoline

RATIONALE

Hyperprolactinemia causes infertility, amenorrhea and oligoamenorrhea. Dopamine inhibits prolactin secretion, so dopamine agonists are used in the treatment of hyperprolactinemia. Cabergoline and bromocriptine are both dopamine agonists. **Bromocriptine** is **short acting**, has to be given frequently and causes intense **nausea and vomiting**. The **recurrence rate** is **high** with bromocriptine as prolactin level starts rising soon after cessation of therapy. **Cabergoline** has **four times higher potency** and **higher selectivity** for D_2 receptors. It causes **tolerable nausea** but can result in hypotension with dizziness. Since hyperprolactinemia does not recur after stopping therapy resulting in complete remission, it is preferred to bromocriptine.

2. *GnRH agonists/GnRH antagonists in metastatic prostate cancer.*

BACKGROUND

Next to lung cancer, prostate cancer is the most frequent cancer occurring in men. Prostate cancer progresses extensively in the presence of androgens. So, androgen deprivation or chemical castration forms the main line of treatment. Androgen deprivation therapy is only palliative and not curative in metastatic cancer and survival rate of chemical castration is higher than estrogen therapy. It improves quality of life, reduces serum levels of prostate specific antigen (PSA) and prevents complications but in many patients chemical castration does not suppress progression of disease. Gonadotropin-releasing hormone (GnRH) stimulates hypothalamus to release LH which stimulates testosterone production.

GONADOTROPIN-RELEASING HORMONE (GnRH) AGONISTS

GnRH agonists are the drugs of choice in metastatic prostatic cancer. Of all the GnRH analogs goserelin is more effective than buserelin and triptorelin. High risk groups should be started with neoadjuvant chemotherapy with GnRH agonists. These agents are effective when given for 4 to 6 months prior to radiotherapy. Chronic administration of GnRH agonists blocks hypothalamic release of FSH and LH. Suppression of LH release from hypothalamus decreases peripheral testosterone levels. GnRH agonists have high efficacy, safety and tolerability with less frequent dosage. They improve both overall survival period and disease free or relapse free period. Long acting preparations are given once in 3 months and triptorelin can be given once in 6 months.

GONADOTROPIN-RELEASING HORMONE (GnRH) ANTAGONISTS

Gonadotropin-releasing hormone antagonists are not preferred as first line treatment in prostate cancer. Similar to GnRH agonists, GnRH antagonists also have good safety index. GnRH agonists and antagonists do not cause testosterone surge. GnRH antagonists are costly and have to be administered more frequently as once monthly therapy. Lower efficacy, frequent administration and higher cost are their disadvantages.

Drug of Choice: Gonadotropin-releasing Hormone Agonists

RATIONALE

Efficacy, tolerability, safety and frequency of administration are all determinants for choosing the first line drug in metastatic carcinoma. Chemical castration is more effective when given along with radiotherapy. **GnRH agonists** are the **drugs of choice** in metastatic carcinoma. Neoadjuvant chemotherapy of GnRH agonists for 4 to 6 months prior to radiotherapy is **very effective**. Goserelin is more effective than buserelin and triptorelin. Since long acting preparations are available, they can be given once in 3 months and in case of triptorelin once in 6 months administration is very effective. This is in contrast to **GnRH antagonists** that have to be administered **once monthly** increasing the cost of overall therapy. Besides GnRH antagonists such as abarelix have **lower efficacy**. GnRH agonists and antagonists have good safety profile and do not cause androgen surge. Since GnRH antagonists have lower efficacy, higher dosage frequency and **high cost** of overall treatment they are not preferred.[107]

3. *Somatostatin/Somatostatin analogs in acromegaly.*

BACKGROUND

Excess of growth hormone synthesis causes acromegaly in adults. Arthropathy, visceromegaly, hypertension and hyperglycemia are few manifestations. Pharmacological therapy is the primary treatment for persistent GH levels. Surgery of microadenomas does not appear to reduce persistent GH levels. Irradiation of microadenomas causes long-term complications.

SOMATOSTATIN ANALOGS

Somatostatin analogs have revolutionized the treatment of acromegaly. Somatostatin analogs are preferred as first line drugs in acromegaly. Octapeptide derivatives such as *octreotide* and *lanreotide* exhibit higher selectivity for somatostatin receptors. They selectively bind to somatostatin SST_2 and SST_5 receptors, reduce GH and IGF-1 levels and do not interfere with glycemic level. They are more potent, more selective and more effective and so preferred.

SOMATOSTATIN

Somatostatin inhibits secretion of GH, TSH and prolactin from pituitary. It also causes dyspepsia, nausea and diarrhea. Duration of action of somatostatin is only about 2 to 3 minutes. Since it does not selectively inhibit GH secretion it is not preferred. Besides, growth hormone level increases drastically on stopping the treatment.

Drug of Choice: Somatostatin Analogs

RATIONALE

Somatostatin analogs are preferred to somatostatin for the treatment of acromegaly. They are more **selective** and **inhibit** SST_2 and SST_5 **somatostatin receptors**. They reduce GH, IGF-1 levels to normal level and do not interfere with glycemic control. Somatostatin is not effective and results in rebound increase in GH hormone level after cessation of therapy.

4. *Octreotide/Lanreotide as the preferred somatostatin analog in acromegaly.*

BACKGROUND

Somatostatin analogs inhibit somatostatin receptors selectively. Hence, they suppress GH and IGF-1 levels more selectively. They do not interfere with insulin secretion and glycemic control.

OCTREOTIDE

Octreotide is a somatostatin analog preferred for the treatment of acromegaly. It has long half-life and selectively binds to SST_2 and SST_5 receptors. Slow release long acting once monthly depot preparation of *octreotide* is available and this biodegradable polymer reduces the frequency of administration. Long acting *octreotide* causes persistent suppression of growth hormone and are administered intramuscularly once a month in the dose of 20 to 30 mg. It is well tolerated and reduces tumor size which rebounds on stopping therapy. It causes nausea, diarrhea, gallstones and inhibition of TSH level but it inhibits insulin release to a lesser extent when compared to somatostatin.

LANREOTIDE

Although lanreotide is long-acting, its duration is shorter than octreotide. Lanreotide is given as deep subcutaneous injection once in 10 to 14 days. It causes sustained reduction in growth hormone secretion than octreotide. Depot formulation leads to more predictable and uniform plasma levels. The clinical efficacy of lanreotide in acromegaly is similar to octreotide but when compared to octreotide, frequent administration is required because its duration of action is shorter and has to be administered once in 10 to 14 days. It has similar safety profile but causes GIT side effects, gallstones and fall in insulin level.

Drug of Choice: Octreotide

RATIONALE

Somatostatin **analogs inhibit** somatostatin **receptors selectively** and so suppress GH and IGF-1 levels more selectively. They **do not interfere** with **insulin secretion** and **glycemic control. Long acting octreotide** is administered **once** in a **month** and causes **persistent suppression** of GH release. It causes **reduction** of **tumor** size. Lanreotide is also equally effective, causes clinical improvement but has to be administered frequently and so less preferred[108] to octreotide. These drugs are well tolerated and have similar side effect profile.

Thyroid and Antithyroid Drugs

1. *Propylthiouracil/Carbimazole in thyroid storm.*

BACKGROUND

It is a rare, extreme status of thyrotoxicosis, triggered by stress, thyroid surgery, severe illness or radioactive iodine. It results in delirium, tachycardia, diarrhea, high fever and unless corrected quickly can result in death. Propranolol is given but should be used with caution in patients with heart failure. Corticosteroids if used, should be tapered gradually once clinical improvement occurs. Aspirin increases T_4 level by displacing it from thyroxine-binding globulin (TBG) so, should be avoided.

PROPYLTHIOURACIL

Propylthiouracil is preferred as it has dual action both in thyroid gland and in periphery. It inhibits iodothyronine synthesis by preventing incorporation of iodine into tyrosine. It also prevents coupling of iodotyrosine residues. When compared to carbimazole, this coupling action is more sensitive to propylthiouracil. It inhibits peroxidase enzyme preventing the oxidation of iodotyrosine residues or iodide. In addition propylthiouracil inhibits the peripheral conversion of thyroxine (T_4) to triiodothyronine (T_3).

CARBIMAZOLE

Carbimazole, a carbethoxy derivative of methimazole acts by getting converted to methimazole. It also inhibits peroxidase enzyme preventing coupling reaction. Similar to propylthiouracil, carbimazole also prevents oxidation of iodide to iodine but it does not alter the rate of peripheral conversion of T_4 to T_3. Since suppression of peripheral T_3 levels is highly beneficial in thyroid storm, propyl thiouracil is preferred to carbimazole in thyroid storm.

Drug of Choice: Propylthiouracil

RATIONALE

Thyrotoxic crisis or thyroid crisis is an emergency due to increased T_3 levels. Propylthiouracil has dual action both within thyroid gland and in periphery. It **inhibits oxidation** of iodide to iodine, **formation** and **coupling** of iodotyrosine residues as well as **inhibition** of **peripheral conversion** of T_4 to T_3. **Carbimazole lacks** the **peripheral** action of propylthiouracil and so is **less effective**. Hence, propylthiouracil is the drug of choice in thyroid storm.

2. *Carbimazole/Radioactive iodine I_{131} in Graves' disease with ophthalmopathy in older age group.*

BACKGROUND

Most common cause of hyperthyroidism is Graves' disease, an autoimmune condition. Incidence is high in women than in men at the ratio of 8:1. More common feature is exophthalmoses due to infiltrative ophthalmopathy. Less common occurrence is pretibial myxoedema or infiltrative dermopathy. Family history of Graves' disease or Hashimoto's thyroiditis is common.

CARBIMAZOLE

Carbimazole is the drug of choice in Graves' disease and has the convenience of once daily administration with improved compliance. Its intrathyroidal and plasma half-life is high hence, it has long duration of action besides it is well tolerated and its adverse effects are lower than propylthiouracil. Response is delayed in those taking fortified iodine preparations or with bigger goiters and recurrence occurs in 50% of patients after cessation of therapy. Agranulocytosis can occur during initial therapy but reversible on stopping the drug.

RADIOACTIVE IODINE I$_{131}$

Radioactive Iodine I$_{131}$ destroys overactive thyroid tissue and normalizes thyroid level. In patients receiving antithyroid drugs I$_{131}$ is ineffective and result in treatment failure. It may be effective if drugs are discontinued 4 days prior to I$_{131}$ administration. Its advantages are its low cost, permanent cure and absence of mortality but disadvantage is a higher risk of delayed hypothyroidism and life-long monitoring. It is contraindicated in patients with exophthalmoses as it worsens this condition in 25% of patients. In older individuals antithyroid drugs are preferred to I$_{131}$.

Drug of Choice: Carbimazole

RATIONALE

Graves' disease is an autoimmune condition with higher incidence in women. **Radioactive I$_{131}$ destroys thyroid tissue** and reduces peripheral thyroxine level. It can be given at an outpatient level. Its advantages are its cheaper cost, simple mode of administration, permanent cure and absence of mortality but most common disadvantage is risk of **life-long hypothyroidism**. Besides, it is not preferred in patients with Graves' **ophthalmopathy** as it can **exaggerate** this **condition**. **Carbimazole** has the convenience of **once daily** administration. Its **intrathyroidal and plasma half-life** is **higher** with **longer** duration of action but recurrence can occur on cessation of therapy in 50% of patients. Agranulocytosis can occur during initial therapy but is reversible on stopping the drug.

3. *Lithium/Iodide for preoperative preparation of thyroid gland before thyroid surgery except in Graves' disease and multinodular goiter.*

BACKGROUND

Thyroidectomy is advised for nodular goiters with high-risk for malignancy. It is also indicated for non-responding uncontrolled thyrotoxicosis during pregnancy. In Graves' disease resection of one full lobe of the gland with partial resection of other lobe is done but

4 g of thyroid tissue should be left out otherwise chances for recurrence will be high.[109] Thiourea and propranolol are given to make the patient euthyroid prior to surgery. For surgery in hyperthyroid status high dose propranolol is given to inhibit thyroid crisis.

IODIDE

Iodide is given preoperatively to reduce the vascularity of thyroid gland and it often causes marked and rapid response within a period of 24 hours. Iodide blocks the release of thyroid hormone into circulation reducing its peripheral level. It also inhibits synthesis of thyroid hormone in gland to a lesser extent. It reduces vascularity making gland firmer and convenient for handling during surgery. Colloid reaccumulates within follicles as cells shrink increasing amount of bound iodine. Continuous administration of iodide for 10 to 15 days results in maximum benefit but preoperative iodide is not indicated in multinodular goiter and should be avoided. Similarly iodide for preoperative preparation in Graves' disease is debatable.

LITHIUM

The adverse effect of lithium when used in bipolar disorder is goiter. Similar to iodide, lithium inhibits hormone release from thyroid gland. Coadministration of lithium 800 to 1200 μg with antithyroid drugs causes euthyroidism. Euthyroidic state is achieved quickly, effectively, safely with no report of side effect[110] but unlike iodide, lithium does not inhibit the synthesis of thyroid hormone. Besides, lithium does not reduce vascularity of the gland and it neither is firm nor easy to handle during surgery.[111] So lithium is less preferred to iodide for preoperative preparation of thyroid gland but lithium is given in nodular goiter as well as in Graves' disease preoperatively.

Drug of Choice: Iodide

RATIONALE

Prior to surgical resection of thyroid gland, conversion of hyperthyroid status to euthyroid state is necessary in order to avoid intra and postoperative thyroid storm. Although thioamides and propranolol are given they take long time to achieve euthyroid state. Iodide and lithium can both inhibit the release of thyroid hormone from thyroid gland. Iodide also interferes with the synthesis of thyroid hormone. Being a highly vascular organ, thyroid gland can be handled more easily if its vascularity is reduced. **Iodides reduce vascularity** thereby making **gland firmer** and **convenient for handling during surgery**. Colloid reaccumulates within follicles of thyroid gland as cells shrink, increasing the amount of bound iodine. Lithium does not share this advantage. Although **Lithium corrects hyperthyroidism quickly, safely** and **efficiently** it **does not reduce vascularity of gland**. In preoperative preparation of multinodular goiter and Graves' disease iodide should be avoided but lithium can be given safely in such patients.

4. *Liothyronine/Levothyroxine in treatment of myxedema coma.*

BACKGROUND

Myxedema coma is a critical state with very high mortality rate up to 60%. It occurs more commonly during winter in elderly due to precipitating factors such as cerebrovascular accidents, pulmonary infection and cardiac failure. Antidepressants, sedatives and opioids can also potentiate this condition. Cardinal features are respiratory depression, hypothermia and loss of consciousness. Paucity of reflexes, bradycardia, dry skin and macroglossia are other features. Intravenous administration of steroids is given before thyroid supplements as co-existing adrenal crisis is common. Parenteral thyroid hormone is advised as the GIT absorptive capacity is minimal.

LEVOTHYROXINE

Levothyroxine has a long half-life and can be administered once daily. Initial loading dose of 300 to 400 µg IV is ideal followed by 50 to 100 µg IV daily. It has slow onset but leads to sustained action reducing incidence of adverse effects. Improvement of CVS, renal, pulmonary and metabolic parameters occur within a week. Serum level of T_4 is easier to monitor but lower doses are required in CAD patients.

LIOTHYRONINE

Liothyronine is used in the preparation of patient with thyroid cancer for I_{131} therapy. It is also used by a few physicians for rapid response in myxoedema coma. Commercially available T_3 is the synthetic form of natural thyroid hormone. It has abrupt onset but rapid termination of effect as it has shorter half-life. It has to be administered every 8 hours to compensate for its rapid termination but this can result in fluctuating plasma levels potentiating its adverse effects. Since such rapid plasma fluctuation increases body temperature as well as oxygen consumption very rapidly, it can cause MI and cardiac arrhythmias in patients with coronary artery disease. Since peripheral conversion of T_4 to T_3 is slow, some clinicians combine T_4 and T_3 but this should be considered only in case of suboptimal response to T_4.

Drug of Choice: Levothyroxine

RATIONALE

Myxedema coma is a critical state with mortality rate up to 60% and occurs more commonly during winter in elderly due to some precipitating factors such as cerebrovascular accidents, pulmonary infection and cardiac failure. Antidepressants, sedatives and opioids can potentiate this condition. Since the oral absorption of T_4 in GIT is minimal, parenteral levothyroxine is advised. Although some physicians prefer coadministration of T_3 and T_4 during initial period, this is not advantageous and **T_3 should be given only during suboptimal response of T_4. T_3 is fast acting** but it causes **high plasma fluctuations** as it has **shorter duration** of action and has to be administered once in 8 hours. Such high fluctuations can potentiate adverse effects such as **cardiac arrhythmias and myocardial infarction in CAD patients. T_4** has **slow onset** and causes much **steady plasma concentration** with minimal plasma fluctuation but requires dose reduction in patients with CAD. Hence, T_4 is preferred to T_3 in the management of myxedema coma.

Corticosteroids

1. *Sudden withdrawal/Gradual withdrawal ideal after prolonged corticosteroid therapy.*

BACKGROUND

Prolonged administration of corticosteroids suppresses hypothalamic–pituitary axis. Most patients are able to recover from such prolonged suppression within few weeks but the recovery may be delayed in a few patients and they may take more than a year. Therapy beyond one week causes dose and time related increase in side effects. Withdrawal of corticosteroids can also cause an exacerbation of the underlying disease.

GRADUAL WITHDRAWAL

Gradual withdrawal allows for the HPA axis to recover from prolonged suppression. To overcome suppression of HPA axis intermediate preparation such as prednisone is used. It is started as single morning dose and then switched over to alternate day therapy. This regimen overcomes daily diurnal fluctuation in plasma concentration of steroids. It is also effective in stabilizing the patient from prolonged HPA axis suppression.

SUDDEN WITHDRAWAL

Sudden cessation causes withdrawal syndrome or acute adrenal insufficiency. Most severe complication of sudden withdrawal is acute adrenal insufficiency, a life-threatening condition that occurs after sudden cessation of high dose steroids. Hyperkalemia, hyponatremia, hypotension, dehydration and vomiting are common symptoms. IV isotonic saline, corticosteroids and 5% dextrose should be given immediately. Hydrocortisone 100 mg bolus followed by 50 to 100 mg once in every 8 hours as continuous infusion is effective and supplements daily cortisol secretion in response to stress to a large extent. Once the patient is stabilized, oral therapy is instituted followed by gradual withdrawal. Another rare complication of sudden withdrawal is glucocorticoid withdrawal syndrome manifesting as pseudotumor cerebri that causes papilledema and increased intracranial pressure. Hence, high dose steroid therapy given for prolonged period should never be stopped abruptly.

Drug of Choice: Gradual Withdrawal

RATIONALE

If glucocorticoid therapy is extended beyond one week it causes variable side effects on cessation of therapy. Long-term therapy of corticosteroids causes absolute suppression of HPA axis and such prolonged suppression of HPA axis results in patient inability to cope up with sudden withdrawal of steroids. Therefore, steroids should only be tapered gradually and should never be stopped suddenly. **Gradual withdrawal** helps patients to **compensate** for the daily **diurnal fluctuations** of steroids. **Sudden cessation** can cause either **steroid withdrawal syndrome** or **acute adrenal insufficiency**. Steroid withdrawal syndrome is a rare condition causing pseudotumor cerebri characterized by papilledema and increased intracranial pressure. Most severe complication of sudden withdrawal is life-threatening acute adrenal insufficiency. IV isotonic saline, corticosteroids and 5% dextrose should be given immediately. Hence sudden withdrawal of steroids should be avoided and steroids should never be stopped suddenly.

2. *Prednisone/Prednisolone in flare-up of osteoarthritis.*

BACKGROUND

Osteoarthritis is degenerative non-inflammatory joint disease of elders. It is characterized by minimal joint effusion, mild inflammation and other articular signs. It is the disease of aging and occurs more frequently in women. Degeneration of cartilage is the predominant feature with minimal inflammation. Triamcinolone can be injected intra-articularly during episodes of flare-up but it should not be done often and should not be repeated more than four times a year.

PREDNISOLONE

Prednisolone is the metabolite of prednisone and preferred in osteoarthritis. These steroids are intermediate acting with similar anti-inflammatory potency. Steroids bind to glucocorticoid receptor and induce transcription of target genes but the effect of steroids will be evident only after some time so, there is a delay before therapeutic benefits are manifested clinically. Since prednisolone is a biologically active 11β-hydroxy derivative of prednisone, it does not require bioactivation so preferred.

PREDNISONE

Prednisone is 11-keto group and gets enzymatically reduced to prednisolone and the reaction is catalyzed by the enzyme 11β-hydroxy steroid dehydrogenase. This enzyme is present mainly in liver and also in adipocytes, bone, eye and skin. Prednisone is not active as such and has to be reduced enzymatically. The time taken for enzymatic bioactivation delays its clinical benefit. Hence, in osteoarthritis flare-up where quick action is required it is not preferred. Prednisone and prednisolone can result in mineralo-corticoid side effects at higher dosages.

Drug of Choice: Prednisolone

RATIONALE

Osteoarthritis occurs more commonly in elderly and corticosteroids are used to manage the flare-up reaction. An intermediate acting steroid with quicker onset is preferred because generally steroids require time for interaction with its receptors and for further transcription reactions. **Prednisone** is **inactive** as such and has to be

enzymatically reduced by11β-hydroxy steroid dehydrogenase **to its metabolically active prednisolone**. Since the **time required** for **enzymatic reduction delays** its **clinical benefit** it is **not preferred. Prednisolone does not require enzymatic reduction**. Hence, it is preferred.

3. *Prednisone/Dexamethasone in rheumatoid arthritis.*

BACKGROUND

Rheumatoid arthritis is a systemic disease with chronic manifestations. Low dose corticosteroids result in prompt anti-inflammatory benefit relieving pain. It delays articular erosion rate hence given as 'bridge therapy' to suppress disease activity. Since it is a chronic condition, prolonged use of steroids can cause side effects. So, they can only be used as 'stabilizing agents' for those not responding to first line drugs. After prolonged therapy steroids need to be tapered before stopping therapy.

PREDNISONE

Low dose prednisone, 5 to 10 mg daily is the most effective therapy and has more selective glucocorticoid activity with minimal mineralocorticoid activity. It has intermediate duration of action with 4 time higher potency than hydrocortisone. Prednisone has effective anti-inflammatory and immunoregulatory activity and leads to weight gain, osteonecrosis, hyperglycemia and increases risk of cataract.

DEXAMETHASONE

Dexamethasone is long-acting corticosteroid with higher anti-inflammatory activity. Its anti-inflammatory potency is 25 times more than prednisone. Hence, its clinical efficacy is superior to prednisone in rheumatoid arthritis. When compared to prednisone, dexamethasone has negligible mineralocorticoid activity. Although it has higher anti-inflammatory potency, it is not preferred for daily treatment since it requires prolonged therapy in a chronic disease. Dexamethasone is a long acting drug that causes prolonged suppression of HPA axis and immune status resulting in higher susceptibility to infections. Side effects profile is similar except for hypertension and other mineralocorticoid effects. Hence, prednisone is preferred to dexamethasone for daily administration.

Drug of Choice: Prednisone

RATIONALE

Low dose corticosteroids result in prompt anti-inflammatory benefit relieving pain. Steroids delay articular erosion rate and given as **'bridge therapy'** to relieve pain and inflammation. **Prednisone** is the preferred drug and given as **low daily dose** of 5 to 10 mg. It is an intermediate acting drug causing **delayed HPA suppression** and **immunosuppression**. The anti-inflammatory action of **dexamethasone** is **25 times more potent** than prednisone. It causes negligible mineralocorticoid activity. In spite of these advantages it is not preferred for prolonged administration as it is **long-acting** causing **sustained inhibition of HPA axis** leading to more severe **immunosuppression** than prednisone.

4. *Methyl prednisolone/Dexamethasone as 'pulse therapy' for acute synovitis in rheumatoid arthritis.*

BACKGROUND

Pulse therapy has been advocated for many years in rheumatic patients for active synovitis. It results in dramatic effect on immunological and clinical parameters and has only temporary benefit on synovitis in patients with active rheumatoid arthritis. Intravenous high dose of steroid is used either once in three days or on alternate days. High dose 'bridge therapy'[112] is effective in patients with active disease during recurrences.

DEXAMETHASONE

Fluorinated steroid, dexamethasone is long acting with 6 to 7 times higher potency. Its binding to glucocorticoid receptors is longer than methyl prednisolone and has negligible mineralocorticoid activity.

It inhibits IL-1, IL-6, and TNF-α as well as T and B cell mediated immune responses.[113] It is less expensive, has higher efficacy with greater immunosuppressive action. Oral dexamethasone 10 mg once weekly for 4 weeks is found to be effective and safe.

METHYL PREDNISOLONE

Methyl prednisolone has strong inhibitory effect on pro-inflammatory mediators of blood, synovial fluid and synovial membrane. It is an intermediate acting agent with duration of action for 12 to 36 hours. It has potent glucocorticoid and minimal mineralocorticoid activity. The onset of action is quicker as it has faster penetration into cell membrane but, when compared to dexamethasone it is less potent with lower clinical efficacy. Oral dose of 1 g is found to be clinically effective without inherent dangers of IV dose.[114]

Drug of Choice: Dexamethasone

RATIONALE

Pulse therapy of steroids is given during acute exacerbations of active rheumatic disease. It is given to reduce pain and inflammation of synovitis in patients with active disease. High dose intravenous injection of steroids is given either on alternate day or once in three days. **Methyl prednisolone** is an intermediate acting agent with **quicker onset** than dexamethasone. It is a potent anti-inflammatory agent but when compared to dexamethasone it has **lesser efficacy** and **moderate immunosuppressive** action. **Dexamethasone** is **long acting** with **superior anti-inflammatory** and **immunosuppressive** action[115] so, it is preferred. Recently oral pulse therapy with dexamethasone has been found to be highly effective.

5. *Clobetasol/Desonide for topical application on face and occluded areas like axilla or groin.*

BACKGROUND

Absorption of topical steroids from skin is determined by structural integrity of skin. Percutaneous absorption is higher through inflamed skin and moderate from intact skin. Occlusive dressing increases percutaneous absorption substantially. Frequent topical administration does not augment relief so it should be avoided. Chronic administration results in tolerance and tachyphylaxis. To reduce the side effects, a least potent topical steroid should be applied for shortest time. Most common side effect is skin atrophy and the incidence higher with a very potent steroid. It suppresses mitotic activity of fibroblasts, inhibits collagen and glycosamino-glycan leading to thinning of elastin fibers on dermis. The upper layer becomes thin, fragmented and often atrophic changes such as ecchymosis, telangiectasis, striae and purpura develop. Resolution can occur after months but long-term use causes irreversible atrophy or scar. Face and occluded areas such as genitals are particularly susceptible as absorption is higher. Absorption range is around 30% in genitals, 7% in face, 4% in arm pit, 1% in forearm and 0.05% in sole. Fluorinated corticosteroids are very highly potent with higher anti-inflammatory action and as topical agents their degree of absorption from the site of application is very high. So they are not indicated for topical use on face and occluded areas due to high risk of scarring.

DESONIDE

Desonide is low potent steroid, indicated for topical application on face, axilla or groin. It is not a fluorinated corticosteroid hence it is least potent with minimal local absorption. It inhibits phospholipase A_2 so has anti-inflammatory action, is also antipruritic and local vasoconstrictor. Although low potent as 0.05% ointment it should not be used for more than 2 weeks. The amount of desonide applied on face should not exceed 2.5 'finger tip units' which is the amount squeezed from finger tip to 1st crease of finger. It is relatively safe but can cause pruritus, erythema, irritation, indurations or edema.

CLOBETASOL

Clobetasol is a most potent topical fluorinated corticosteroid available as of now. So incidence of skin atrophy or scarring is high.

Hence, it should never be used for topical application on face, axilla or groin.

Drug of Choice: Desonide

RATIONALE

Fluorinated corticosteroids are highly potent and although they have higher clinical efficacy as anti-inflammatory agent, their ability to get absorbed even on topical administration is very high. They can cause skin atrophy very frequently resulting in scarring of skin. Absorption from face, groin and axilla is high. Even single administration of high potent **fluorinated** agent such as **clobetasol** can result in **skin thinning** lasting for three days.[116] **Desonide** is **non-fluorinated,** so **least potent.** It is **safer** for **application** on **face and occluded areas** such as groin but still the quantum of application **should not exceed 2.5 fingertip units**.

6. *Prednisone/Prednisolone as anti-inflammatory agent in those with hepatic failure.*

BACKGROUND

Glucocorticoids are the most potent anti-inflammatory agents used in therapy. They do not alter the underlying disorder but often cause dramatic and temporary relief. Immune responses of lymphocytes are also profoundly altered by corticosteroids. So they are used in a variety of conditions ranging from urticaria to transplantation rejection. They reduce release of chemo attractive and vasoactive factors critical for inflammation and reduce secretion of proteolytic, lipolytic enzymes inhibiting leucocytic chemotaxis. They also inhibit lipotropin secretion and reduce expression of cytokines mediating inflammation. The double bond between C_1 and C_2 selectively increases glucocorticoid activity but does not in any way interfere with mineralocorticoid activity of these agents. Prednisolone and prednisone have an additional double bond between C_1 and C_2 so they have equal efficacy as glucocorticoids and anti-inflammatory agents. They have intermediate duration of action with minimal mineralocorticoid activity.

PREDNISONE

Prednisone is an inactive prodrug and should be de-esterified to be an active compound. It contains 11-keto group and is reduced by 11β-hydroxysteroid dehydrogenase to prednisolone its active metabolite. This reduction is catalyzed predominantly in liver, also in bone, skin, adipocytes and eye. In liver failure it cannot be used as it cannot be converted to its active metabolite. The administration of corticosteroids in liver disease is controversial but is beneficial in autoimmune hepatitis.

PREDNISOLONE

Unlike prednisone, prednisolone is active as such and does not need activation in liver. It is not an ester moiety and has 80 to 100% bioavailability with peak plasma level of 1 hour. Its plasma half-life is 2 to 3 hours but its duration of action extends from 18 to 36 hours. It does not need de-esterification in liver so can be given in autoimmune hepatitis.

Drug of Choice: Prednisolone

RATIONALE

Prednisone and prednisolone are intermediate acting steroids with similar clinical efficacy. While **prednisolone** is **active as such prednisone** is **inactive** and **requires enzymatic reduction in liver**. Prednisone is an inactive prodrug and has to be de-esterified into prednisolone in liver. Hence in conditions such as **hepatic failure**, where there is **impairment of enzymatic activity** it is prudent to use an active drug like prednisolone rather than its inactive prodrug.

7. *Fludrocortisone/Hydrocortisone in Addison disease.*

BACKGROUND

Primary adrenal insufficiency is caused by absence or dysfunction of adrenal cortex where the deficiency of cortisol is a characteristic feature along with deficiency of ACTH. Hyperkalemia, hyponatremia and volume overload occur in Addison disease. Fatigue, anxiety, anorexia, mental irritability, weight loss and vomiting are common symptoms. Orthostatic hypotension and hypoglycemia are the most disturbing features.

HYDROCORTISONE

Hydrocortisone is the drug of choice in Addison disease. An oral dose of 15 to 30 mg in divided doses is effective in most patients. It is short acting and given more than once daily to mimic normal steroid level. To simulate diurnal fluctuation two thirds of dose is given in morning and one third in afternoon but it does not substitute for increase in serum glucocorticoid level in morning. It is quickly absorbed, rapidly acting and its blood level is easier to monitor.

FLUDROCORTISONE

Fludrocortisone is potent mineralocorticoid with sodium retaining property. It is a slower acting steroid and is given at the daily dose of 0.05 to 0.3 mg orally. It has intermediate duration of action with 125 time higher mineralocorticoid potency. If given in early stages it can cause severe hypokalemia and cardiac abnormalities. It is not used in mild disease but if symptoms progress, it is added to hydrocortisone.

Drug of Choice: Hydrocortisone

RATIONALE

In Addison disease, **hydrocortisone**, a glucocorticoid, is the preferred drug. It is given twice daily, once in morning and in the evening to **mimic** the **normal diurnal fluctuation** of steroid but this does not effectively supplement the increased requirement during early morning. **Fludrocortisone** is **slow acting** steroid with intermediate duration. Although its mineralocorticoid capacity is 125 times more than hydrocortisone, it is not preferred because as a potent mineralocorticoid it can cause **severe hypokalemia** and **cardiac abnormalities** if given early in this condition. However, if the condition progresses fludrocortisone should be combined with hydrocortisone.

1. *Neutral Protamine Hagedorn (NPH)/Glargine as suitable insulin for therapy.*

BACKGROUND

The amount of insulin required to reduce rabbit fasting blood glucose level to 45 mg/dL is called one unit. Most insulin preparations are available at neutral pH and are stable at room temperature. Insulin preparations are classified as short, intermediate and long acting preparations. NPH is dispensed at neutral pH while glargine is dispensed at acidic pH. Duration of action depends on the amount of absorption from site of injection and by its rate of dissociation from zinc.

GLARGINE

Glargine is available in acidic pH of 4.0 as clear solution with stable insulin hexamer. At neutral pH of subcutaneous space it aggregates causing prolonged and definitive absorption resulting in sustained peakless action, reducing the incidence hypoglycemia. Besides, due to its prolonged action it can be given as once daily dose. It does not accumulate on repeated injections and can be given at any time of day. It should not be mixed with other insulin preparations at neutral pH as it is acidic. Glargine reduces risk of nocturnal and severe hypoglycemia by 40 to 60%. Unlike NPH it provides clinically meaningful sustained reductions in hypoglycemia risk.

NEUTRAL PROTAMINE HAGEDORN (NPH)

Neutral protamine hagedorn (NPH) is mixture of protamine and zinc with insulin. It contains protamine zinc insulin and crystalline zinc insulin in the ratio of 1:2. It is also known as isophane as this 1:2 ratio results in equivalent amounts of protamine and zinc. It is a turbid suspension with zinc and protamine in phosphate buffer at neutral pH. Insulin dissociates gradually from zinc thereby prolonging its duration of action. Onset of action is 2 to 4 hours and total duration of action is from 10 to 20 hours. Hence, it is more often given twice daily with short acting insulin. It does not maintain a peakless action and so the incidence of hypoglycemia is high.

Drug of Choice: Glargine

RATIONALE

Hypoglycemia is a major risk of insulin administration. **Glargine** is a **long acting** preparation given **once daily** and available in **acidic pH**. In neutral pH of subcutaneous space it aggregates and is absorbed very slowly. Hence, it results in **sustained peakless action** and compared to NPH, it **reduces** the **risk** of **nocturnal as well** as **severe hypoglycemia** by 40 to 60%.[117] It does not accumulate on repeated injections so can be administered at any time of day. **NPH** is available at neutral pH and its duration is from 10 to 20 hours necessitating twice daily administration. The **risk of hypoglycemia is high**[118] with NPH and so, it is not preferred.

2. *Glulisine/Regular insulin in patients with gastroparesis.*

BACKGROUND

Intake of food is minimal and irregular in patients with gastroparesis. Gastroparesis occurs commonly in hypothyroidism, cortisol deficiency and uncontrolled diabetes mellitus. Early satiety or postprandial fullness and abdominal distension are frequent symptoms. This often results in postprandial hypoglycemia as insulin is administered prior to meal.

GLULISINE

The amino acid lysine at position B_{29} is replaced by glutamic acid and asparagine at B_{23} position is replaced by lysine in insulin molecule of glulisine. These changes result in rapid dissociation from polymer to monomer form and such rapid dissociation results in rapid onset and quick termination of action. In addition to effective control of HbA₁C, glulisine reduces risk of hypoglycemia. In gastroparesis it can be administered after food depending on the quantity consumed and its dose can be altered accordingly.

REGULAR INSULIN

Regular or native insulin has slow absorption from the site of administration. At neutral pH it dissociates slowly from hexamer to monomer so absorption is delayed. Hence, it is administered 30 to 45 minutes prior to food to control postprandial hyperglycemia. The amount of carbohydrates consumed during early meal should be more to prevent hypoglycemia but it can create problem in patients with gastroparesis as absorption is often erratic.

Drug of Choice: Glulisine

RATIONALE

Gastroparesis is often associated with uncontrolled diabetes mellitus. It is characterized by early satiety or postprandial fullness and abdominal distension. Absorption of food is often erratic leading to postprandial hypoglycemia. **Glulisine** is **quickly absorbed**, has **quick onset** and **rapid termination** of action. It is usually administered 15 minutes before food but in patients with **gastroparesis** its **administration can be delayed** and can be given **after food** altering the dose according to the amount consumed. Therefore, it is preferred in patients with gastroparesis. **Regular insulin** should be administered at least **30 to 45 minutes before food** as it takes more time for the onset of action. In individuals who consume less food due to early satiety as **in gastroparesis** it **results in hypoglycemia** hence, it is not preferred.

3. *(Basal-bolus)/(Split-mixed) regimens as preferred regimen in type-I diabetes mellitus.*

BACKGROUND

Insulin does not control postprandial hyperglycemia if given as single daily injections. Multiple injections of complex regimens are necessary to achieve euglycemia. In addition, the therapeutic end points should be monitored carefully to assess insulin effect. Periodic assessment of HbA$_1$C will establish the overall control of blood glucose. Besides, self monitoring of fasting and postprandial blood glucose should be advised.

BASAL-BOLUS REGIMEN

Basal dose of insulin suppresses hepatic glycogenolysis, proteolysis and lipolysis but supplemental dose is required during each meal to control rise in blood glucose level. Multiple injections per day effectively manage basal and postprandial hyperglycemia. Glargine is given either once or twice daily along with supplemental short acting insulin which is administered prior to each meal. It mimics physiologic insulin replacement strategy as it maintains basal plasma level. This provides background insulin coverage over which rapid acting analogs act.

SPLIT-MIXED REGIMEN

Time required for peak action is delayed in intermediate acting insulin preparations. So they are given with short acting preparations to reduce postprandial hyperglycemia. Rapidly acting insulin analogs or regular insulin can be combined with NPH. They can be mixed in same syringe as they are available in neutral pH. Split-mixed regimens of NPH and regular insulin is available as 70%, 30% combination. Disadvantage is that regular insulin interacts with zinc in NPH and loses its potency. Insulin lispro should not be combined with NPH as it loses its stability. Mixture of neutral protamine hagedorn and lispro is available for clinical use. This split mixture is given as pre-breakfast and pre-supper administration. Most often pre-supper administration is insufficient to control nocturnal hyperglycemia. So it is split into regular insulin as pre-supper dose and the next dose of NPH at bed time. It does not maintain basal plasma insulin level to suppress lipolysis or glycogenolysis.

Drug of Choice: Basal-Bolus Regimen

RATIONALE

Euglycemic control cannot be achieved through single daily dose of either long acting or short acting insulin preparation. Insulin has to be administered as multiple daily injections as complex regimens. A **basal** level of plasma **insulin suppresses hepatic glycogenolysis, proteolysis** and **lipolysis. Glargine** provides **peakless basal level** in plasma that exerts an effective protection as it **mimics normal physiological** level providing background coverage of insulin. Additional **supplemental short acting insulin** analogs should be given **prior to each meal** to control postprandial hyperglycemia. **Split-mixture regimen** contains NPH and either regular insulin or other short acting insulin analogs but it is **less effective** in **controlling nocturnal hyperglycemia**. Besides it does not inhibit lipolysis, hepatic glycogenolysis or proteolysis as it does not provide background insulin coverage and does not maintain basal plasma insulin level.

4. *Insulin/Oral hypoglycemic agents for management of diabetes mellitus in hospitalized patients.*

BACKGROUND

Prevalence of diabetes mellitus in hospitalized patients without prior diagnosis is 30%. Stress due to illness is associated with insulin resistance and glucose intolerance. Stress induces release of cytokines and secretion of counter regulatory hormones such as steroids and adrenaline. Surgery induces stress and can result in ketoacidosis in an already diabetic patient. IV dextrose and glucocorticoids used for therapy can potentiate risk of diabetes mellitus. Irrespective of severity of disease, hyperglycemia causes poor outcome in such patients.

INSULIN

Insulin is the drug of choice for management of hyperglycemia in such patients. IV Insulin is the only option for critically ill patients with edema or variable BP. It can be given through subcutaneous administration if the patient is stable. Various insulin regimens are available for effective management of glucose level. Basal/bolus regimen is preferred and prevents wider fluctuations in blood glucose preventing the onset of both hypo and hyperglycemia and speedening up the recovery.

ORAL HYPOGLYCEMIC AGENTS

Oral hypoglycemic agents have only limited value in the treatment of hyperglycemia. They are less potent and in the presence of erratic absorption result in irregular control. Besides they may increase the incidence of adverse events in hospitalized patients. Fluid retention or edema induced by thiazolidinediones can aggravate heart failure. Similarly metformin is contraindicated for patients with liver or kidney dysfunction. Hence, oral hypoglycemic agents are not preferred in hospitalized patients.

Drug of Choice: Insulin

RATIONALE

Illness and surgery stimulate stress mediated release of cytokines, inflammatory mediators as well as counter regulatory hormones such as adrenaline, growth hormone and steroids. During hospital stay glucocorticoids and IV dextrose are often used, elevating blood glucose level. **Oral hypoglycemic agents** are not preferred as they are **less potent** due to **improper absorption** and often exacerbate adverse events. In critically ill patients IV insulin is preferred and in stable patients subcutaneous administration is effective. Various insulin regimens are available for therapy but basal/bolus regimen is preferred.

5. *Glyburide/Glipizide as suitable sulfonylurea for therapy in elderly patients.*

BACKGROUND

Second generation sulfonylureas are most potent insulin releasers widely used in therapy. They bind with sulfonylurea receptors (SUR) on beta cells of pancreas and inhibit closure of ATP mediated K^+ channel causing membrane depolarization thereby increasing intracellular calcium level and leading to insulin release. Sulfonylureas additionally increase insulin level by inhibiting insulin clearance by liver.

GLIPIZIDE

Glipizide, a second generation sulfonylurea is given as single dose. It is less potent, given 30 minutes before food and has shorter duration of action than glyburide. It is metabolized to inactive compounds and to be avoided in liver dysfunction. Incidence of hypoglycemia is minimal with glipizide and it does not inhibit the physiological compensatory mechanisms required for the recovery from hypoglycemia. Hence, it is ideal drug in elderly. It neither blunts the compensatory mechanism for hypoglycemia nor causes secondary failure.

GLYBURIDE

Glyburide is 2nd generation sulfonylurea, highly potent when compared to 1st generation. Among sulfonylureas it has greatest affinity for SUR and has potent insulinotropic action. Its binding to SU receptors on cardiac myocytes and vascular smooth muscle prevents the protective 'ischemic preconditioning' and increases cardiac risk. The half-life of glyburide is 1 to 2 hours but its biologic effects extend up to 24 hours because it is metabolized into active metabolites that have potent hypoglycemic action. It is unique and binds not only to SUR on β cell but also gets sequestrated within cell, prolonging its pharmacological action. Glyburide causes prolonged hypoglycemia as it blunts the compensatory mechanisms. Elderly persons are more susceptible for glyburide induced risk of hypoglycemia. It should not be used in kidney and liver dysfunction as it can prolong hypoglycemia. Secondary failure due to down regulation of SUR on pancreatic β cell is common.

Drug of Choice: Glipizide

RATIONALE

Second generation sulfonylureas are 100 times more potent than first generation sulfonylureas. They bind to sulfonylurea receptors on beta cells of pancreas. **Glyburide** not only binds with SUR on β cell but also gets sequestrated within cell and so exerts **longer duration** of action. Its active metabolites are also responsible for its prolonged action and results in **late onset hypoglycemia** especially during later part of day. Elderly patients are more sensitive to this side effect. Besides it **blunts the normal compensatory responses** that occur during hypoglycemic attack. Glyburide also interacts with SU receptors in cardiac myocytes and vascular smooth muscle **preventing** the protective **'ischemic preconditioning'** reflex. On **chronic administration** it causes secondary failure of therapy. Hence, glyburide is not preferred. **Glipizide** is **less potent** with **shorter duration** of action so **lessens** the risk of **hypoglycemia**. Besides, it does not blunt the compensatory responses to hypoglycemia and does not cause secondary failure on chronic use. Hence, glipizide is preferred to glyburide especially in elderly patients.

6. *Metformin/Thiazolidinediones for obesity induced insulin resistance.*

BACKGROUND

One of the important lifestyle risk factors causing diabetes mellitus is obesity. Insulin resistance is directly proportional to the extent of visceral obesity. Fat deposited in mesenteric and omental areas directly influence the resistance to insulin. Influence of subcutaneous fat is very minimal in determining insulin insensitivity. Those with increased visceral fat are called 'metabolically obese' and are highly prone. Physical exercise greatly influences visceral fat and determines the onset of diabetes. Many mechanisms are involved in development of obesity induced insulin resistance such as increase in free fatty acid levels and its oxidation in skeletal muscle. Adipokines, adiponectin favor insulin action and resistin inhibits insulin action. Imbalance and abnormal levels of these adipokines contribute to its pathophysiology. Release of tissue necrosis factor-α and IL-6 from macrophages will also impair insulin signaling.

METFORMIN

Insulin sensitizer metformin promotes insulin action without facilitating its release. It is the first line drug and inhibits hepatic gluconeogenesis and lipogenesis. It stimulates adenosine monophosphate mediated protein kinase activity in liver. It promotes peripheral uptake of glucose and inhibits intestinal glucose absorption. In obese individuals it reduces triglycerides, postprandial and fasting glucose level. It interferes with calcium mediated absorption of vitamin B_{12}-intrinsic factor complex. It causes anorexia, abdominal discomfort, diarrhea and vomiting in 20% of patients.

THIAZOLIDINEDIONES

Thiazolidinediones bind to peroxisome proliferator-activated gamma (PPARγ). PPARγ are mainly found in adipocytes and involved in lipid and glucose metabolism. It causes differentiation of adipocytes promoting uptake of circulating fatty acids. Shift of lipid stores from nonadipose to adipose tissues improves insulin sensitivity. Most common side effects of thiazolidinediones are edema-induced weight gain. They also cause an increase in overall weight gain and body adiposity. If given along with insulin, the incidence of weight gain and edema is doubled. Besides they increase risk of fractures, worsen macular edema and cardiac problems.

Drug of Choice: Metformin

RATIONALE

Obesity is an important lifestyle factor responsible for diabetes mellitus. Insulin resistance is directly proportional to the extent of visceral obesity and fat deposited in mesenteric and omental areas directly influence the resistance. Metformin and thiazolidinediones are insulin sensitizers effective in promoting peripheral utilization of glucose. They **both reduce hepatic gluconeogenesis** and reduce plasma free fatty acid levels. Additionally **metformin** causes **anorexia** and inhibits intestinal absorption of glucose. Hence, it is more suitable for obese patients. Most common side effects of **thiazolidinediones** are **edema and weight gain**. Thiazolidinediones

increase overall **weight** gain and body adiposity. The intensity of weight gain and edema is doubled if coadministered with insulin. Besides they increase risk of fractures, worsen macular edema and cardiac problems.

7. *GLP-1 agonist/DPP-4 inhibitors in diabetes mellitus.*

BACKGROUND

Compared to IV glucose, oral glucose evokes 3 to 4 fold increase in insulin release. This is due to the capacity of oral glucose in releasing gut hormones or 'incretins', glucagon like peptide 1(GLP-1) and glucose dependent insulinotropic peptide 1 (GIP1). While GIP1 secretion is retained GLP-1 secretion is impaired in type 2 diabetes. Administration of GLP-1 in type 2 diabetes patients stimulates insulin release. Insulinotropic action is glucose dependent so does not cause release of insulin at fasting state. In addition GLP-1 also has other extra pancreatic and pancreatic effects. It inhibits release of glucagon, preserves integrity of islet cells by inhibiting apoptosis and markedly inhibits feeding by central action and by delaying gastric emptying time.

DIPEPTIDYL PEPTIDASE-4 (DPP-4) INHIBITORS

The incretins GLP-1and GIP are proteolyzed by dipeptidyl peptidase as well as endopeptidases. DPP-4 inhibitors such as sitagliptin, alogliptin, linagliptin and saxagliptin inhibit these enzymes prolonging the action of GLP-1and GIP1. DPP-4 inhibitors prolong the duration endogenous incretins augmenting their action. They cause more insulin release, better control of postprandial and fasting blood glucose. They can be administered orally as they are well absorbed and are more convenient to patients. They are equieffective to GLP-1 analogs, safe with no consistent side effects. Unlike GLP-1 analogs they do not cause nausea and do not result in weight loss. Nasopharyngitis is frequent but pancreatitis and allergic reactions such as anaphylaxis, angioedema and Stevens-Johnson syndrome are also reported but the frequency of such serious allergic reactions is unclear. They may be due to elevated substance P and neuropeptide Y, the substrates of DPP-4.

GLP-1 ANALOGS

GLP-1 analogs exenatide and liraglutide are available for therapy. They are metabolically more stable than GLP-1 as they are not rapidly degraded. They are parenteral preparations and have to be administered subcutaneously. They are not metabolized by DPP-4 so their duration is longer than native GLP-1. GLP-1 analogs along with insulin releasers sulfonylureas cause hypoglycemia. Dose dependent nausea is the main side effect but it may subside on continuation of therapy. They are less favored due to risk of necrotizing or hemorrhagic pancreatitis.

Drug of Choice: DPP-4 Inhibitors

RATIONALE

Oral administration of glucose releases insulin more effectively due to action of incretins or gut hormones. Glucagon like peptide-1 (GLP-1) and glucose dependent insulinotropic peptide 1 (GIP1) are important incretins that stimulate insulin release. **GLP-1 analogs** inhibit **release** of **glucagon** preserve integrity of islet cell by inhibiting its apoptosis. Besides, it reduces food intake by acting centrally and by delaying gastric emptying. Insulinotropic action is glucose dependent so they do not release insulin at fasting state but the native GLP-1 is metabolized very quickly by dipeptidyl peptidase enzyme. When compared to GLP-1, its analogs exenatide and liraglutide have longer half-life as they are not metabolized by DPP-4 **but** they **cause intense nausea** and have a **high risk** for necrotizing or **hemorrhagic pancreatitis**. **DPP-4 inhibitors** inhibit metabolism of endogenous GLP-1 and GIP1 augmenting their efficacy and prolonging their duration of action. Hence, DPP-4 inhibitors cause more insulin release and better control of postprandial and fasting blood glucose levels. Frequent side effect is nasopharyngitis but in a few it can cause serious allergic reactions. They are **safe** with **no consistent side effects**. Hence, they are preferred.

8. *Sitagliptin/Linagliptin as DPP-4 inhibitors in patients with renal dysfunction.*

BACKGROUND

Most often diabetes mellitus and nephropathy coexist in many patients. DPP-4 inhibits metabolism of incretins, GLP-1 and GIP1 prolonging their action. DPP-4 inhibitors result in long lasting inhibition of the enzyme DPP-4. They increase the circulating GLP-1 to around 100% from 20%. The therapeutic efficacy and toxicity profile of all DPP-4 inhibitors is almost similar.

LINAGLIPTIN

Linagliptin has similar efficacy and toxicity profile as sitagliptin. Its daily dose is 5 mg, not metabolized and excreted primarily through bile. Unlike sitagliptin, it favorably alters lipid profile and reduces plasma LDL-C because structurally it contains xanthine ring and so has antioxidant property. Since it is not mainly excreted through kidney, it can be given in renal dysfunction.

SITAGLIPTIN

Sitagliptin is a competitive inhibitor and inhibits 95% of enzyme for 12 hours. GLP-1 and GIP1 levels increase by two folds following its administration. Given as monotherapy at 100 mg/day, sitagliptin improves HbA_1C by 0.5 to 1.4%. In some patients it causes serious allergic reactions and predispose to nasopharyngitis. It is mainly excreted through kidney, so, dose reduction by at least 50% in renal dysfunction is required.

Drug of Choice: Linagliptin

RATIONALE

Almost all DPP-4 inhibitors result in similar glycemic control and have same toxicity profile. Most often **nephropathy coexists** with diabetes mellitus and **except linagliptin** all **other DPP-4 inhibitors** are mainly **excreted** through **renal route**. Hence, all DPP-4 inhibitors except linagliptin require dose reduction as per creatinine clearance in renal dysfunction.[119] **Linagliptin** is not metabolized and is mainly **excreted** through **bile**. So, it is preferable in patients with renal dysfunction. Besides, xanthine nucleus in its structure promotes its antioxidant property reducing LDL-C.

9. *Regular insulin/Short acting insulin analogs for intravenous administration in the management of diabetic ketoacidosis.*

BACKGROUND

Diabetic ketoacidosis is life-threatening emergency needing immediate attention. It has very poor prognosis in older patients with 20% mortality rate but only 5% in younger patients. Generally occurs in type I but can also occur in type II under stress, trauma or sepsis. Plasma glucose > 350 mg/dL, pH < 7.3, ketones > 1.8, hyperphosphatemia, hyperkalemia, hyponatremia, increased urea and creatinine are diagnostic features. Hyperkalemia occurs due to shift of intracellular potassium to extracellular fluid. Correction of acidosis and reduction of osmolality as well as normalization of blood glucose, restoration of tissue perfusion and plasma volume are also vital for patient's survival. Therapy includes fluid replacement, administration of potassium and sodium bicarbonate. Regular insulin, insulin analogs like glulisine and lispro are approved for intravenous use.

REGULAR INSULIN

Regular insulin is preferred to glulisine for treatment of ketoacidosis. It is stable and can be given undiluted either directly into vein or as infusion. This is convenient to administer loading dose as well as maintenance dose. Insulin inhibits entry of free fatty acids into liver reducing ketone synthesis, increasing pH leading to correction of acidosis. It reduces gluconeogenesis, glycogenolysis, hyperglycemia and hyperosmolality. A loading dose of 0.1 unit/kg is followed by continuous infusion of 0.1 unit/kg/hour. Once ketoacidosis is controlled therapy is continued by subcutaneous insulin. Basal insulin with rapid acting insulin is given subcutaneously prior to first meal.

Intravenous infusion of regular insulin should be discontinued one hour after SC injection. Glargine with glulisine is preferred to NPH with regular insulin for continuation.

SHORT ACTING INSULIN ANALOGS

Although IV glulisine is approved, it is not used in therapy of ketoacidosis. Glulisine rapidly dissociates from polymer to monomer stage and acts quickly. Hence, glulisine causes more rapid reduction of plasma glucose and ketones necessitating continuous monitoring of blood glucose. Further, it causes rapid shift of extracellular potassium into cells lowering plasma potassium resulting in dangerous hypokalemia, hence glulisine is not preferred. Besides, it is stable only in 0.9% sodium chloride and can be given only with normal saline.

Drug of Choice: Regular Insulin

RATIONALE

Intravenous administration of insulin is preferred to subcutaneous or intramuscular route as rapid reduction of plasma glucose and ketones is required in diabetic ketoacidosis. Insulin reduces entry of free fatty acids into liver reducing ketone synthesis. It also reduces gluconeogenesis, glycogenolysis, hyperglycemia and hyperosmolality. Regular insulin is preferred as it is short acting, more stable and can be given either directly into vein or as an intravenous infusion. This is convenient to administer loading dose and maintenance dose. Glulisine rapidly dissociates from polymer to monomer stage and acts more rapidly than regular insulin. Hence, it causes rapid reduction in plasma glucose level and rapid shift of extracellular potassium into cells increasing the risk of dangerous hypokalemia[120] necessitating continuous monitoring of blood glucose and serum potassium to avoid hypoglycemia and hypokalemia. Besides, it is stable only in normal saline and should be diluted in normal saline before administration. So, regular insulin is preferred to short acting insulin analogs.

10. *Liraglutide/Exenatide as GLP-1 analog.*

BACKGROUND

The native peptide GLP-1 is rapidly proteolyzed by dipeptidyl peptidase (DPP) but GLP-1 analogs are metabolically more stable and not metabolized by DPP. GLP-1 analogs induce satiety and cause weight loss as they delay gastric emptying.

LIRAGLUTIDE

Liraglutide is soluble fatty acid acylated GLP-1analog resistant to DPP-4 metabolism. It is long acting with duration of action for 12 hours so, can be given once daily as monotherapy. Mild renal impairment does not affect estimated treatment index of liraglutide as it is not excreted by glomerular filtration. Since, liraglutide is mainly metabolized by plasma and tissue endopeptidases its pharmacokinetics is not altered by mild renal impairment.[121] Liraglutide improves satiety, decreases body weight so reduces cardiovascular risk such as hypertension, proteinuria and progressive renal disease associated with obesity. As the efficacy of liraglutide is not altered in mild renal impairment, unlike exenatide it does not increase the incidence of end stage renal disease. It causes nausea and rarely pancreatitis is noted in patients taking liraglutide.

EXENATIDE

Exenatide is resistant to metabolism by DPP-4 with half-life of 2.4 hours. It is given as subcutaneous injection twice daily as its duration of action is only 6 hours. Its actions are similar to GLP-1 in reducing glucagon release and promoting gastric emptying. It reduces food intake and causes weight loss with sustained reduction in HbA_1C. It is mainly cleared by glomerular filtration and so should be avoided in renal dysfunction. It causes intense nausea and a higher risk of hemorrhagic or necrotizing pancreatitis. Besides it is found to be nephrotoxic and causes renal impairment in many patients. Exenatide is often associated with higher incidence of end stage renal disease. It prolongs gastric emptying, delays absorption of many drugs including antibiotics.

Drug of Choice: Liraglutide

RATIONALE

Liraglutide and exenatide are the two GLP-1 analogs used in therapy. Unlike native GLP-1 they are not inhibited by dipeptidyl peptidase. **Exenatide** is **short acting** and has to be administered **twice daily**. It causes **intense nausea** and increased incidence of **pancreatitis**. Besides it is found to be associated with renal impairment and acute renal failure as reported by FDA through post-marketing surveillance. **Liraglutide** is **long acting**, can be administered **once daily** and has **better therapeutic efficacy** when compared to exenatide. It is mainly metabolized by plasma and tissue endopeptidases and not excreted through glomerular filtration. Hence, it can be administered safely in mild renal impairment. Since the safety and efficacy of liraglutide is not altered by renal dysfunction, it is preferred to exenatide.

11. *Acarbose/Miglitol as alpha glucosidase inhibitors to reduce intestinal absorption of carbohydrates.*

BACKGROUND

Polysaccharides in food should be converted to monosaccharides by enzyme α-glucosidase present in intestinal brush border for better absorption. Inhibitors of α-glucosidase prevent breakdown of polysaccharides to monosaccharides inhibiting the absorption of disaccharides, starch and dextrin and reducing the postprandial rise in glucose. They also release GLP-1 into circulation that adds to its glucose lowering effect. They should be taken in the beginning of meals for better therapeutic benefit. They are both potent inhibitors of alpha-amylase, glucoamylase and sucrase and minimal inhibitors of isomaltase but do not inhibit lactase or trehalase

ACARBOSE

Acarbose binds to intestinal disaccharides 1000 times more than with sucrose. It is started at the dose of 50 mg twice daily and gradually increased to 100 mg thrice daily. Acarbose acts locally on intestinal α-glucosidase as it is minimally absorbed. Since it is a tetrasaccharide only as little as 2% is absorbed from intestine. It causes flatulence, abdominal bloating and diarrhea that are dose dependent but does not cause hypoglycemia when given alone. Flatulence is due to bacterial action on undigested carbohydrates reaching lower intestine. When combined with insulin secreto-gogues or insulin it can cause hypoglycemia. Acarbose induced hypoglycemia should be countered with glucose and not sucrose.

MIGLITOL

Miglitol has similar clinical efficacy and started at the dose of 25 mg thrice daily. Adverse effects are similar to acarbose and it does not cause hypoglycemia as monotherapy. Since it has structural simi-larity with glucose it is absorbed into circulation. It is not metabo-lized and excreted unchanged through renal route. Hence, it should not be given in patients with compromised renal function.

Drug of Choice: Acarbose

RATIONALE

The enzyme α-glucosidase is present in intestinal brush border and is responsible for the breakdown of polysaccharides to monosaccharides for effective absorption of glucose. Inhibitors of α-glucosidase prevent breakdown of polysaccharides to mono-saccharides inhibiting the absorption of disaccharides, starch and dextrin. These drugs reduce the rate of postprandial rise in glucose by reducing intestinal absorption of carbohydrates. Although the efficacy of acarbose and miglitol is similar, **Acarbose** is **not absorbed** and can be given safely in mild renal impairment. **Miglitol** is **structurally similar to glucose** and **absorbed** into circulation. Although not metabolized and mainly excreted through kidney it should be avoided in renal failure. They result in flatulence, abdominal bloating and diarrhea. If given alone they do not cause hypoglycemia but can result in hypoglycemia if coadministered with insulin secretogogues or insulin. **Hypoglycemia induced by α-glucosidase inhibitors should be treated with glucose and not sucrose.**

12. *Sodium glucose transporter 2 (SGLT2) inhibitors/Dipeptidyl peptidase-4 (DPP-4) inhibitors as monotherapy in diabetes mellitus.*

BACKGROUND

Type 2 diabetes mellitus is a progressive condition creating difficulty in tight glycemic control. Uncontrolled diabetes is usually treated with combination therapy. Addition of an insulin sensitizer with insulin secretogogue is a traditional combination but monotherapy is more convenient to patients and improves their compliance. Newer targets are being exploited for better control of glycemic index.

DIPEPTIDYL PEPTIDASE-4 INHIBITORS

Dipeptidyl peptidase inhibitors inhibit the metabolism of GLP-1 and GIP1. They do not have direct action and their action is secondary to increased GLP-1 level. They increase insulin release, decrease glucagon release and inhibit glycogenolysis. They can be used both for monotherapy and as adjuvant with other drugs. DPP-4 inhibitors reduce HbA_1C by 0.8% when given as monotherapy. Common side effect is nasopharyngitis although a few cases of pancreatitis are reported. They have better efficacy and safety and are suitable for monotherapy.

SODIUM GLUCOSE TRANSPORTER 2

Sodium glucose transporter 2 is expressed in proximal convoluted tubule. It promotes reabsorption of glucose from tubular lumen into renal epithelial cells. It is a high efficacy symporter that reabsorbs sodium and glucose in the ratio of 1:1. SGLT2 inhibitors inhibit the reabsorption promoting urinary excretion of glucose. These agents promote the loss of urinary glucose by 50 to 100 g per day. Canagliflozin and dapagliflozin are the two SGLT2 available for therapy but these agents increase the incidence of urinary tract infections and genital infections. Intravascular volume contraction and hypotension can also occur due to excessive glycosuria. By reducing hyperglycemia SGLT2 inhibitors prevent formation of glycation products reducing long-term complications of diabetes like nephropathy and retinopathy. In patients with diabetes there is either reduced insulin secretion or insulin resistance. SGLT2 inhibitors neither promote insulin secretion nor improve insulin action actively. Hence, they are more suitable for combination therapy rather than monotherapy. While canagliflozin increases LDL-C dapagliflozin causes breast and bladder cancer.

Drug of Choice: Dipeptidyl Peptidase-4 (DPP-4) Inhibitors

RATIONALE

Sodium glucose transporter 2 is expressed in proximal convoluted tubule and facilitates reabsorption of glucose from tubular lumen into renal epithelial cells. It is a high efficacy symporter and promotes reabsorption of sodium and glucose in the ratio of 1:1. SGLT2 inhibitors inhibit the reabsorption promoting urinary excretion of glucose. These agents promote the loss of urinary glucose by 50 to 100 g per day. By reducing hyperglycemia **SGLT2 inhibitors prevent formation of glycated products**. This **reduces long-term complications** of diabetes such as nephropathy and retinopathy. In patients with diabetes there is either low insulin secretion or high insulin resistance. **SGLT2 inhibitors neither actively promote insulin secretion nor improve insulin action**. Hence, they are **more suitable for combination therapy** rather than monotherapy. Besides they have higher toxicity profile. DPP-4 inhibitors facilitate insulin release by inhibiting GLP-1 metabolism and so can be given as monotherapy. Besides they have better efficacy and safety. Hence DPP4 inhibitors are more suitable for monotherapy.

Estrogens and Progestins

1. *Tamoxifen/Raloxifene for prevention and treatment of osteoporosis in high-risk postmenopausal women.*

BACKGROUND

Tamoxifen and raloxifene are selective estrogen receptor modulators (SERM). They are agonist-antagonists and have antiestrogenic or partial estrogenic activity. They are used as alternative for replacement of estrogen at high-risk hypogonadal women and they provide beneficial effects of estrogen during postmenopausal period in women.

RALOXIFENE

Raloxifene has antiresorptive property as it is an estrogen agonist in bone. It has high affinity towards ERα and ERβ receptors and binds to both estrogen receptors. It reduces plasma low-density lipoprotein-cholesterol (LDL-C) and total cholesterol levels but does not alter high-density lipoprotein-cholesterol (HDL-C) levels. It inhibits proliferation of ER positive breast cancer cells, reducing the risk of breast cancer by 50% but does not modulate ER-negative cancer cells. The risk of endometrial carcinoma is minimal as it does not induce endometrial proliferation. It causes hot flushes, leg cramps and increased incidence of deep vein thrombosis.

TAMOXIFEN

Tamoxifen exerts estrogenic, antiestrogenic or mixed actions depending on the tissues. It reduces size of breast tumor by inhibiting proliferation of breast cancer cells but it facilitates proliferation of uterine endometrium potentiating risk of uterine cancer. It does not increase the risk of fractures as it has agonistic antiresorptive activity in bone. Although it reduces LDL-C and lipoprotein (a) it does not influence HDL-C or triglycerides. It increases the risk of venous thromboembolism, nausea, cataract and hot flushes.

Drug of Choice: Raloxifene

RATIONALE

Tamoxifen and raloxifene are called selective estrogen receptor modulators (SERM) and are agonist-antagonists as they have antiestrogenic or partial estrogenic activity and suitable for prevention and treatment of osteoporosis in high risk postmenopausal women. **Tamoxifen** exerts estrogenic, antiestrogenic or mixed actions depending on the tissues. It **inhibits proliferation** of breast cancer cells and it also exerts **antiresorptive property** in bone but **induces** endometrial proliferation increasing the risk of **endometrial cancer**. **Raloxifene** is **more selective** to bone **without inducing endometrial proliferation**. Therefore, it does not increase the risk of endometrial carcinoma. Besides, it inhibits proliferation of breast cancer cells and reduces the incidence of invasive breast cancer by 50%. Hence, raloxifene is preferred to tamoxifen for osteoporosis.

2. *Levonorgestrel/Ulipristal as emergency contraceptive.*

BACKGROUND

Emergency or postcoital contraception is followed after unprotected intercourse. Inhibition of ovulation, gamete survival and implantation are the possible mechanisms. Since its efficacy is inferior to standard methods it should not be advocated frequently.

ULIPRISTAL

Ulipristal is a selective progesterone receptor modulator and 19-norprogesterone derivative. It is a progesterone agonist and highly potent in inhibiting ovulation by suppressing LH action. Even after LH surge it blocks ovulation preventing implantation of fertilized egg. It is effective as a single dose of 30 mg up to five days after intercourse and so preferred. It is more versatile than levonorgestrel it can be taken till 120 hours after intercourse and it is also a weak glucocorticoid antagonist. It causes abdominal pain and headache.

LEVONORGESTREL

Levonorgestrel is progesterone used specifically as postcoital pill to prevent conception. Levonorgestrel is most effective if taken at 0.75 mg within 72 hours of intercourse. Second dose of levonorgestrel should be repeated after 12 hours for complete benefit. Another regimen is to take 1.5 mg of levonorgestrel as single agent within 72 hours but it is less effective than ulipristal if given 72 hours after intercourse. So, it is not preferred.

Drug of Choice: Ulipristal

RATIONALE

Emergency or postcoital contraception is given to prevent pregnancy following unprotected intercourse. **Ulipristal** is a **selective modulator** and partial agonist of progesterone. It suppresses ovulation even after LH surge. Besides, it also prevents implantation of fertilized egg in uterine endometrium. It is effective as a **single dose**, highly versatile and acts as contraceptive **up to 5 days (120 hours)**. It is weak antagonist of glucocorticoid. **Levonorgestrel** should be given in **2 doses** at an **interval of 12 hours** and **within 72 hours** of unprotected intercourse. It is **not effective after 72 hours** and its efficacy is inferior to ulipristal. Hence, it is not preferred.

3. *Monophasic/Multiphasic formulation of combined pills as effective oral contraceptives.*

BACKGROUND

Estrogen-progesterone combination pills are the most effective contraceptive pills. They inhibit ovulation by suppressing mid-cycle LH surge and pituitary GnRH response. Release of FSH from pituitary during follicular phase is inhibited by estrogens. Progesterone renders the cervical mucus viscous preventing penetration of sperm. They increase uterine contractility and make endometrium unsuitable for implantation. Combination pills have ethinyl estradiol as estrogen component and 19-nortestosterone as progestin component. Newer preparations such as desogestrel contain progestin with less androgenic activity and drospirenone that blocks androgenic and mineralocorticoid activity. In 28 day menstrual cycle they are administered for the first 21 days. Biphasic and triphasic combinations contain different levels of estrogen and progestin and newer preparations contain lower amount of hormones to reduce side effects.

MONOPHASIC PILLS

In monophasic pills the quantity of estrogen or progesterone remains same throughout the cycle. Monophasic pills have similar contraceptive efficacy to triphasic pills. They do not increase accidental pregnancy rates or incidence of bleeding. There are considerable evidences for safety and efficacy of monophasic pills. Sequential order is not required so they improve compliance. They do not mimic hormonal pattern of normal menstrual cycle but still preferred.

MULTIPHASIC PILLS

Triphasic combination contains three different doses of estrogen or progestin. Some preparations have two different doses of estrogen while others have same dose. Most often the preparations contain three increasing doses of progesterone. Progesterone dose is low during first phase and increases in second and third phase. Doses and number of days of each phase may vary as (6 + 5 + 10) or (7 + 7 + 7) or (7 + 9 + 5) in each preparation. Triphasic pills, if not taken on required sequential order result in contraceptive failure and can also result in breakthrough bleeding. Hence, triphasic formulation has no advantage in efficacy over monophasic pills.

Drug of Choice: Monophasic Pills

RATIONALE

Combined pills contain both estrogen and progesterone and are more efficient than other formulations in preventing pregnancy. Most of the preparations contain ethinyl estradiol as estrogen and levonorgestrel/norethindrone/norgestimate as progestin. Newer preparations have either desogestrel as progestin with less androgenic activity or drospirenone, a progestin with antiandrogen and antimineralocorticoid activity. Most recent preparations contain lesser amount of hormones to reduce the incidence of side effects. Triphasic preparations contain three different doses of hormones for each phase of single menstrual cycle. The doses and number of days in each phase may vary for each preparation. Generally in all preparations, the dose of progestin increases from first to third phase. In monophasic pills the amount of estrogen and progesterone remains same throughout the cycle. There is **no adequate evidence to prove the superiority of multiphasic pills in terms of contraceptive efficacy, rate of breakthrough bleeding** and **accidental pregnancy rates. Muliphasic pills, if not taken in required sequential order**, can **lead to contraceptive failure or breakthrough bleeding**. In areas with low literacy rates the risk is high if the user does not take pills in the required sequential order. **Monophasic pills** are preferred due to their **safety, efficacy** and **better compliance**.

4. *Minipill/Combined pill as oral contraceptive.*

BACKGROUND

Fertility returns back after stopping oral contraceptives within a period of 2 months. Sometimes multifetal pregnancy occurs due to rebound increase in fertility. Pregnancy occurring during use of contraceptives should be terminated because sex hormones are teratogenic to fetus and can cause malformations. Combined and mini pills can both suppress mid cycle luteinizing hormone (LH) surge inhibiting ovulation. They induce thick cervical mucus secretion hostile to sperm penetration.

COMBINED PILL

The efficacy rate of combined pills is very high with only 0.3% failure rate. They contain both estrogen and progesterone that act through multiple mechanisms. They inhibit follicle-stimulating hormone (FSH) and mid cycle LH surge and have potent antiovulatory activity. The hormone combination makes endometrium most unsuitable for nidation thereby preventing conception. Headache, nausea, spotting or breakthrough bleeding are minor side effects. They also cause mood swings, glucose intolerance, weight gain, chloasma, thromboembolism and hypertension. They also increase the risk of cancer. Recent contraceptive preparations contain low dose of hormones so they result in minimal side effects.

MINI PILL

Mini pill contains only progesterone and therefore has only minimal efficacy with higher failure rate. It suppresses midcycle LH surge, inhibits ovulation and alters cervical mucus. Since the failure rate is around 3% it is most unpopular contraceptive formulation. Episodes of breakthrough bleeding and irregular erratic spotting occur frequently. Headache, acne, reduced HDL-C and increased LDL-C levels are frequent side effects. It does not cause thromboembolism, nausea, hypertension or breast tenderness as it does not contain estrogen. Due to its poor efficacy and higher failure rates it is not preferred.

Drug of Choice: Combined Pill

RATIONALE

Combined pills contain estrogen and progestin and have higher efficacy rate with lower failure rate. They **act by multiple mechanisms**. They inhibit the gonadotropin release from pituitary. They also inhibit FSH and mid cycle LH surge. They are antiovulatory in nature and alter endometrium so that it is unsuitable for implantation. Although they cause mild to severe side effects, they are preferred as they are **highly effective** in preventing pregnancy with **lower failure rate**. **Mini pill** is **progesterone alone pill** with **high**

failure rate. Although it causes minimal side effects it is not preferred due to its high failure rate.

5. *3-Ketodesogestrel/Depot medroxy progesterone acetate as long acting progesterone contraceptive.*

BACKGROUND

Many long acting contraceptive preparations contain progesterone. They are highly effective as intramuscular injection when given as oily preparation as its absorption is delayed. It is also available as subdermal implants that can be removed surgically after few years. These reduce the need for daily doses of hormonal contraceptives, so are very convenient to use. They inhibit ovulation, alter cervical mucus and also act on uterine endometrium.

3-KETODESOGESTREL

3-ketodesogestrel (etonogestrel) is progestin-impregnated rods and implanted subdermally. It is a metabolite of desogestrel and slowly releases progestin for about 3 years. Amount of progesterone released is little higher than that is needed to suppress ovulation. After removal of implant ovulation returns back within a period of 6 weeks. Subdermal implants are preferred because of effective contraception for many years. It may cause weight gain and breakthrough bleeding intermittently in some women.

DEPOT MEDROXY PROGESTERONE ACETATE

Depot medroxy progesterone acetate has efficacy up to three months. It is either given as intramuscular or subcutaneous injection for effective contraception. It causes total amenorrhea and complete alteration of normal menstrual pattern but has black box warning in label for decreased bone density as it induces osteoporosis.

Drug of Choice: 3-Ketodesogestrel

RATIONALE

Long acting progesterone preparations are used as contraceptive as they have higher efficacy. Besides they can be administered once in a few months or years and need not be given daily. They are either administered as intramuscular or subcutaneous injection. Subdermal implant of progesterone is available recently. **Depot medroxy progesterone acetate** is given as IM or SC injection with duration of action of about **3 months**. Although it provides contraception it causes **total amennorhea** with completely **altered menstrual pattern**. Besides, it has a **black box** warning for **reduced mineral bone density**. **3-ketodesogestrel** (etonogestrel) is **subdermal implant** containing progestin-impregnated rods. It is effective **for 3 years** and releases progesterone slowly. Progesterone released is a little higher and **ovulation returns back within 6 weeks of** surgical **removal of implant**. It is preferred because of its higher efficacy and longer duration of action.

6. *Unopposed HRT/Combined HRT as suitable hormone replacement therapy.*

BACKGROUND

Hormone replacement therapy (HRT) is given for postmenopausal women and in women who have had hysterectomy. This is given to prevent urogenital atrophy, vasomotor symptoms and bone fractures. Vasomotor symptoms such as chills, hot flashes, paresthesia and excessive sweating occur in menopause due to decline in ovarian function. Increased incidence of fractures due to weak and thin bones such as trauma fracture of hip and compression fracture of vertebrae is also common after menopause. Incidence of cardiovascular disease increases rapidly after menopause.

COMBINED HORMONE REPLACEMENT THERAPY

Combined HRT includes both estrogen as well as progestin for therapy. Addition of progestin in HRT reduces the risk of endometrial carcinoma. It causes migraine, breast tenderness, alopecia and fluid retention. It reduces the risk of ovarian cancer but increases the risk of breast cancer. So unopposed HRT in such women reduces progesterone induced side effects.

UNOPPOSED HORMONE REPLACEMENT THERAPY (HRT)

Unopposed HRT includes estrogen without progesterone in therapy. Estrogen is very effective in alleviating most symptoms of menopause. Estrogen reduces vasomotor symptoms, fractures and vaginal dryness. It promotes vasodilatation, reduces LDL-C so reduces cardiovascular disease. It reduces bone fractures and causes modest but sustained reduction in bone pain. It improves post menopausal depression and glycemic control but unopposed HRT does not reduce risk of colorectal cancer or myocardial infarction and increases the risk of breast cancer, ovarian and endometrial cancer. Lower dose of estrogen reduces the adverse effects when compared with high dose. It also increases risk of stroke, pancreatitis, gallstones and lowers seizure threshold.

Drug of Choice: Combined Hormone Replacement Therapy (HRT)

RATIONALE

HRT is given to postmenopausal women and women who have undergone hysterectomy to treat postmenopausal symptoms such as vasomotor symptoms, fractures and vaginal dryness. **Unopposed HRT** with estrogen alone **reduces** postmenopausal **symptoms**, improves glycemic control and depression **but increases risk of endometrial, colorectal, ovarian** and **breast cancers**. The incidence of breast cancer is not altered with **combined HRT** but the risk of **endometrial cancer is reduced**. Hence, it is preferred to unopposed HRT. Unopposed HRT can be given to reduce progesterone induced side effects.

1. *Spironolactone/Flutamide in hirsutism.*

BACKGROUND

Hirsutism is characterized by virilization in females with alopecia, clitoromegaly and deep voice. It can be familial or idiopathic or secondary to polycystic ovarian syndrome (PCOS). Higher level of androgens may not always be detectable in patients with hirsutism but they have elevated levels of dihydrotestosterone metabolite, androstenediol. Excessive androstenediol is produced by skin and hirsutism has a familial predisposition. Fifty-percent of women with PCOS have elevated levels of serum or free testosterone. In women with deficiency of 21-hydroxylase, the secretion of cortisol is low. This leads to compensatory increase in ACTH secretion causing adrenal hyperplasia and hirsutism. Cushing syndrome, acromegaly, ovarian tumors and porphyria can all result in hirsutism.

FLUTAMIDE

Flutamide is an androgen antagonist inhibiting the binding of testosterone to its receptors. It is given as 250 mg/day for one year followed by 125 mg/day for maintenance. It is used along with GnRH analog to inhibit the gonadotropin release from pitutary; if used alone, it is less effective as it increases testosterone secretion by stimulating LH. It improves hirsutism by reducing male pattern baldness, acne and change of voice. Since flutamide is teratogenic it should be prescribed only to nonpregnant women. It inhibits symptoms of hirsutism better than spironolactone but prolonged use of flutamide can result in hepatotoxicity.

SPIRONOLACTONE

Spironolactone, the potassium sparing diuretic is a weak androgen receptor antagonist. It is also a weak inhibitor of testosterone synthesis. Very often it causes gynecomastia in males and this adverse effect of spironolactone is utilized in therapy for masking the symptoms of hirsutism. It is less effective than flutamide and can cause hyperkalemia. It is contraindicated in women of reproductive age group and during pregnancy.

Drug of Choice: Flutamide

RATIONALE

Hirsutism can be familial or secondary to certain conditions such as steroidogenic enzyme deficiency, PCOS, ovarian tumor, Cushing syndrome, acromegaly and porphyria. **Flutamide**, the androgen antagonist is effective when given along with GnRH analogs as this combination **inhibits** the LH mediated secretion of testosterone. When compared to spironolactone it inhibits all symptoms of hirsutism like voice change, acne and male pattern baldness but it can cause hepatotoxicity. **Spironolactone**, the potassium sparing diuretic is less effective. It is a weak androgen antagonist. Since it has tendency to **cause hyperkalemia** it should be monitored during spironolactone administration. They are both contraindicated in reproductive age group.

2. *Aromatase inhibitors (AI)/Selective estrogen receptor modulator (SERM) in gynecomastia.*

BACKGROUND

Unilateral or asymmetrical enlarged and palpable male breast is called gynecomastia. It is common among obese or tall teenagers and in athletes who use anabolic steroids. In around 60% of boys pubertal gynecomastia can occur but subsides within one year. Unusual firmness, asymmetry or retraction of nipple indicate higher chance of malignancy. It may be induced by certain drugs like spiranolactone. Persistent and painful gynecomastia requires therapy for about 9 to 12 months.

SELECTIVE ESTROGEN RECEPTOR MODULATOR

Selective estrogen receptor modulator (SERM) or selective estrogen receptor modulators are effective in true glandular gynecomastia so preferred to aromatase inhibitors (AIs). Among the SERM, raloxifene is found to be more effective than tamoxifen. Oral dose of raloxifene is 60 mg daily and has to be continued for many months. It directly inhibits proliferation of breast cells suppressing further increase in size. It does not cause osteoporosis as it increases bone mass reducing bone loss.

AROMATASE INHIBITORS

The synthesis of estrogens from androgens by aromatase enzyme is inhibited by AI. Aromatase inhibitor inhibits the conversion of testosterone to estradiol and androstenedione to estrone. Aromatase is present in breast and its inhibition by AI decreases estrogen levels inhibiting the growth of breast tissue as the primary stimulus, estrogen is reduced. Examestane, a third generation AI is very potent and can be administered orally. As 'suicide substrate' it irreversibly inhibits aromatase decreasing estrogen synthesis. It is usually well tolerated but can cause muscle cramps, diarrhea and arthralgia. Osteoporosis induced clinical fractures and visual disturbances are serious side effects. It delays fusion of epiphysis and can increase the overall height. Hence, aromatase inhibitors should be avoided for long-term therapy in adolescents.

Drug of Choice: Selective Estrogen Receptor Modulator (SERM)

RATIONALE

Gynecomastia is common among obese or tall teenagers and in athletes who use anabolic steroids. True glandular gynecomastia is often painful and necessitates treatment. Selective estrogen receptor modulators (**SERMs**) are antagonist and partial agonists of estrogen. They are preferred to AI in true glandular gynecomastia. Raloxifene is more effective than tamoxifen. It **inhibits proliferation** of **breast cells** and **does not cause osteoporosis** as it acts as agonist in bone. **Aromatase inhibitors** are very effective as they directly **inhibit synthesis** of **estrogen** by suppressing the enzyme aromatase required for conversion of testosterone to estradiol and androstenedione to estrone. In adolescent boys AI cause **impaired fusion of epiphysis** increasing height. Further it augments osteoporosis and so not preferred.

3. *Testosterone cypionate/Testosterone undecanoate in male hypogonadism.*

BACKGROUND

Deficient testicular secretion of testosterone causes male hypogonadism. Hypogonadotropic hypogonadism is due to reduced secretion by pituitary but hypergonadotropic hypogonadism results due to testicular pathology. In children it presents as delayed puberty and in adults as decreased libido. Therapy with testosterone is helpful in both types of male hypogonadism but it should be administered only when serum levels of testosterone is low. Testosterone cypionate and undecanoate are esters of testosterone. They have more androgenic activity and lesser anabolic steroid activity. Esterification of testosterone at 17α OH group makes it more lipophilic.

TESTOSTERONE UNDECANOATE

Testosterone undecanoate is a depot preparation with longer action. It can be administered at the dose of 1000 mg by slow intramuscular injection (IM) injection. It is followed by 1000 mg after 6 weeks and same dose repeated every 3 months. It improves exercise endurance, sense of well being and physical vigor. It has a favorable pharmacokinetics and does not cause plasma fluctuations as it is released slowly with no bizarre plasma fluctuation[122] so it is preferred. Testosterone undecanoate has an excellent profile of safety and efficacy. It is available as testosterone undecanoate in oil. This oily preparation enters into lymphatics bypassing hepatic metabolism.

TESTOSTERONE CYPIONATE

Testosterone cypionate is cheaper than undecanoate and the usual dose is 200 mg. It is a lipophilic compound available as oil base intramuscular injection every 2 weeks. Hydrolysis of the ester in vivo releases testosterone into circulation. Increasing the dose to reduce frequency of administration does not improve symptoms. Infrequent doses cause poor therapeutic outcome due to wider plasma fluctuation. It does not mimic physiological dosing and causes fluctuation in testosterone levels. Besides testosterone is higher than normal during initial period but decreases subsequently and such steady decline in its levels affect mood and stability of patient. It can cause benign prostatic hypertrophy or aggravate pre-existing angina. It also increases erythrocytosis, sleep apnoea, nocturnal awakenings and acne.

Drug of Choice: Testosterone Undecanoate

RATIONALE

Male hypogonadism is treated with testosterone only when its plasma levels are low. The aim of therapy is to mimic normal physiological fluctuations of testosterone as undue fluctuations not only alter mood or stability of patient but also increase cardiovascular risk, BPH and erythrocytosis. Testosterone **undecanoate** is **slowly released** from its depot preparation and **provides sustained plasma level** for about 6 weeks. It is safe and effective with favorable pharmacokinetics. Testosterone cypionate has to be administered as intramuscular injection every two weeks causing **wide plasma fluctuations**. After each injection, the level of testosterone is **high initially increasing the risk for cardiovascular disease, BPH and erythrocytosis**. After few days it **declines slowly** causing **depressed mood** and **altered stability**. Hence, it is not preferred.

Agents Affecting Mineral Ion Homeostasis and Bone Turnover

1. *Alendronate/Risedronate in osteoporosis.*

BACKGROUND

Bisphosphonates have very strong affinity for bone surface that undergoes remodeling. They do not cross membranes as they are negatively charged and enter bone matrix through endocytosis and remain there till bone remodeling is completed. They exert direct inhibitory effect on osteoclasts preventing hydroxyapatite dissolution. The main mechanisms of bisphosphonates are inhibition of osteoclastic apoptosis and inhibition of cholesterol biosynthetic pathway. Bisphosphonates are administered either once in a month or given every week.

ALENDRONATE

Alendronate is an oral bisphosphonate administered at a dose of 70 mg. It is either given as effervescent formulation or oral tablet once a week. The effervescent formulation is swallowed after it is dissolved in water for 5 minutes and stirred for few seconds before drinking to prevent esophageal irritation. Alendronate is effective in reducing both vertebral and nonvertebral fractures. Besides it is superior in efficacy to risedronate in reducing nonvertebral fractures, so preferred. It causes greater bone mineral density and larger reduction in bone turnover. If continued beyond 5 years it causes 'chalk stick' shaft or subtrochanteric femur fracture.

RISEDRONATE

The dose of risedronate is 35 mg and effective when given once a week but it has inferior efficacy and causes lesser bone mineral density. It is similar to alendronate and reduces both vertebral and non vertebral fractures but the effect of alendronate in decreasing the incidence of nonvertebral fractures is superior. Its upper gastrointestinal tract (GIT) tolerability and safety profile are similar to alendronate.

Drug of Choice: Alendronate

RATIONALE

Bisphosphonates reduce bone resorption, promote bone formation and they promote apoptosis of osteoclasts. Oral bisphosphonates should be given on empty stomach to increase its bioavailability. The patient should be advised to be in upright position to prevent esophageal irritation and heart burn. Alendronate has more efficacy than risedronate and has higher potential in improving bone mineral density and prevents bone turnover to a greater degree.[123] Although these drugs prevent vertebral and nonvertebral fractures, Alendronate has better efficacy in preventing nonvertebral fractures. Hence, it is preferred to risedronate. Safety profile of risedronate including upper GIT tolerability is similar to alendronate but its efficacy is inferior. Hence, it is not a preferred oral bisphosphonate. These drugs should not be continued beyond 5 years as they promote shaft or subtrochanteric fracture of femur.

2. *Parenteral bisphosphonates/Oral bisphosphonates for osteoporosis in patients with active upper GIT disease.*

BACKGROUND

Reduction of bone integrity that occurs due to loss of osteoid bone causes osteoporosis. Although rate of formation of bone is normal, rate of resorption is increased. Therapy with high dose glucocorticoid increases the chances of osteoporosis. Pharmacological therapy is indicated in those with bone density T scores less than 2.5 and those osteopenic patients with T scores between 2.0 and 2.5 are given prophylactic therapy. Bisphosphonates are the first line drugs in the treatment of osteoporosis. They inhibit osteoclasts-induced bone resorption, increase bone density and reduce the incidence of nonvertebral and vertebral fractures.

PARENTERAL BISPHOSPHONATES

Zoledronate and pamidronate are intravenous third generation bisphosphonates that can be given to patients who are unable to tolerate oral bisphosphonates. They are also indicated in osteoporosis for patients with acute upper GIT problems when given as intravenous infusions they can cause acute phase reactions that usually are common after first dose but subside after few days. They are given as infusion either once in six months or once in a year.

ORAL BISPHOSPHONATES

Risedronate, alendronate and ibandronate are few orally acting bisphosphonates. They have very limited oral bioavailability due to poor oral absorption. The bioavailability of risedronate and alendronate is less than 1%. So they are given on empty stomach half an hour before breakfast with 200 mL of water and the water used should either be filtered or tap water but not mineral water. Effervescent formulations should be dissolved in water and stirred well before drinking and the patient should remain in upright position to reduce risk of esophagitis. Oral bisphosphonates causes esophageal irritation and increase risk of esophageal cancer. The risk is higher in patients with active upper GIT disease and so it is not indicated in such patients. Besides, repeated courses are needed as their effect wanes off after discontinuation of the drug.

Drug of Choice: Parenteral Bisphosphonates

RATIONALE

Bisphosphonates are the first line drugs in therapy of osteoporosis. Oral and parenteral forms of bisphosphonates are available for therapy. **Oral bisphosphonates** are more **convenient** to patients

but should not be given to those with active upper GIT disease as they **cause severe esophagitis, increasing the risk of esophageal cancer.** Besides to improve their bioavailability they need to be given on empty stomach further aggravating the pre-existing GIT problem. Hence in such patients, parenteral bisphosphonates are preferred. They can be given once in 6 or 12 months but can result in acute phase reactions.

3. *Zoledronate/Pamidronate as parenteral bisphosphonate.*

BACKGROUND

Zoledronate and pamidronate are parenteral bisphosphonates available for therapy and are indicated in those who are unable to tolerate oral bisphosphonates. They are also indicated in active upper GIT problem where oral formulations are contraindicated. FDA has issued warning for osteonecrosis following use of bisphosphonates.

ZOLEDRONATE

Zoledronate can be administered once in 6 months with no loss of efficacy. It is given prophylactically to breast or prostate cancer patients receiving hormonal therapy to prevent osteoporosis and to reduce hypercalcemia induced by malignancies. In around 42% of patients, first dose of zoledronate can cause acute phase response characterized by flushing, chills, musculoskeletal pain, diarrhea and vomiting. When compared to pamidronate it is more potent with higher long term efficacy and safety. Dizziness, edema, headache, ocular inflammation and fatigue occur but are transient and resolve after few days. It may still recur after subsequent doses. Zoledronate causes severe hypocalcemia and hypocalcemia induced seizures. It can induce renal toxicity, so should be given slowly over a period of 15 minutes. At low doses of 5 mg, the chances of osteonecrosis and renal toxicity are minimal.[124] Zoledronate has longer duration of action and can be given once in 12 months.

PAMIDRONATE

Pamidronate causes cytokine release resulting in flushing, joint pains and nausea. These reactions occur commonly if drug is given in high concentration at faster rate. The symptoms are much more severe with pamidronate than with zoledronate. Although the symptoms subside after some time they can recur during subsequent injection. Pamidronate has lower long-term efficacy with similar adverse effects and has to be given once in 6 months.

Drug of Choice: Zoledronate

RATIONALE

Parenteral bisphosphonates cause acute phase response characterized by flushing, chills, musculoskeletal pain and vomiting. These reactions subside after few days but recur after subsequent injection. Since pamidronate causes cytokine release the symptoms are more severe when it is infused. **Zoledronate** is **more potent** than pamidronate with **long-term efficacy** and safety[125] **but** it can **cause** severe **hypocalcemia** triggering seizures and **renal toxicity** necessitating monitoring of renal parameters. If given at a low dose of 5 mg the risk of osteonecrosis and renal toxicity is greatly reduced.

4. *Bisphosphonates/Calcitonin in Paget disease.*

BACKGROUND

Disorganized formation of osteoid with high turnover of bone is the characteristic feature of Paget disease. Increased osteoclastic activity of the involved bone causes lytic lesions in bone making it vascular, deformed and weak with yearly increase in size by 1 cm. It is polyosteotic and involves many bones in majority of patients but in 28% it involves single bone with monoosteotic presentation. The frequently affected bones are femur, pelvis, humerus, skull and vertebrae. Pain and degenerative arthritis, fragile bones assuming bowed shape, warmth due to vasodilatation, headache and deafness in case of skull involvement are common.

BISPHOSPHONATES

Bisphosphonates are the first line drugs for the treatment of Paget disease. Zoledronate is the drug of choice and given as single intravenous dose of 5 mg. In majority of patients, it normalizes serum alkaline phosphatase level within 6 months. In 98% of patients, it normalizes alkaline phosphatase level within a period of 2 years. Zoledronate results in greater and complete response with longer median duration. It can cause acute phase reaction, hypocalcemia triggered seizures or renal toxicity. Oral bisphosphonates used in this condition are alendronate and risedronate. Alendronate is given daily for 2 months while risedronate is given daily for 6 months. The effect of oral bisphosphonates lasts only for 2 years and they need to be repeated again. Oral therapy is devoid of antigenicity and much cheaper but can cause esophageal irritation.

CALCITONIN

In hypercalcemia due to bone resorption calcitonin reduces plasma calcium. In Paget disease, patients have high bone turnover, although calcitonin reduces bone resorption patients become refractory, due to down regulation of receptors. Long-term therapy causes profound reduction in serum alkaline phosphatase but such prolonged therapy is always associated with development of antibodies. Calcitonin is reliable, skeletal analgesic but many patients develop resistance to it.

Drug of Choice: Bisphosphonates

RATIONALE

Disorganized formation of osteoid with high turnover of bone forms the basis of Paget disease. The osteoclastic activity of the involved bone is increased causing lytic lesions resulting in deformed, weak and vascular bone. **Bisphosphonates** are first line drugs in the treatment of Paget disease. Parenteral zoledronate reduces serum alkaline phosphatase considerably when given as single 5 mg dose. In about 98% of patients it **normalizes the serum alkaline phosphatase level** within a period of 2 years. Zoledronate results in greater and complete response with longer median duration. **Calcitonin** is very **effective** during **initial period** but **requires prolonged administration** for a significant **reduction** in serum alkaline phosphatase level. Patients become refractory to its effects after some time due to down regulation of receptors and development of antibodies. Calcitonin is reliable, skeletal analgesic but many patients develop resistance to it. Hence, it is unsuitable in the treatment of Paget disease.

5. *Doxercalciferol/Cinacalcet in secondary hyperparathyroidism.*

BACKGROUND

Secondary hyperparathyroidism often occurs in those with chronic kidney disease. It develops in patients with vitamin D deficiency due to renal dysfunction which reduces the synthesis of 1, 25 dihydroxycholecalciferol. This along with hypophosphatemia causes reduction in ionic calcium level and as a compensatory mechanism parathyroid gland is enlarged.

CINACALCET

Cinacalcet is a calcimimetic or calcium sensor mimetic, that lowers parathyroid hormone level. It inhibits PTH secretion by acting as calcium on calcium sensor receptors. It is effective in secondary hyperparathyroidism due to chronic renal disease. It is available as 30, 60 and 90 mg and started at 30 mg per day with maximum dose up to 250 mg. 50% of patients with secondary hyperparathyroidism are resistant to vitamin D analogs. Cinacalcet is preferred to calcitriol for secondary hyperparathyroidism. Hypocalcemia is the main side effect and can be minimized by starting with low dose.

DOXERCALCIFEROL

Doxercalciferol suppresses renal disease induced hyperplasia of parathyroid gland. It is an analog of vitamin D or calcitriol, more effective and safer than calcitriol. The affinity of doxercalciferol to vitamin D receptor is comparable to calcitriol and it causes minimal hypercalcemia and hypercalciuria when compared to calcitriol. Patients with renal disease develop resistance to doxercalciferol and it is very expensive. Besides it has low efficacy when compared to cinacalcet.

Drug of Choice: Cinacalcet

RATIONALE

The most common cause of secondary hyperparathyroidism is chronic renal disease. **Cinacalcet** is a **calcimimetic** or calcium sensor mimetic which is effective in lowering parathyroid hormone (PTH) levels. It mimics the action of calcium on calcium sensor receptors and inhibits the secretion of PTH. It can cause hypocalcemia but this risk can be minimized by starting cinacalcet at lower doses. **Doxercalciferol** is a vitamin D analog that helps in suppressing the hyperplasia of parathyroid gland due to chronic renal disease. Since 50% of patients with chronic renal disease develop **resistance** to doxercalciferol it is **less effective than cinacalcet** in the treatment of secondary hyperparathyroidism due to chronic renal disease. Besides doxercalciferol is **expensive** and causes **hypercalcemia** and hypercalciuria.

6. *Ibandronate/Teriparatide for postmenopausal osteoporosis.*

BACKGROUND

Estrogen deficiency during menopausal period increases the risk of osteoporosis where generalized fragility of bones with loss of trabecular bone due to lack of estrogen is a common feature and results in type I form of primary osteoporosis during menopause.

TERIPARATIDE

Teriparatide, an analog of parathormone stimulates production of collagenous matrix and increases the mineral density of bones. In postmenopausal women, it reduces the risk of vertebral and nonvertebral fractures. Except in distal radius, it improves bone density in most of the bones. Although it does not improve cortical bone density, it improves axial bone mineralization. Women with a history of single or multiple fractures due to osteoporosis are most benefited. Chalk stick fractures associated with bisphosphonates is improved by teriparatide. But higher dose of teriparatide has the potential to increase the risk of osteosarcoma. It has a **black box** warning for osteosarcoma so contraindicated in Paget disease.

IBANDRONATE

Ibandronate, the bisphosphonate is used for prevention and treatment of osteoporosis. It inhibits bone resorption and promotes bone formation. It is administered orally at the dose of 150 mg once in every month reducing the incidence of vertebral fractures but not nonvertebral fractures. Ibandronate can cause esophagitis, heart burn and hypercalcemia.

Drug of Choice: Teriparatide

RATIONALE

Lack of estrogen during menopause results in type I primary osteoporosis characterized by loss of trabecular bone. **Teriparatide, an** analog of parathormone **stimulates** the production of **collagenous bone matrix** and **increases bone density**. Although it does not improve cortical bone mineralization it improves mineralization of axial bone. Ibandronate inhibits bone resorption and promotes bone formation. **Teriparatide reduces** the risk of **vertebral** and **nonvertebral** fractures while **ibandronate reduces** only **vertebral** fractures and **not nonvertebral** fractures. Hence, **teriparatide** is preferred in post menopausal osteoporosis but it has a **black box** warning for **osteosarcoma**.

Environmental Toxicology

Section Outline

Chelating Agents

1. *Calcium disodium ethylenediaminetetraacetic acid (EDTA)/ Succimer in chronic lead poisoning in children with blood level above 45 μg/dL.*

BACKGROUND

Lead is a divalent or tetravalent ion and primarily found in divalent form. Chronic exposure to even small quantities of lead causes major unwanted effects. Lead substitutes for calcium or zinc in many proteins altering their structure resulting in inappropriate activation of proteins and subsequent inhibition of function. Ninety-nine percent of absorbed lead binds with hemoglobin and distributes in soft tissues, accumulates in liver and tubular epithelium of kidney but gets distributed and deposited mainly in bone, teeth and hair. Small quantities of lead may deposit in basal ganglia and gray matter of brain. During pregnancy when calcium levels decrease lead reenters circulation from bone crossing placenta and enters into fetal circulation affecting the developing neural system. Chronic exposure causes lead palsy, intestinal spasms and encephalopathy. It inhibits biosynthesis of heme causing microcytic hypochromic anemia. It causes glomerulosclerosis, proximal tubular nephropathy and inhibits glomerular filtration rate (GFR).

SUCCIMER

Succimer has good bioavailability with highly selective chelating property without affecting other metals. Unlike calcium disodium EDTA it does not bind and chelate zinc, iron or copper and because of this property, its toxicity profile is lower. It binds with lead and favors its urinary excretion thereby reducing the plasma concentration. Being hydrophilic it reduces accumulation of lead and promotes immediate excretion. Hence, it is preferred in the treatment of chronic lead poisoning in children.

CALCIUM DISODIUM EDTA

Calcium disodium EDTA is effective only in acute poisoning and not in chronic poisoning. Lead competes with calcium for binding with EDTA and the chelated lead gets excreted. In chronic poisoning lead accumulates in bone and in other places like teeth, hair and as the concentration in plasma is reduced it is mobilized from bone, its storage site. Such mobilization increases its redistribution into other places like brain and liver. This potentiates risk for encephalopathy. At physiological pH, EDTA is highly ionized and neither accumulates intracelullarly nor enters brain. Therefore, calcium disodium EDTA should never be given in chronic lead poisoning. It is given as IM or IV and local anesthetics are added with IM formulation as it is painful. Adequate fluids should be given to prevent nephrotoxicity and to maintain renal function.

Drug of Choice: Succimer

RATIONALE

Chronic lead poisoning in children is characterized by cognition and learning impairment, decreased school performance and changes in behavior. It also causes lead palsy, intestinal spasms and at high doses encephalopathy. Lead inhibits biosynthesis of heme causing microcytic hypochromic anemia. Initially lead accumulates in soft tissues like kidney and liver. On chronic exposure it accumulates in bone, hair and teeth. Lead crosses blood-brain barrier (BBB) and accumulates in brain. Calcium disodium EDTA is effective in acute lead poisoning. It chelates lead and promotes its excretion but in **chronic poisoning** once calcium disodium EDTA reduces the plasma concentration of **lead** it is **mobilized** from its storage site, mainly bone into plasma to maintain equilibrium. This potentiates the risk of **lead encephalopathy**[126] as lead from plasma enters brain and gets sequestered there. Being highly **ionized,**

calcium disodium EDTA does not cross BBB to chelate lead that has accumulated in brain. **Succimer chelates plasma lead** and being **hydrophilic** it **reduces** accumulation of lead promoting its immediate excretion. Hence, it is more beneficial in chronic poisoning. Besides succimer is **more selective** and does not chelate other metals like iron, copper and zinc but **calcium disodium EDTA** is **nonspecific** and chelates these ions. Hence, the toxicity profile of succimer is lower compared to calcium disodium EDTA. So, succimer is preferred in chronic lead poisoning.

2. *Succimer/Dimercaprol for lead encephalopathy in combination with calcium disodium EDTA.*

BACKGROUND

Very high blood levels of lead above 70 µg/dL increases risk of lead encephalopathy. Children exposed to high doses suffer from cognition impairment and irritability as lead affects interaction between glial cells and neurons inhibiting synaptic transmission. It causes delirium, ataxia, vertigo, impaired learning and neurobehavioral changes.

DIMERCAPROL + CALCIUM DISODIUM EDTA

Being ionic calcium disodium EDTA does not cross BBB to chelate lead in brain. Dimercaprol is lipophilic crosses BBB and chelates the lead accumulated in brain and should be given first. It is given as deep intramuscular injection as it has poor oral bioavailability. IM formulation contains peanut oil and it should be avoided in persons allergic to peanuts. Dose of intramuscular dimercaprol is 4 to 5 mg/kg every 4 hours for 5 days. Dose of calcium disodium EDTA is 50 mg/kg per day in 4 to 6 divided doses and it is given to reduce plasma levels of lead.

SUCCIMER + CALCIUM DISODIUM EDTA

Succimer is chemically similar to dimercaprol but has two additional carboxylic acids and this structural change modifies its bioavailability, mechanism of chelation and distribution. Unlike dimercaprol, succimer is orally acting with selective chelation of metals. It is not lipophilic but hydrophilic and promotes quicker excretion of metals. It does not cross BBB as it is not lipophilic so does not chelate lead in brain. Although succimer is similar to dimercaprol it is less toxic and orally effective. Since calcium disodium EDTA is also ineffective as it does not enter brain succimer cannot be combined with it for lead encephalopathy.

Drug of Choice: Dimercaprol + Calcium Disodium EDTA

RATIONALE

Very high blood levels of lead above 70 µg/dL increases the risk of lead encephalopathy. Children exposed to high doses suffer from cognition impairment and irritability. Lead affects interaction between glial cells and neurons inhibiting synaptic transmission causing delirium, ataxia, vertigo, impaired learning and neurobehavioral changes. **Calcium disodium EDTA is highly ionized** and **does not cross BBB** and **cannot chelate the lead accumulated in brain**. **Dimercaprol is lipophilic** and enters CSF and **chelates lead in brain**. In lead encephalopathy both calcium disodium EDTA and dimercaprol are used. While calcium disodium EDTA promotes reduction of plasma lead, dimercaprol chelates lead accumulated within brain. Although structurally similar to dimercaprol, **succimer is hydrophilic** and not lipophilic so **does not enter** CSF and **does not chelate lead in brain**. Hence, it cannot be used in lead encephalopathy.

3. *Acidification/Alkalinization of urine during dimercaprol therapy.*

BACKGROUND

Dimercaprol is also known as antiarsenical war gas or British antilewisite (BAL). Structurally it has sulfydryl groups that form chelation complexes with metals. Dimercaprol is used in arsenic, mercury, gold, copper and nickel poisoning. It forms a stable complex with metals in the ratio of 2:1 with 2 parts of dimercaprol. Since heavy metals bind to sulfydryl groups of essential enzymes in tissues inhibiting them, BAL should be given immediately after exposure to metals to prevent such inhibition. It provides SH groups to which the metals bind instead of tissues forming chelation complex. It is not effective in reactivating the already bound SH enzyme so, should not be delayed.

ALKALINIZATION OF URINE

Large number of drugs used in therapy is either weak acid or weak base. Weak acids are unionized in acidic urine and so are reabsorbed in kidney. Weak bases are unionized in alkaline urine and are reabsorbed in kidney. Weakly acidic drugs are ionized in alkaline urine and are not reabsorbed and excreted. Sodium bicarbonate, potassium citrate and sodium citrate alkalinize urine. Dimercaprol-metal complex is stable in alkaline urine and does not dissociate. Therefore, alkalinization favors excretion of metal chelator complex thereby preventing nephrotoxicity and the dissociation of metals from dimercaprol. Hence, urine should be alkalinized if dimercaprol is used as chelating agent.

ACIDIFICATION OF URINE

Ascorbic acid, ammonium chloride and citric acid are some of the acidifying agents. In acidic urine the SH-metal binding of dimercaprol-metal complex is highly labile. Dimercaprol will be dissociated from the metal complex increasing free metal concentration. Dissociated metals arsenic or mercury enters renal tissue aggravating nephrotoxicity. Arsenic damages renal capillaries, glomerulus and tubules causing severe renal toxicity. Mercury causes tubular necrosis reducing GFR resulting in acute renal failure. Hence, acidic urine will aggravate nephrotoxic potential of dimercaprol-metal complex.

Drug of Choice: Alkalinization of Urine

RATIONALE

Dimercaprol or BAL is used as chelating agent for arsenic, mercury and gold poisoning. It provides SH groups for binding with metals preventing interaction of metals with essential enzymes in body. **Dimercaprol-metal complex dissociates in acidic urine** as the SH group metal interaction is highly **labile** in acid urine. This releases metals that enter renal tissue causing **nephrotoxicity**. **Metal-chelator complex** is more **stable** in **alkaline urine** and is **excreted**, sparing renal tissue. In order to prevent dissociation of metals from dimercaprol in acidic urine alkalinizing agents should be used to prevent nephrotoxicity.

4. *Penicillamine/Trientine in Wilson's disease.*

BACKGROUND

Hepatolenticular degeneration or Wilson's disease is a rare autosomal recessive disorder and is due to diminished excretion and excessive accumulation of copper. It affects adenosine triphosphatase, the copper transporting enzyme in liver resulting in improper function of this enzyme causing excessive copper deposition in brain and liver. In young adults it presents as neuropsychiatric disease while in adults it causes liver disease. Kayser-Fleisher brownish or gray-green ring in descemet membrane of cornea is the characteristic feature.

PENICILLAMINE

Penicillamine is less potent and more toxic chelating agent used in Wilson's disease. It has good oral bioavailability, cheaper and required in low doses for chelation. Since it is relatively stable it is well absorbed and almost totally metabolized by liver. It is given in the dose of 1 to 2 g per day in four divided doses on empty stomach. To determine if dose of penicillamine is adequate urinary copper should be monitored. Pyridoxine should be coadministered as penicillamine causes its deficiency. Early treatment is necessary to prevent neurologic and hepatic involvement. It causes cutaneous lesions like maculopapular lesions, urticaria and dermatomyositis. It inhibits hematopoietic system causing agranulocytosis, aplastic anemia or leucopenia. Reversible hematuria and proteinuria may progress to a more severe nephrotic syndrome. Zinc supplements inhibit intestinal absorption of copper but cause hepatotoxicity.

TRIENTINE

Trientine is also an alternative copper chelating agent but less effective than penicillamine. It is effective orally and generally reserved for patients who are unable to tolerate penicillamine. It should be given on empty stomach at the dose of 2 g/day in 2 to 4 divided doses. Since it causes deficiency of iron, short courses of iron is necessary during therapy but both should not be coadministered and should be given at the gap of 2 hours.

Drug of Choice: Penicillamine

RATIONALE

Hepatolenticular degeneration or Wilson's disease is rare autosomal recessive disorder due to diminished excretion of copper, leading to its excessive accumulation. In young adults it presents as neuropsychiatric disease and as liver disease in adults. Kayser-Fleisher brownish or gray-green ring in descemet membrane of cornea is present in all patients. It affects adenosine triphosphatase, the copper transporting enzyme resulting in improper function of this enzyme. This causes excessive copper deposition in brain and liver. **Penicillamine chelates copper** and **promotes** its **excretion**. It can be administered orally but is **less potent** and **toxic**. It causes cutaneous reactions, leucopenia, agranulocytosis and aplastic anemia. It should be given on empty stomach and pyridoxine supplementation is necessary to overcome its deficiency. **Trientine** is an alternative and generally **reserved** for patients who are unable to tolerate penicillamine as it is less effective and causes iron deficiency. Trientine and iron should not be coadministered and should be given with a gap of 2 hours between each other.

5. *Deferoxamine/Deferiprone for chronic iron intoxication.*

BACKGROUND

Ingestion of more than 40 to 60 mg/kg elemental iron causes acute iron toxicity resulting in hematemesis, acidosis, diarrhea and hypotension, metabolic acidosis, intestinal perforation, peritonitis and sepsis leading to death. Potentially toxic serum iron level is above 500 µg/dL and toxic level is above 1000 µg/dL. Chronic iron overload can occur due to frequent therapeutic blood transfusion.

DEFEROXAMINE

Drug of choice is iron chelator deferoxamine that has high affinity for ferric iron and it removes iron from ferritin, hemosiderin and to a lesser extent transferrin. Vin-rose appearance is characteristic due to deferoxamine-iron complex in urine. It does not chelate iron from cytochromes or hemoglobin and is highly selective. It has poor oral bioavailability so should be given IM and in severe poisoning through IV. Rapid bolus should be avoided as it causes hypotension but can be given as constant infusion. Prolonged infusion beyond 36 to 48 hours causes acute respiratory distress syndrome. It can cause anaphylaxis, pruritus, rash, tachycardia, fever, dysuria or diarrhea.

DEFERIPRONE

Deferiprone is oral iron chelating agent with selective affinity to ferric iron. It is rapidly absorbed from upper GIT within 5 to 10 minutes and forms complex with iron in the ratio of 3:1. This complex is stable over wide range of pH with minimal binding to copper or zinc. Deferiprone is not preferred due to its lower long-term safety and many drug interactions. It causes arthralgia, elevation of liver enzymes, headache and blood dyscrasias. **Black box** warning has been issued for agranulocytosis, neutropenia and serious infection. It interacts with ferric fumarate, ferric gluconate, iron-dextran and iron-sucrose.

Drug of Choice: Deferoxamine

RATIONALE

Iron overload occurs due to frequent blood transfusion. One such condition is thalassemia patients who receive frequent therapeutic blood transfusions. Drug of choice is iron chelator **deferoxamine** that has **high affinity** for ferric iron and selectively removes iron bound to ferritin as well as hemosiderin. It is a **parenteral** iron chelating agent and should not be given as rapid bolus dose as it can cause severe hypotension and prolonged infusion beyond 36 to 48 hours causes acute respiratory distress syndrome. Although **deferiprone** forms **complex** with iron as 3:1 ratio stable in wide range of pH with deferiprone 3 parts and iron 1part, it is **not preferred** due to its multiple drug interactions and **questionable long-term safety**. Besides, it has **black box** warning on its label for agranulocytosis, neutropenia and severe infection.

Respiratory System

56   Antitussives, Mucolytics, Pharmacotherapy of Bronchial Asthma and Chronic Obstructive Pulmonary Disease

1. *Salmeterol/Formoterol for nocturnal asthma in combination with inhalational corticosteroids.*

BACKGROUND

Salmeterol and formoterol are long acting β_2 agonists and used for prevention of nocturnal asthma. Salmeterol is a partial agonist and formoterol is a complete agonist. They improve exercise tolerance and prevent exacerbations of asthma thereby reducing symptoms in chronic asthma. They should not be repeated within a period of 12 hours as they provide effective bronchodilatation for 12 hours. Long acting β_2 agonists should never be used alone because they do not treat the underlying chronic inflammation. Prolonged adminis-tration of long acting β_2 agonists as monotherapy is imprudent as it increases the risk of fatal asthmatic attacks. More often long acting β_2 agonists causes intense bronchoconstriction probably through phospholipase-C mediated stimulation. Inhalational cortico-steroids should always be combined with long acting β_2 agonists because, as anti-inflammatory agents corticosteroids significantly reduce the mortality.

FORMOTEROL

Formoterol has immediate onset of action and has a higher affi-nity for β_2 receptors. It is highly lipophilic and is a long acting drug and concentrates within the lipid bilayer of plasma membrane. It is gradually released and results in prolonged stimulation of beta receptors. It can be used for exercise induced acute exacerbations as it has quick onset of action. Formoterol is also used as a drug for maintenance. The adverse effects are hypokalemia, tachycardia, tremor and hyperglycemia. Although tolerance develops for tremor and tachycardia, the rate of development of tolerance is higher for formoterol. Since it has quick onset and higher rate of tolerance for adverse effects it is preferred.

SALMETEROL

Salmeterol is highly lipophilic and has additional anti-inflamma-tory action. Although it has a prolonged duration of action, the onset of action is slow even through inhalational route. Hence, it cannot be used for acute exacerbation. Generally it is well tolerated but can cause hypokalemia, tachycardia, tremor and hyperglyce-mia. Tolerance develops for tremor and tachycardia.

Drug of Choice: Formoterol

RATIONALE

Long acting β_2 agonists such as salmeterol or formoterol is never used for monotherapy and should always be combined with inhalational corticosteroids for maintenance therapy as they do not have anti-inflammatory activity. They are effective in prevent-ing nocturnal attacks as they are long acting but should not be administered within a gap of 12 hours between each dose as it causes exaggerated stimulation of sympathetic system. **Salmeterol** has **delayed onset** of action but **formoterol** has **immediate onset** of action. Besides **formoterol** can be given for **exercise induced acute exacerbations** but salmeterol ca not be given for the same. In view of the above, although both drugs are equi-effective with similar adverse effects, formoterol is preferred to salmeterol.

2. *Salmeterol/Albuterol as adjunct for treatment of mild exacerbations of asthma.*

BACKGROUND

Minimal signs of airway dysfunction occur in mild exacerbations and short acting β_2 agonists are generally very effective in this condition. They can be administered through inhalational route but require frequent administration as they are short acting. Since exacerbation can also occur in patients who are already on oral corticosteroids therapy, addition of β_2 agonists for one week is suitable.

ALBUTEROL

Albuterol is a short acting β_2 agonist and drug of choice for mild exacerbations as it is very effective, safe and inexpensive. Therefore, it is most suitable for 'rescue therapy' as it has an immediate onset of action when given through inhalational route. It results in selective bronchodilatation without cardiac stimulation because it does not act on β_1 receptors. It causes bronchodilatation within 15 minutes through inhalational route and the action persists for 3 to 4 hours. The S-enantiomer of albuterol provokes inflammation but the R-enantiomer causes bronchodilatation. Hence, it is available as a purified preparation of R- isomer in the form of metered dose inhaler. It relaxes airway smooth muscle and improves airflow providing relief and improvement of symptoms. The required number of puffs varies depending on the severity of symptoms but a minimum of 20 minutes gap should be given between each puff. Minimum clinical improvement after 4 puffs necessitates additional inhalational steroids.

SALMETEROL

Compared to albuterol, the duration of action of salmeterol is longer. It has 50 times greater selectivity than albuterol to β_2 receptors. Its onset is considerably slow even when administered through inhalational route. Hence, it is not suitable for immediate management of exacerbations of asthma.

Drug of Choice: Albuterol

RATIONALE

Albuterol is a **short acting** β_2 agonist while **salmeterol** is a **long acting** and more **selective** β_2 agonist. **Albuterol** has **immediate onset** of action when given through inhalational route so it is **preferred** in acute exacerbations. It is **safe, inexpensive, very effective** but additional treatment is required in patients who do not respond to 4 puffs at 20 minute intervals. Salmeterol is a long acting drug and has a slow onset of action even when administered through inhalational route. Therefore, it is not preferred for acute situations and only indicated in maintenance therapy.

3. *Fluticasone propionate/Beclomethasone dipropionate as inhalational steroid in bronchial asthma.*

BACKGROUND

Airway inflammation, an important component of bronchial asthma is due to inflammatory mediators such as histamine, eicosanoids, leukotrienes and cytokines. Steroids inhibit recruitment of mast cells, eosinophils, neutrophils, lymphocytes and macrophages at the site of inflammation.

FLUTICASONE PROPIONATE

Fluticasone propionate is a potent locally acting agent with not demonstrable systemic effect. Virtually zero (<1%) oral bioavailability is the unique feature of fluticasone due to its minimal absorption and high presystemic metabolism in gut as well as liver. Lack of systemic effect through intranasal route is its main advantage and at half the dose its clinical efficacy is equivalent to beclomethasone. Its mean residence time at the site of action is higher and around 5 hours. Hence, it causes significant increase in peak expiratory flow rate (PEF) with no systemic benefit. This drug does not cause significant difference in morning and urinary cortisol level.

BECLOMETHASONE DIPROPIONATE

Beclomethasone dipropionate is a prodrug and rapidly hydrolyzed to monopropionate. It is deposited primarily in nasal passages if given as aqueous or aerosolized form. Since only 2% is deposited in nasal passages and remaining drug is swallowed and forms the basis for its low clinical efficacy through this route.[127] Most of the drug is swallowed, enters systemic circulation and suppresses nocturnal cortisol after 1 year of continuous use but the systemic absorption of drug deposited in nasal passages is almost negligible because it undergoes presystemic first-pass metabolism in lung. Mean residence time at site of action and peak expiratory flow rate (PEF) of beclomethasone is lower than fluticasone.

Drug of Choice: Fluticasone Propionate

RATIONALE

Inhalational corticosteroids are potent anti-inflammatory agents and preferred in bronchial asthma. Beclomethasone and fluticasone do not cause significant difference in morning and urinary cortisol level. Beclomethasone dipropionate is a prodrug and rapidly hydrolyzed to its active monopropionate form. Its systemic absorption is minimal but only 2% is deposited primarily in nasal passages when given as aqueous or aerosolized form and remaining drug is swallowed minimizing its mean residence time and lowering PEF. **Fluticasone** propionate has **higher clinical efficacy** even at 50% of dose and results in higher PEF. Its **mean residence time is around 5 hours** and its **systemic absorption is lower than 1%**.[128] Hence, fluticasone is preferred to beclomethasone.

4. *Inhalational/Systemic route as effective route of administration for β_2 agonists in bronchial asthma.*

BACKGROUND

β_2 agonists act through activation of Gs mediated adenylcyclase pathway and cause bronchodilatation through direct stimulation of β_2 receptors resulting in rapid reduction of airway resistance improving airflow. Substitution in terminal amine of phenyl ethylamine causes selective β_2 action. Terbutaline, salbutamol or albuterol are few examples of selective β_2 agonists. Salmeterol, arformoterol and formoterol are few long acting β_2 agonists as they are not metabolized by catechol-o-methyl transferase or COMT.

INHALATIONAL ROUTE

Inhalational route is preferred for β_2 agonists in bronchial asthma as the drug is selectively delivered to target organ. The onset is rapid as the drug is delivered directly and it improves airflow. Since low doses are adequate for therapeutic benefit side effects are minimal. Direct delivery to site of action minimizes first pass metabolism but drug delivery depends on mucociliary clearance and aerodynamic filtration. Presence of cough or sneeze also determines the extent of delivery of a drug. Nasal hair removes drug particles above 15 μm and so larger particle size is ineffective. Particles of 10–15 μm are deposited in nasopharynx and do not reach smaller airways. Inhalational route offers rapid onset, equivalent activity and minimal systemic effects.

SYSTEMIC ROUTE

Systemic route is not preferred for administration of β_2 agonists in bronchial asthma as higher dose is required to circumvent pre-systemic first pass metabolism. Besides, it results in tachycardia, tremor, anxiety, excessive sweating, insomnia and agitation through this route. Hypokalemia secondary to insulin release is a potentially dangerous side effect and these side effects are due to unwanted stimulation of extrapulmonary beta receptors.

Drug of Choice: Inhalational Route of Administration

RATIONALE

In bronchial asthma **inhalational** delivery of β_2 agonists is **preferred** as it is **directly delivered** to its **site of action** resulting in **immediate onset** of action. Small doses result in optimal therapeutic benefit with minimal systemic side effects.[129] The **particle size less than 10 μm** of drug influences the delivery of drug to smaller airways. **Systemic** administration of β_2 agonists is not preferred due to **high incidence of side effects**. Hypokalemia is the potentially dangerous side effect. They also result in tachycardia, tremor and anxiety. Side effects are mainly due to stimulation of extrapulmonary beta receptors.

5. *Pressurized metered-dose inhalers (pMDI)/Dry powder inhaler (DPI) as suitable route of drug delivery in bronchial asthma.*

BACKGROUND

Inhalational route of drug delivery is the most preferred route in bronchial asthma and it is possible to deliver drugs through inhalational route by several methods. Large volume spacer chambers and nebulizers are not portable and are used in infants and small children who cannot be trained to use inhalational device. Portable small nebulizers or soft mist inhalers are currently available. Dry powder inhaler and pressurized metered dose inhalers are easy to carry.

DRY POWDER INHALER

Dry powder inhaler is environmentally safer as no propellant is used. It is also breath activated but has a far greater deposition in lower respiratory tract. Nearly 30 to 60% particles are of smaller size and easily enter into lungs. Rotahaler, turbuhaler, diskhaler and accuhaler are few forms of DPI. Its main advantage is that very minimal coordination is required for its use and a steady full inspiration required to empty capsule and the delivery depends on inspiratory rate. This creates problems in children although 55% of children learn to use it correctly. Delivery depends on air turbulence due to inhalation so minimal coordination is required. Even though some experience irritation due to dry powder, DPI is still preferred by many patients.

PRESSURIZED METERED DOSE INHALER

Propellant is placed in canister to propel drugs from pressurized metered dose inhalers. Freon or chlorofluoro carbon was the propellant used earlier in canister but is now replaced by 'ozone' friendly hydrofluoroalkane to propel the drug. These canisters are portable, convenient and capable of delivering 100 to 400 doses but patients need to be taught about using this device as it is breath activated. Breath holding for 10 seconds improves the delivery of drug from canister and particle size influences the delivery of drug into small airways. Glyceryl trinitrate and ergotamine can also be delivered through pMDI. Eighty percent of the delivered drug deposits in mouth, 10% remains in canister, 1% is exhaled and only 9% reaches lungs.

Drug of Choice: Dry Powder Inhaler (DPI)

RATIONALE

In bronchial asthma inhalational route of drug delivery is the most preferred route and many types of appliances are available for this route of delivery. **Dry powder inhaler** is preferred as it is **devoid of propellant** use, results in far **greater drug delivery** up to **lower respiratory tract** and requires **minimal coordination** for use and the delivery of drug depends on air turbulence caused by inspiration. **Pressurized metered dose inhaler** is less preferred as it **requires** a **propellant** and needs **greater coordination** creating problem in many patients. Since **breath holding** for 10 seconds is necessary for higher therapeutic benefit this **maneuver** is **difficult** for **children**. However, DPI can cause irritation in some patients due to inhalation of dry powder.

6. *Ipratropium bromide/Tiotropium bromide in the treatment of chronic obstructive pulmonary disease (COPD).*

BACKGROUND

Anticholinergic agents such as ipratropium and tiotropium bromide are quaternary ammonium compounds and superior to β_2 agonist in COPD. They both have selective actions on the respiratory tract and are given through inhalational route. Ipratropium blocks all three muscarinic receptor subtypes namely M_1, M_2 and M_3 while tiotropium selectively blocks M_1 and M_3 subtypes with a lower affinity to M_2 receptors. Although well tolerated minimal rebound occurs on stopping therapy. Being anticholinergics, they reduce mucus secretion causing thick viscid mucus.

TIOTROPIUM BROMIDE

Among the three muscarinic receptors, M_2 subtype receptor is an autoreceptor and stimulation of this autoreceptor inhibits neuronal release of acetylcholine. Although tiotropium binds to all three receptor subtypes, it quickly dissociates from M_2 receptor subtype. Besides, it has prolonged binding with M_1 and M_3 receptors increasing its therapeutic benefit preventing M_3 mediated bronchoconstriction. Tiotropium is given once daily as it is a long acting anticholinergic drug. It reduces the disease exacerbations but does not inhibit disease progression. Loss of efficacy does not occur for a period of 1 year and it improves lung function if given for a four year period. Unlike ipratropium, tiotropium does not cause paradoxical bronchoconstriction.

IPRATROPIUM BROMIDE

Ipratropium blocks the M_2 autoreceptors along with other muscarinic subtypes. So, it increases the amount of acetylcholine released at postganglionic sites thereby counteracting its beneficial blockade on M_1 and M_3 receptors. Ipratropium has slow onset and has to be given three to four times a day. Bronchoconstriction can occur due to hypotonic solution and additives present in nebulizer.

Drug of Choice: Tiotropium Bromide

RATIONALE

Atropine substitutes, ipratropium bromide and tiotropium bromide have more selective actions on respiratory tract than atropine and are administered through inhalational route. Ipratropium blocks all three muscarinic receptor subtypes. Hence, ipratropium counteracts its beneficial effect on M_1 and M_3 receptors. **Ipratropium has slow onset** and has to be given **three to four** times a day. **Paradoxical bronchoconstriction** is sometimes caused due to hypotonic solution and other additives present in nebulizer. Given **once daily, tiotropium** antagonizes M_1 and M_3 receptors for a prolonged period while its association with M_2 receptors is for a shorter period. This potentiates the therapeutic efficacy of tiotropium. Unlike ipratropium, **tiotropium does not cause paradoxical bronchoconstriction**. Hence, tiotropium bromide is preferred to ipratropium bromide in the treatment of COPD.

7. *Theophylline/Doxofylline in bronchial asthma.*

BACKGROUND

Theophylline and doxofylline are methylxanthines and are related to caffeine and cause bronchodilatation by inhibiting phosphodiesterase enzyme. They have no added significance over inhaled β_2 agonists in bronchial asthma due to their poor safety profile. Therefore, they are used mainly during asthma exacerbations. In addition to bronchodilatation they have anti-inflammatory and immunomodulatory action. In spite of their bronchoprotective action they have restricted role in bronchial asthma. They are both nonselective weak inhibitors of phosphodiesterase enzyme (PDE).

DOXOFYLLINE

Doxofylline has more stable plasma concentration than theophylline and therefore requires monitoring only in patients with hepatic dysfunction. It has similar pharmacodynamic profile and causes minimal adenosine antagonism. Therefore, it has minimal toxicity profile when compared to theophylline. Since it does not block central and cardiac adenosine receptors, it does not cause seizures or arrhythmias. It is superior in improving PEFR and causes lesser GIT side effects. Unlike theophylline it does not interfere with sleep pattern and CNS function.

THEOPHYLLINE

Theophylline increases cyclic AMP by inhibiting PDE enzyme and is inexpensive. It suppresses inflammation by increasing IL-10 release, anti-inflammatory cytokine and inhibits the survival of granulocytes, the mediators of chronic inflammation. Theophylline promotes apoptosis of granulocytes and T lymphocytes and inhibits pro-inflammatory gene transcription. Further it recruits histone deacetylase-2 to inhibit the inflammatory response. It antagonizes cardiac and CNS adenosine receptors causing arrhythmias and seizures. It has very narrow therapeutic index and has to be monitored very closely. Due to inhibition of PDE4, it causes headache, nausea, vomiting, tremor, insomnia, restlessness, abdominal discomfort and diuresis. Behavioral problems and difficulty in learning are frequent side effects of theophylline. It is less effective in improving peak expiratory flow rate (PEFR) than doxofylline.

Drug of Choice: Doxofylline

RATIONALE

Methylxanthines have no added significance over inhaled β_2 agonists in bronchial asthma. Theophylline and doxofylline are nonselective weak inhibitors of phosphodiesterase enzyme (PDE). **Theophylline** is **cheaper**, suppresses inflammation by increasing release of IL-10, and inhibits chronic inflammation promoting apoptosis of granulocytes and T lymphocytes. Theophylline also inhibits pro-inflammatory gene transcription. When compared to doxofylline the **efficacy** of theophylline in improving PEFR is **lower**. Besides, theophylline has **narrow therapeutic index,**[130] blocks central and cardiac adenosine receptors resulting in **seizures** and **cardiac arrhythmias. Doxofylline is more effective**[131] with minimal toxicity profile as it **does not antagonize adenosine receptors**. It has more **stable plasma concentration** and requires monitoring only in patients with hepatic dysfunction.

8. *Codeine/Dextromethorphan as antitussive in chronic idiopathic cough.*

BACKGROUND

Asthmatic, nonasthmatic and eosinophilic cough have specific lines of treatment. The antitussives are not effective in treating these conditions. Generally postviral cough usually resolves on its own and may not need medication but chronic cough occurs frequently and is due to airway hyperesthesia. Codeine and dextromethorphan are equipotent antitussives. They are both very effective in chronic idiopathic cough.

DEXTROMETHORPHAN

Dextromethorphan does not act through opioid receptors. It elevates threshold for cough centrally but does not inhibit peripheral ciliary activity. Unlike codeine, it neither has opioid mediated analgesic action nor result in addiction. In addition, it acts by blocking central N-methyl D-aspartate (NMDA) receptors. Dextromethorphan is suitable for long-term administration due to minimal side effects. Hence, it is better than codeine in chronic idiopathic cough.

CODEINE

Codeine raises the threshold of cough center and also has additional peripheral action. It acts on peripheral cough receptors present in airways. It is methyl morphine and gets demethylated to morphine. Unlike morphine, has minimal affinity to μ receptors. When compared to morphine, its action is more selective on cough center. Constipation is its main side effect and is contraindicated in asthmatics. Prolonged use of codeine results in addiction and dependence in chronic cough.

Drug of Choice: Dextromethorphan

RATIONALE

Chronic idiopathic cough is often troublesome to patients and is usually treated with antitussives. Although codeine is the standard antitussive, it is demethylated to morphine and can result in sedation and addiction. **Chronic** administration of **codeine frequently** results in **constipation**. On the other hand **dextromethorphan** is **equally effective**, causes only **mild GIT** side effects. Hence, it is preferred to codeine as an antitussive.

9. *N-acetylcysteine/Bromhexine as mucolytic.*

BACKGROUND

Increased secretion of mucus occurs in bronchial asthma, COPD and cystic fibrosis. Constant irritation causes excessive mucus secretion in chronic bronchitis. Elastase and proteinase released due to neutrophil activation and chymase released from mast cells cause copious secretion. Since inflammation stimulates mucus secretion, anti-inflammatory agents inhibit its production. Inhalational corticosteroids are anti-inflammatory agents and reduce production of mucus. Mucolytic agents reduce the viscosity of mucus promoting their expectoration.

N-ACETYLCYSTEINE

N-acetylcysteine is a derivative of cysteine and used as mucolytic. It is rapidly and completely absorbed and reversibly bound to plasma proteins. It is very effective and has both direct and indirect mucolytic activity. Direct action decreases viscoelastic property of sputum increasing volume of thin mucus. The thiol groups in N-acetylcysteine reduce the disulfide linkages that bind glycoproteins to albumin and IgA. Loss of disulfide bridges breaks down mucus protein into smaller units reducing viscosity and elasticity of mucus facilitating its expectoration. Indirectly N-acetylcysteine also facilitates mucociliary clearance. It has additional anti-inflammatory and antioxidant property.

BROMHEXINE

Bromhexine is derived from vasicine the alkaloid obtained from *adhatoda vasika*. It is both mucokinetic and mucolytic increasing production of thin mucus causing release of lysosomal enzymes and depolymerizing the mucopolysaccharides. It has lower efficacy than N-acetylcysteine as it is neither an antioxidant nor an anti-inflammatory agent.

Drug of Choice: N-acetylcysteine

RATIONALE

Increased secretion of mucus occurs in chronic bronchitis, bronchial asthma, COPD and cystic fibrosis. Activation of neutrophils releases elastase and proteinase that increase production of mucus. Another secretogogue of mucus is chymase released from mast cells. Since inflammation stimulates mucus secretion, anti-inflammatory drugs inhibit the production of mucus. Mucolytic agents reduce the viscosity of mucus promoting their expectoration. **N-acetylcysteine** reduces viscosity and elasticity of mucus **facilitating** its **expectoration** and **mucociliary clearance**. It has **additional anti-inflammatory and antioxidant property.**[132] **Bromhexine** is a mucolytic increasing production of thin mucus but it is **less effective** as mucolytic agent as it is **devoid of anti-inflammatory action**[133] and is not a potent antioxidant.

Gastrointestinal Tract

CHAPTER
57
Acid Peptic Disease and Gastroesophageal Reflux Disease

1. *Proton pump inhibitors (PPIs)/H₂ Blockers for short-term management in peptic ulcer.*

BACKGROUND

Duodenal ulcers are at least five times more common than gastric ulcer and occur due to impaired mucosal defense factors or excessive aggressive factors. Gastrin is a potent inducer of acid secretion while mucus helps to protect gastric mucosa. Somatostatin inhibits acid secretion while prostaglandins increase mucus secretion.

PROTON PUMP INHIBITORS

Proton pump inhibitors inhibit acid secretion by blocking the final step of synthesis. As irreversible inhibitors they bind covalently to H^+K^+ ATPase inactivating it. Secretion of acid resumes only after new H^+K^+ ATPase is synthesized, so their action is long lasting, promoting healing of ulcer by inhibiting acid environment. Though their half-life is less than two hours their action exceeds 24 hours. 90% duodenal ulcer heals after 4 weeks therapy and gastric ulcer requires 8 weeks therapy. PPIs are safe for short therapy but longer therapy causes B_{12}, calcium and iron deficiency.

H₂ BLOCKERS

Gastric histamine secreted by enterochromaffin like cells lies closer to parietal cells. Histamine acts as a mediator in stimulating H^+K^+ ATPase for acid secretion. Histamine diffuses into parietal cells stimulates acid secretion by activating H_2 receptors. H_2 receptor antagonists bind reversibly with H_2 receptors and prevent its activation. This reduces the stimulation of $H^+K^+ATPase$, the proton pump, inhibiting acid secretion. However, unlike PPIs, H_2 blockers do not block final step of acid secretion. The production of acid still continues through other factors such as gastrin and acetylcholine so the healing rate of ulcer with H_2 blockers is only around 85% even with long-term therapy. Hence, H_2 blockers are not preferred to PPIs in the treatment of peptic ulcer.

> **Drug of Choice: Proton Pump Inhibitors (PPIs)**

RATIONALE

Impaired mucosal defense factors or excessive aggressive factors cause peptic ulcer. Gastrin is the most potent inducer of acid secretion while prostaglandins mediated mucus secretion helps to protect gastric mucosa. $H^+K^+ATPase$ or proton pump is the final step involved in the synthesis of acid. **Proton pump inhibitors** covalently bind to $H^+K^+ATPase$ and cause **irreversible inhibition**. Secretion of acid resumes only after new $H^+K^+ATPase$ is synthesized. Hence, blockade of proton pump reduces acid environment for longer time facilitating healing of ulcers. Although its half-life is less than 2 hours its effect persists for around 24 hours. PPIs cause 90% healing of duodenal ulcer after 4 weeks therapy and 90% healing of gastric ulcer after 8 weeks therapy. Prolonged use results in deficiency of vitamin B_{12}, calcium and iron so long-term use should be avoided. **Histamine mediates stimulation of $H^+K^+ATPase$ enzyme through H_2 receptors**. H_2 blockers bind to H_2 receptors and prevent their activation. **In spite** of this **blockade proton pump** can **still** be **stimulated** by other mediators such as acetylcholine or gastrin. Besides they are less effective in promoting the healing of ulcers. Hence, H_2 blockers are less preferred in the treatment of peptic ulcer.

2. *Omeprazole/Pantoprazole as suitable proton pump inhibitor (PPI) for therapy.*

BACKGROUND

PPIs suppress $H^+K^+ATPase$ or proton pump involved in gastric acid secretion. They inhibit basal secretion as well as acid secretion stimulated by other factors. They are mainly activated in acidic medium of gastric canalicular cells. Hence, they are given as enteric coated tablets to prevent their degradation in stomach. Enteric coating promotes their absorption in intestine in alkaline medium. They get absorbed into systemic circulation and enter gastric canaliculi and are activated in acidic environment forming an intermediate sulfenamide moiety. They bind covalently to sulfhydryl groups of $H^+K^+ATPase$ pump inhibiting its function. Secretion of acid resumes only after new $H^+K^+ATPase$ pump is synthesized. They cause flatulence, constipation, nausea, headache, arthralgia and abdominal pain.

PANTOPRAZOLE

Several doses of PPIs are required for maximum acid suppression if given orally, because all $H^+K^+ATPase$ pumps are not activated at the same time. Hence, it requires 2 to 5 days for 70% of acid suppression through oral route. However, intravenous administration reduces 80 to 90% of acid secretion within one hour. Pantoprazole is approved for intravenous administration in acute conditions. It is less acid labile and has better bioavailability and effective both orally as well as through intravenous administration. It does not inhibit CYP2C19 and does not interfere with the antiplatelet activity of clopidogrel. Since it does not result in many drug interactions it is preferred to omeprazole.

OMEPRAZOLE

Omeprazole is not approved for intravenous administration in acute conditions. It is given through oral route and is more acid labile with only 50% oral bioavailability. It is both an enzyme inducer and inhibitor causing many drug interactions. It inhibits CYP2C19 decreasing metabolism of drugs such as phenytoin and disulfiram. It stimulates CYP1A2 augmenting metabolism of theophylline, imipramine and others. Clopidogrel is a substrate and is converted to its active form by CYP2C19. Omeprazole inhibits antiplatelet activity of clopidogrel by competing for this enzyme and coadministration increases cardiovascular risk of clopidogrel in few patients. Prolonged use causes B_{12} deficiency and interferes with absorption of iron, ampicillin and ketoconazole. Besides, omeprazole causes hypergastrinemia and rebound hypersecretion of acid.

Drug of Choice: Pantoprazole

RATIONALE

PPIs cause prolonged suppression of acid secretion and it resumes only after synthesis of new $H^+K^+ATPase$ pump is synthesized. Hence, they provide long-term benefit in peptic ulcer. Since all $H^+K^+ATPase$ pumps are not activated at the same time several doses of PPIs are required for maximum acid suppression when given through oral route. Since **omeprazole** is **not approved** for **IV administration** it is **not suitable** in **acute** conditions. It is highly acid labile with poor oral bioavailability so given in enteric coated form. It is both enzyme inducer and inhibitor resulting in many drug interactions. It **inhibits activation** of **clopidogrel potentiating** its **cardiovascular risk**. It causes rebound acid secretion due to hypergastrinemia, B_{12}, iron deficiency and interferes with bioavailability of ampicillin and ketoconazole. **Pantoprazole** is more **acid stable** with better oral bioavailability and available as enteric coated form. It is **effective both** through **oral** or **IV** route, **does not** result in many drug interactions and **does not interfere with antiplatelet activity of clopidogrel**. It does not cause **hypergastrinemia** and so preferred.

3. *Triple therapy/Quadruple therapy as anti H. pylori regimen.*

BACKGROUND

The gram negative rod *H. pylori* causes gastritis leading to gastric and duodenal ulcer. If left untreated this may progress to adeno-carcinoma or gastric B-cell lymphoma. Since *H. pylori* is involved in pathogenesis of peptic ulcer its eradication forms main line of therapy. Eradication of *H. pylori* is difficult and combination therapy is more suitable as single drug is ineffective. Several regimes have been tried to eradicate *H. pylori*, to promote healing and to relieve dyspepsia. 14 days therapy is available for uncomplicated *H. pylori* associated peptic ulcer. Since single antibiotic therapy promotes microbial resistance other drugs are added. Additional 2 to 4 weeks therapy is required for complicated and large ulcers.

QUADRUPLE THERAPY

Triple therapy contains two antibiotics and an acid suppressive agent and given twice daily for 14 days. Acid suppressive agent can either be PPI or H$_2$ blocker although PPI is preferred. Frequently used and effective antibiotics are amoxicillin and clarithromycin. Metronidazole/tinidazole with clarithromycin is given to penicillin allergic patients. Quadruple therapy contains bismuth compounds as an additional component such as colloidal bismuth subcitrate (CBSC). Either citrate or salicylate salts are commonly used. Bismuth has antisecretory, antimicrobial and anti inflammatory action but black staining of tongue and dark stools occurs during its use. It is due to bismuth sulfide formed due to reaction between the bacilli and drug. It is taken as 120 mg tablets on empty stomach before each major meal and again at bed time. It detaches the *H. pylori* organisms attached to gastric epithelial cells into lumen. The antibiotics act on the detached *H. pylori* bacteria and destroy them. Quadruple regimen is very effective in case of clarithromycin resistance.

TRIPLE THERAPY

Triple therapy is very effective in eradicating 90% of the harmful bacteria but resistance to clarithromycin is very high and this reduces the efficacy of therapy. In areas where clarithromycin resistance is minimal it is still the first line drug. Dose of amoxicillin is 1 g and clarithromycin is 500 mg along with PPI twice daily. Resistance to clarithromycin is attributed to mutations in *H. pylori* preventing its binding with antibiotic.

Drug of Choice: Quadruple Therapy

RATIONALE

H. pylori is involved in pathogenesis of peptic ulcer and its eradication forms main therapy. Since eradication of *H. pylori* is difficult by single drug, combination therapy is followed. If given as a single drug, antibiotics develop microbial resistance so other drugs are added. **Triple therapy** contains **amoxicillin** and **clarithromycin** along with **PPI**. In patients allergic to penicillin group metronidazole or tinidazole is added and therapy is given twice daily for 14 days. Dose of drugs is clarithromycin 500 mg + amoxicillin 1 g along with PPI twice daily. Since **resistance** to **clarithromycin** is **high** it is **not preferred**. In **quadruple therapy bismuth compounds** are **added**. At the dose of 120 mg on empty stomach before each major meal and again at bed time, it has antisecretory, antimicrobial and anti-inflammatory action. It detaches *H. pylori* organisms attached to gastric epithelial cells into lumen. The antibiotics act on the detached *H. pylori* bacteria and destroy them. It can cause black tongue or dark stools due to formation of bismuth disulfide. Quadruple therapy is **effective in overcoming clarithromycin resistance** and is **very effective** where resistance to this antibiotic is prevalent.

4. *Systemic/Nonsystemic antacids in therapy of peptic ulcer.*

BACKGROUND

Efficacy of antacid is expressed in terms of milliequivalents of its capacity to neutralize acid. It is the amount of 1NHCl brought down within 15 minutes to pH 3.5. Antacids have better efficacy in neutralizing gastric acid as suspension than as powder. They increase gastric pH and do not reduce or interfere with acid secretion but increase in pH beyond 4 causes reflex gastrin secretion and rebound acidity.

NONSYSTEMIC ANTACIDS

Nonsystemic antacids are not absorbed and are devoid of systemic side effects. Magnesium and aluminum combination is most effective because aluminum reduces GIT motility while magnesium facilitates motility of gut. Aluminum is slow acting and magnesium is fast acting and the combination is very useful. Magaldrate is hydroxymagnesium aluminate complex and has both Mg^{2+} and Al^{3+}. At gastric pH it is rapidly converted to magnesium and aluminium hydroxide and provides sustained effect. Since they are poorly absorbed, they are safer than systemic antacids.

SYSTEMIC ANTACIDS

Sodium salts such as sodium bicarbonate and sodium citrate are systemic antacids. They are called systemic as they are absorbed through systemic circulation. Both are very effective, rapidly acting with quick neutralization of acid. Sodium bicarbonate releases carbon dioxide that provides symptomatic relief but if large amount of sodium is absorbed it results in dangerous systemic alkalosis. Sodium overload also causes edema increasing the risk of renal and cardiac dysfunction. Carbon dioxide causes belching, flatulence and abdominal distension.

Drug of Choice: Nonsystemic Antacids

RATIONALE

Efficacy of antacid is expressed in terms of milliequivalents of its capacity to neutralize acid and it is the amount of 1NHCl brought down within 15 minutes to pH 3.5. Antacids are more effective as suspensions. Sodium in **sodium** containing preparations is absorbed into systemic circulation, so they are called systemic antacids. Although they are very effective and act rapidly, they are not preferred as they are **absorbed** into **systemic circulation** causing alkalosis. Carbon dioxide released from sodium bicarbonate causes belching, flatulence and abdominal distension. **Nonsystemic antacids** are **safer** as they are **not absorbed** and are usually combined as single preparation. **Magaldrate** is **hydroxymagnesium aluminate complex** that dissociates in gastric pH to form magnesium and aluminium ions. **Magnesium** is **fast acting** and promotes bowel motility while **aluminum** is **slow acting** and delays motility. Given together they compensate each other's action and provide sustained benefit.

5. *H_2 blockers/PPI in stage II and III of GERD.*

BACKGROUND

Gastroesophageal reflux disease (GERD) is associated with severe erosive esophagitis. Stage I is characterized by uncomplicated heart burn with less than three episodes per week. Antacids or H_2 blockers with diet and lifestyle modification is adequate for relief. Stage II is characterized by more frequent episodes and heartburn with or without esophagitis. It progresses to stricture formation or heart burn or Barrett's metaplasia in stage III. Squamous epithelium is replaced with columnar epithelium in Barrett's metaplasia and it has a huge risk for development of adenocarcinoma. Pathogenesis of GERD is due to acid reflux from stomach into esophagus.

PROTON PUMP INHIBITOR (PPI)

Proton pump inhibitors are more effective than H_2 blockers in stage II and III. Since they suppress acid synthesis, the main causative factor they are very effective. Healing rate of PPI is 80% after 4 weeks and 90% after 8 weeks of therapy. PPI is effective even in patients with stricture and reduce need for esophageal dilatation. Optimal dose is decided by the dose required for relief of symptoms and by esophageal pH but most often Barrett's metaplasia is resistant to therapy with PPI.

H_2 BLOCKERS

The cure rate of H_2 blockers is only around 50 to 75% in GERD stage II or III as they only modulate the secretion of gastric acid through H_2 receptor antagonism. Since they do not block synthesis of acid, they are less effective than PPI. GERD is a chronic condition requiring long-term therapy and PPI are less suitable for prolonged therapy. Hence, to maintain symptomatic remission PPI can be switched over to H_2 blockers. Step down should be attempted after one full course with PPI as it is first line therapy.

Drug of Choice: Proton Pump Inhibitor (PPI)

RATIONALE

Gastroesophageal reflux disease or GERD is associated with severe erosive esophagitis. Stage I is characterized by uncomplicated heart burn with less than three episodes per week. Antacids or H_2 blockers with diet and lifestyle modification is adequate for relief. Stage II is characterized by more frequent episodes, heartburn with or without esophagitis and progresses to stricture formation or heart burn or Barrett's metaplasia in stage III that creates a huge risk for development of adenocarcinoma. **PPIs** are the **first line** drugs for stages II and III but most often Barrett's metaplasia is resistant to therapy. As agents inhibiting acid synthesis PPI is very effective in GERD as it is mainly due to acid reflux into esophagus. **Cure rate** ranges from **80** to **90%** with PPI. Comparatively **H_2 blockers** are **less effective** as they only decrease acid secretion by modulating proton pump. Their **efficacy** and **cure rate** is **lower** than PPI. However, they can be effective for **step down therapy** to maintain symptomatic remission. Since GERD is a chronic condition, **PPIs** are **not suitable for long-term therapy.**

6. *PPI monotherapy/(PPI + H_2 blockers coadministration) for suppressing nocturnal acid breakthrough in GERD.*

BACKGROUND

Unrelenting chronic symptoms of GERD is a great threat for adenocarcinoma. Frequent relapse need to be treated otherwise it will cause permanent mucosal damage which is directly related to the amount of acid contact time with mucosa. Acidic gastric fluid of pH less than 4.0 is highly injurious to esophageal mucosa. The gastric distension due to vasovagal reflex triggers lower esophageal sphincter relaxation.

PPI + H_2 BLOCKERS COADMINISTRATION

H_2 blockers are very effective in reducing the nocturnal acid secretion. They predominantly reduce basal acid secretion than total acid secretion. Hence, they are more effective than PPI in suppressing nocturnal acid secretion. H_2 blockers with PPI should not be coadministrated at the same time because they interfere with the efficacy of PPI. Inhibition of nocturnal acid secretion forms basis of their use in stress ulcers prevention. In patients receiving PPI, H_2 blockers should be given as evening dose. Evening dose of H_2 blockers effectively reduces nocturnal acid.

PPI MONOTHERAPY

PPI offer adequate control in 90% of patients with heart burn even in stages II and III. Complete resolution of heart burn occurs in around 50% of patients treated with PPI. The cure rate of esophagitis is around 80% following once or twice daily dose of PPI. Lying down in supine posture opens esophageal sphincter increasing acid reflux and such patients are more prone for nocturnal acid breakthrough with severe symptoms. More than two thirds of patients with GERD are prone for nocturnal acid breakthrough. These patients are often refractory to treatment with monotherapy of PPI. Even twice daily dose of PPI is unable to reduce the nocturnal acid breakthrough. They should undergo endoscopy to rule out Barrett's metaplasia or erosive esophagitis.

Drug of Choice: PPI + H_2 Blockers Coadministration

RATIONALE

Gastric distention due to vasovagal reflex triggers lower esophageal sphincter relaxation. Acidic gastric fluid of pH less than 4.0 is highly injurious to esophageal mucosa. The cure rate of esophagitis is around 80% following once or twice daily dose of PPI. But even twice daily dose of PPI is unable to reduce the nocturnal acid breakthrough which occurs in more than two thirds of patients with GERD. **When compared to PPI, H_2 blockers reduce basal secretion** hence, **effectively** control **nocturnal acid secretion**. When given as an **additional evening dose** in persons taking single morning dose of PPI, they are effective in **preventing nocturnal acid breakthrough** thereby **promoting healing of ulcers** and this forms the basis of their use in prevention of stress ulcers. However, both H_2 blockers and PPI should not be administered at the same time as H_2 blockers interfere with the efficacy of PPI.

7. *Famotidine/Cimetidine for long-term maintenance to suppress nocturnal acid secretion in peptic ulcer.*

BACKGROUND

Mucosal defense factors are mucin, bicarbonate, prostaglandin and nitric oxide. Aggressive luminal factors that damage mucosa are pepsin and gastrin. Duodenal ulcers are more common and antrum is common site for gastric ulcer. It is more common in men than in women frequently occurring above 50 years. Peptic ulcer is chronic and recurrence can occur within one year in most of the patients. Proton pump inhibitors promote healing of ulcers more rapidly than H_2 blockers but they are unsuitable for long-term therapy as they result in B_{12} and iron deficiency. H_2 blockers are suitable for maintenance of symptomatic remissions. Cimetidine, ranitidine, famotidine and nizatidine are the H_2 blockers used in therapy.

FAMOTIDINE

Famotidine results in longer duration of action than cimetidine as it binds tightly with H_2 receptors. It has a low affinity to subtypes of CYP450 so it has a lower propensity to cause drug interactions. It is not antiandrogenic and does not cause gynecomastia so is safer in men. In women, it neither interferes with estrogen metabolism nor prolactin secretion. It causes minimal side effects such as mild dizziness or headache so preferred.

CIMETIDINE

Cimetidine is hydrophilic well absorbed with around 80% bioavailability. About two thirds of drug is excreted unchanged while one third is metabolized. It requires reduction of dose in renal impairment as it is mainly excreted through kidney. Cimetidine inhibits CYP2D6, CYP1A2 and CYP2C9, the subtypes of CYP450. Hence, it increases the plasma levels of drugs that are substrates for these enzymes. It is antiandrogenic and inhibits binding of testosterone to androgen receptors. In addition it also inhibits cytochrome that hydroxylates estrogen inhibiting its metabolism. In men it results in impotence, gynecomastia and reduced sperm count. It increases prolactin level and causes galactorrhea in women, so not preferred. It causes rashes, headache, dry mouth, dizziness and transient elevation of liver enzymes. Hence, it is not preferred.

Drug of Choice: Famotidine

RATIONALE

H_2 blockers are preferred for long-term therapy in maintenance of symptomatic remission. They reduce basal secretion of acid and so are very effective in inhibiting nocturnal acid secretion. **Cimetidine** has good oral bioavailability but is a short acting drug. It interferes with binding of testosterone to its receptors causing **impotence, gynecomastia** and reduced sperm count in **men**. In **women**, cimetidine interferes with estrogen metabolism, **increases prolactin** level causing **galactorrhea**. Further, it inhibits many subtypes of CYP450 resulting in many drug interactions. **Famotidine** has **lower propensity** to cause **drug interactions**, is **devoid of antiandrogenic action**, causes minimal side effects and so preferred.

CHAPTER
58
Antiemetics and Disorders of Bowel Motility

1. *Alvimopan/Methylnaltrexone in postoperative paralytic ileus due to exogenous opioid administration.*

BACKGROUND

Neurogenic, hormonal and inflammatory mechanisms are involved in pathogenesis of paralytic ileus. Neurogenic response is mainly due to surgical stress following bowel manipulation and inhibitory neural reflexes are stimulated leading to reduced bowel motility. Inflammatory response causes recruitment of macrophages, mast cells and neutrophils. These release inflammatory mediators including opioid peptides that reduce motility. Proinflammatory cytokines also decrease motility. Hormonal response due to corticotropin release factor induces inflammatory mediators. Local hormones nitric oxide, substance P and calcitonin gene related peptide are released. Administration of opioids during pre or postoperative period can cause paralytic ileus. Incidence of postoperative ileus with fentanyl as anesthetic is less than 1%. They stimulate μ receptors in gut causing non-propulsive disorganized motility and also reduce acetylcholine release potentiating the risk for paralytic ileus.

ALVIMOPAN

Alvimopan is a selective μ receptor antagonist that targets peripheral opioid receptors. It has longer duration of action, usually well tolerated and can be administered orally. It antagonizes selectively μ opioid receptors in gut, so are effective in inducing motility. It has 200 times more affinity to peripheral opioid receptors compared to central receptors. Its potency is 6 times higher than naloxone in inhibiting the peripheral opioid receptors. It accelerates the time required for recovery of GIT function postoperatively. By blocking the opioid receptors it improves motility increasing the transit time. One dose of 12 mg prior to surgery followed by once daily dose is ideal but should not exceed 15 doses. It has **black box warning** for potential risk of myocardial infarction on long-term use.

METHYLNALTREXONE

Methylnaltrexone is similar to alvimopan as a peripheral opioid antagonist. Although it enhances GIT transit time it does not accelerate ileum recovery time. It is given subcutaneously and its duration of action is shorter than alvimopan. It is more effective in the treatment of opioid induced constipation in cancer patients.

Drug of Choice: Alvimopan

RATIONALE

One of the main reasons for postoperative paralytic ileus is administration of opioids during perioperative period of surgery. They are used as preanesthetic medication and for postoperative analgesia. This stimulates the peripheral opioid μ receptors resulting in non-propulsive disorganized motility. The incidence of postoperative paralytic ileus with fentanyl as anesthetic is very minimal and less than 1%. **Alvimopan** is a **selective peripheral opioid antagonist** blocking the action of opioid μ receptors in gut. Its selectivity for peripheral opioid μ receptors is 200 times higher than central opioid μ receptors. It can be administered **orally**, has **long duration** of action enabling for **once daily dosage** and accelerates the time taken for recovery by promoting GIT transit time. The **total** number of **doses** should **not exceed 15 times** as it has **black box warning** for **myocardial infarction** on **long-term use.**[134] Methylnaltrexone has similar mechanism of action but has **lesser efficacy**, has **short duration** of action and has to be administered **subcutaneously.**

2. *Racecadotril/Octreotide in secretory diarrhea due to neuroendocrine tumors.*

BACKGROUND

Diarrhea is the second leading cause of morbidity and mortality due to infectious diseases. Standard therapy of diarrhea involves anti diarrheal agents and antibiotics. Replacement of fluid and electrolytes form the main line of therapy. Alteration of normal microflora is responsible for antibiotic induced diarrhea. Probiotic preparations containing nonpathogenic bacteria are given to recolonize gut. Many components are involved in regulation of intestinal fluid secretion. Endogenous opioid peptide enkephalin stimulates delta opioid receptors reducing cAMP. The enzyme enkephalinase that degrades enkephalins is also an important regulator. Vasoactive intestinal peptide and prostaglandins E_2 increase cAMP levels inducing water and electrolyte secretion in the gut. Neuroendocrine tumors such as carcinoid cause secretory diarrhea. Ideal antidiarrheal agent should decrease fluid secretion by intestinal mucosa. It should have rapid onset, limited constipating effect with low abuse potential. It should have high therapeutic index and minimal CNS side effects.

OCTREOTIDE

Octreotide, an analog of somatostatin is effective in acute secretory diarrhea and in neuroendocrine tumors such as gastrinoma and carcinoid. It inhibits secretion of 5HT as well as peptides like VIP, insulin and secretin. Octreotide can be given at 50 to 100 µg subcutaneously 2 to 3 times daily. Long acting once a month preparation of octreotide is given in acromegaly. It causes significant and consistent reduction in volume as well as frequency of stools. It is a highly potent, effective antisecretory agent with minimal need for fluid replacement. It improves consistency of stools and reduces the duration of diarrhea.

RACECADOTRIL

As enteric neurotransmitters enkephalins inhibit the intestinal secretion but do not affect motility of gut in spite of reducing intestinal secretion. Racecadotril inhibits enkephalinase increasing enkephalins levels and reducing intestinal secretions. Hence, racecadotril is effective in acute secretory rotavirus induced diarrhea. Since it does not interfere with motility it is less likely to cause constipation. It is rapidly acting and causes quick resolution of symptoms in acute diarrhea but it is weak antisecretory so it does not reduce frequency, volume and stool consistency. Besides, racecadotril increases frequency and requirement of more fluid replacement. Hence, racecadotril is less preferred than octreotide.

Drug of Choice: Octreotide

RATIONALE

Standard therapy of diarrhea involves antidiarrheal agents, antibiotics with replacement of fluid and electrolytes. Enkephalins decrease cAMP inhibiting water and electrolyte secretion in the gut. Vasoactive intestinal peptide and prostaglandins E_2 increase cAMP levels. **Octreotide** is an analog of somatostatin is highly potent, inhibits secretion of 5HT as well as peptides like VIP, insulin and secretin. It causes **significant** and **consistent reduction in volume** as well as **frequency** of stools **improving consistency** of stools and reducing duration of diarrhea. As a strong antisecretory agent, it reduces the frequency and amount of fluid replacement. **Racecadotril increases enkephalins** level **and inhibits fluid secretion** so **useful in secretory diarrhea**. It does **not affect the motility** of intestine. Since it is a **weaker antisecretory** agent it **does not reduce frequency, volume** of stool and its **consistency**.[135] Hence, octreotide is more effective than racecadotril in acute secretory diarrhea due to neuroendocrine tumors.

3. *Loperamide/Alosetron in diarrhea dominant irritable bowel syndrome (IBS) in women.*

BACKGROUND

IBS is a chronic disorder with frequent remissions and exacerbations. It is characterized by intermittent abdominal cramps with changes in stool frequency or consistency and is often accompanied by severe pain due to 'visceral hyperalgesia'. Pain in irritable bowel syndrome does not occur at night during sleep. Pain is usually relieved by defecation and if symptoms persist beyond three months it confirms diagnosis. IBS is either diarrhea dominant or constipation dominant or both symptoms mixed. Fecal incontinence or frequent watery stools occur more than 3 times per day.

ALOSETRON

Serotonin is mainly involved with pain sensation and gastrointestinal motility. $5HT_3$ receptors are involved in emesis and increased gastric motility. Alosetron is a $5HT_3$ antagonist and blocks gastrointestinal motility and has been approved for treatment of IBS with predominant diarrhea in women. It causes significant improvement in global rating resulting in adequate relief reducing stool frequency. It improves stool consistency and reduces fecal urgency but it can cause severe constipation so it is contraindicated in constipation dominant IBS. Occasionally alosetron can cause ischemic colitis, so has to be used with caution. It is reserved only for those who do not benefit from other routine antidiarrheal agents.

LOPERAMIDE

Loperamide is more potent than morphine as antidiarrheal agent. It acts on opioid receptors reduces intestinal motility and increases anal sphincter tone. It has antisecretory activity and promotes absorption of intestinal fluids. Although it improves stool consistency and reduces stool frequency as well as urgency it is not approved in IBS as it causes side effects on long term use. So it is not preferred since IBS is a chronic condition. Randomized trials are yet to confirm the efficacy of diphenoxylate and loperamide.[136]

Drug of Choice: Alosetron

RATIONALE

IBS is often accompanied by severe pain due to 'visceral hyperalgesia'. Pain is very severe but neither occurs at night nor disturbs sleep. Since serotonin is mainly involved with pain sensation and gastrointestinal motility **alosetron, 5HT$_3$ antagonist** can be used. It decreases **gastrointestinal motility reducing stool frequency** as well as **urgency** and **improving consistency**. Alosetron is approved for treatment of IBS with predominant diarrhea in women.[137] Since it causes **severe constipation** it is **contraindicated** in **constipation dominant IBS**. Alosetron can cause **ischemic colitis**, so **reserved** for **resistant IBS** not responding to usual antidiarrheal agents. **Loperamide** has antisecretory activity as it acts on opioid receptors and reduces intestinal motility by increasing anal sphincter tone. It causes **side effects on long-term** use, so not preferred.

4. *Tricyclic antidepressants (TCAs)/Selective serotonin reuptake inhibitors (SSRIs) in IBS.*

BACKGROUND

Multivarious etiological factors such as stress, psychological factors, autonomic neuropathy and serotonin imbalance are involved in pathogenesis of IBS. Pathogenesis involves visceral hypersensitivity and dysregulation of central pain perception. Antidepressants increase central pain threshold, hence they are beneficial in IBS. Chronic use of SSRIs and TCAs in IBS causes habituation and should be discouraged.

TRICYCLIC ANTIDEPRESSANTS

Tricyclic antidepressants such as nortriptyline, imipramine and desipramine are the most effective agents in patients with severe pain as they have analgesic and neuroregulatory properties. TCAs modulate visceral sensitivity, bowel motility and pain perception and their antidepressant activity is useful in relieving stress and psychological component. They normalize the altered sleep pattern, reduce anxiety and improve mood. They are started at low therapeutic doses and increased gradually if pain does not improve. They are effective in both constipation and diarrhea dominant type of IBS.[138] They provide benefit on account of their anticholinergic action, neuropathic effect and regulation of GI transit. They reduce abdominal pain and flatulence besides normalizing frequency of defecation.

SELECTIVE SEROTONIN REUPTAKE INHIBITORS

SSRIs are less effective than TCAs in the management of visceral pain in IBS. Unlike TCAs, they are tried only in constipation dominant IBS and not in diarrhea dominant IBS as they cause diarrhea. Fluoxetine causes overall sense of well being as it is an anxiolytic, but its action is short lived, does not improve abdominal pain and has minimal impact in improving bowel symptoms.

Drug of Choice: Tricyclic Antidepressants (TCAs)

RATIONALE

Stress, psychological factors, autonomic neuropathy and serotonin imbalance are some of the major factors involved in pathogenesis of IBS. Visceral hypersensitivity and dysregulation of central pain perception are major factors causing severe unbearable pain. Antidepressants increase central pain threshold and modify psychological components but prolonged use can cause habituation and should be avoided. **TCAs** nortriptyline, imipramine and desipramine are more effective than SSRI fluoxetine as they **modulate visceral sensitivity, bowel motility** and **pain perception** and also **normalize altered sleep pattern, reduce anxiety, improving mood.** They are **effective** in **both constipation dominant** as well as **diarrhea dominant** IBS as they have **antidepressant** effect. In addition their neuropathic effect, anticholinergic effect and modulator activity on GI transit time are probably the reasons behind their beneficial effect. SSRIs cause diarrhea hence tried in constipation dominant IBS. When compared to TCAs the efficacy of **SSRIs** is minimal. They cause **short lived sense of well being** but are **not** beneficial in **altering the bowel movements** probably due to lack of anticholinergic action. Hence, TCAs are preferred to SSRIs in the management pain and bloating sensation in IBS.

5. *Stimulant laxatives/Bulk forming laxatives for constipation.*

BACKGROUND

Principal determinant of stool volume and consistency is its fluid content. It depends upon the balance between intestinal absorption as well as secretion and ingestion of water. Absorption of nutrients and large quantity of water occurs mainly in small intestine and large intestine does not influence nutrient absorption but contributes to absorption of water. Pathogens and neurohumoral mechanisms alter motility and absorptive capacity. Decreased motility and increased absorption causes impacted or inspissated feces.

BULK FORMING LAXATIVES

Fiber content of diet decides the bulk, hydration and softness of feces. Fiber in diet does not undergo enzymatic digestion and reach colon unchanged. Bulk forming laxatives either contain fiber or increase bacterial mass by fermentation through colonic bacterial action causing higher volume of stool promoting evacuation. Fiber present in laxative stimulates colonic epithelium after breaking down into short chain fatty acids whose prokinetic action contributes to evacuation. Insoluble fibers are poorly fermentable, absorbs water increasing bulk of stool. Such preparations are more preferable as they are effective. Bulk forming laxatives are contraindicated in obstructive lesions and in megacolon.

STIMULANT LAXATIVES

Stimulant laxatives have powerful direct stimulant action on intestinal epithelium and stimulate enteric neurons, enterocytes and intestinal smooth muscle. They increase intestinal motility through accumulation of electrolyte and water. The main mechanisms are activation of nitric oxide cGMP and prostaglandins cAMP pathway, inhibition of Na^+K^+ ATPase and stimulation of platelet activating factor. These laxatives result in water and electrolyte depletion causing severe hypokalemia. Since they can stimulate pregnant uterus they are contraindicated during pregnancy. Long-term use causes atonic nonfunctioning colon and so not preferred.

Drug of Choice: Bulk Forming Laxatives

RATIONALE

Principal determinant of stool volume and consistency is its fluid content and the balance between intestinal absorption of water or fluid as well as intestinal secretion and ingestion of more water or fluids form the primary basis for the bulk of stool. Fiber content of diet decides the bulk, hydration and softness of feces. Fiber in diet does not undergo enzymatic digestion and reaches colon unchanged. **Bulk forming laxatives** either contain fiber or **increase bacterial mass** through fermentation by colonic bacteria and also **break down** the **fiber content** into **small chain fatty acids**. The **prokinetic** action of short chain fatty acids stimulates intestinal epithelium and increased bacterial mass causes higher volume of stool promoting evacuation. Although bulk forming laxatives are **unpalatable** and need to be given in larger quantity they are **preferred** to stimulant laxatives[139] as **they do not cause severe water and electrolyte depletion**. Stimulant laxatives directly stimulate enteric neurons, enterocytes and intestinal smooth muscle and increase motility. They are very powerful laxatives and cause depletion of water and electrolytes frequently causing hypokalemia.

6. *Chenodeoxycholic acid/Ursodeoxycholic acid in biliary cirrhosis.*

BACKGROUND

Primary biliary cirrhosis is due to autoimmune destruction of hepatic bile ducts. It is a chronic progressive condition with insidious onset mostly in women and often coexists with other autoimmune conditions such as celiac disease, Sjogren's syndrome and autoimmune thyroiditis. Pruritus and excessive day time somnolence with elevated liver enzymes are present. Bile acids increase bile flow and also inhibit synthesis of cholesterol, facilitate intestinal excretion of cholesterol, promote absorption of lipids and fat soluble vitamins A, D, E and K. They undergo enterohepatic circulation as 95% is reabsorbed in terminal ileum. It comprises mainly chenodeoxycholic acid the minor component is ursodeoxycholic acid. The salts of taurine and glycine conjugates of bile acid are called bile salts.

URSODEOXYCHOLIC ACID

Ursodeoxycholic acid is dehydroxylated bile acid and hydrophilic in nature and epimerization of chenodeoxycholic acid forms ursodeoxycholic acid. It decreases biliary lipid secretion altering the concentration of bile acid. It reduces the cholesterol content of bile and makes it less lithogenic. It also has cytoprotective and immunomodulatory action on hepatocytes. It slows down progression of disease if given in early stage and facilitates long term survival, protecting hepatocytes and causes minimal side effects. It reduces risk of esophageal varices and delays need for hepatic transplantation. It leads to higher response rates and reduces the risk of recurrent colorectal adenoma. Side effects are minimal and tolerable such as weight gain and diarrhea so it is preferred.

CHENODEOXYCHOLIC ACID

Chenodeoxycholic acid acts mainly by inhibiting synthesis of hepatic cholesterol. Unlike ursodeoxycholic acid it does not influence cholesterol absorption in intestine. By decreasing LDL-C receptors in liver it increases plasma level of LDL-C. It is more toxic and long term therapy increases hepatic aminotransferase level. Since this condition is chronic requiring prolonged therapy it is not suitable. It also causes diarrhea and potentiates gastric and esophageal ulcers so not preferred.

Drug of Choice: Ursodeoxycholic Acid

RATIONALE

Primary biliary cirrhosis is a chronic progressive condition with insidious onset. It often coexists with other autoimmune conditions such as celiac disease and Sjogren's syndrome. **Ursodeoxycholic**

acid decreases biliary **lipid secretion reducing** the **cholesterol content of bile**. Since it is an immunological condition **immuno-modulatory** action of ursodeoxycholic acid confers **cytoprotective** effect **on hepatocytes slowing** down the **progression** of disease **facilitating** long-term **survival**. Prolonged therapy **reduces** the risk of **recurrent** colorectal **adenoma**. It causes minimal and tolerable side effects such as weight gain and diarrhea. It is preferred due to these advantages. **Chenodeoxycholic acid** acts mainly by inhibiting synthesis of hepatic cholesterol. On long-term therapy it **increases** plasma level of **LDL-C** and the level of hepatic **aminotransferase**. Since this condition requires prolonged therapy, it is not preferred.

7. *Cholestyramine/Rifampin in pruritus in primary biliary cirrhosis.*

BACKGROUND

Cholestatic pruritus occurs commonly in primary biliary cirrhosis. The main causative factor of pruritus is bile salts that are deposited in skin. Bile salts degranulate mast cells to release histamine that causes pruritus. Seventy percent of patients with primary biliary cirrhosis suffer from pruritus. Since liver conjugates bile to make it more water soluble-liver diseases can cause pruritus.

CHOLESTYRAMINE

Cholestyramine binds with bile salts preventing their absorption in terminal ileum. It is the first line drug in management of pruritus associated with biliary cirrhosis. It is given as 4 g with fruit juice or water 3 times per day. Improvement is seen after two weeks of therapy as the level of bile salts is reduced. It has very unpleasant taste hence the patient compliance is very poor. It can cause constipation, malabsorption and reduces bioavailability of many drugs. Digoxin, thyroxine and oral contraceptives should be taken at least 4 hours earlier.

RIFAMPIN

Rifampin is an enzyme inducer and induces phase I and II biotransformation enzymes. It induces cytochrome CYP3A4 and conjugating enzymes like UGT1A1 and SULTA1. It thereby enhances metabolism of bilirubin and its breakdown products. The antimicrobial property of rifampin has an additional role in relieving pruritus. Rifampin helps in modifying the synthesis of secondary bile acids in intestinal lumen thereby it helps in reducing the synthesis of hepatotoxic lithocholic acid. Further it competes with and reduces the uptake of bile acids by hepatocytes. It is effective at a daily dose of 300 mg twice daily. Although very effective, it is associated with hepatotoxicity and hemolytic anemia. Thrombocytopenic purpura and renal failure are other complications of rifampin. It is reserved as second line drug due to its efficacy and multiple mechanisms.

Drug of Choice: Cholestyramine

RATIONALE

Cholestatic pruritus occurs commonly in primary biliary cirrhosis as the main causative factor of pruritus is bile salts that get deposited in skin. The incidence of pruritus in patients with primary biliary cirrhosis is 70%. Bile salts degranulate mast cells to release histamine that causes pruritus. **Cholestyramine** is the first line therapy as it **binds** with **bile salts preventing** their **absorption** in terminal ileum reducing its serum level. Improvement is seen after two weeks of therapy as the level of bile salts is reduced,[140] but it has highly unpleasant taste and has to be given at a high dose for two weeks which reduces patient's concordance to treatment. **Rifampin** is an **enzyme inducer** and **induces** the **metabolism of bile salts**. It also prevents synthesis of **hepatotoxic** lithocholic acid in intestinal lumen. Further, it competes with and reduces the uptake of bile acids by hepatocytes. Since it is highly hepatotoxic, causes blood dyscrasias and renal failure it is reserved as second line drug, although it is highly effective with multiple mechanisms.

8. *Metoclopramide/Domperidone as antiemetic agent in children and elderly.*

BACKGROUND

Neuronal areas such as nucleus tractus solitarius, area postrema and central pattern generator within medulla comprise brainstem vomiting center. They are stimulated by four different factors or afferent stimuli to induce emesis. Sight, smell or emotion induce vomiting through stimulation of amygdala. Histamine and cholinergic system mediated by vestibular fibers also stimulate emesis. Stimulation of $5HT_3$ receptors from GIT through afferent vagal fibers induces vomiting. Chemoreceptor trigger zone (CTZ) is located in medulla area postrema outside blood-brain barrier (BBB). It is rich with $5HT_3$, opioid, dopamine D_2 and neurokinin NK1 receptors. Chemotherapeutic drugs, toxins, acidosis, uremia and radiation therapy stimulate CTZ.

DOMPERIDONE

Domperidone is a selective D_2 blocker with inferior prokinetic action. Its efficacy is modest as it does not modulate the action of other receptors. Hence, domperidone does not have significant peripheral action on GIT motility. It blocks D_2 receptors of CTZ but does not cross BBB to block central D_2 receptors. Therefore, domperidone does not cause Parkinsonism like extrapyramidal side effects. So, unlike metoclopramide it can be safely used in children and elderly.

METOCLOPRAMIDE

Metoclopramide is both prokinetic and antiemetic agent used in vomiting. It is D_2 blocker but antagonizes $5HT_3$ receptors also and facilitates $5HT_4$ receptor agonism. It facilitates GIT movement by stimulating muscarinic cholinergic receptors. D_2 mediates reduction of intragastric and lower esophageal sphincter pressures. D_2 also inhibits motility by suppressing acetylcholine release from myenteric plexus. As D_2 blocker metoclopramide increases lower esophageal sphincter tone reduces emesis peripherally. D_2 blockade in CTZ and vomiting center accounts for centrally mediated antiemetic action. As a prokinetic it facilitates antral and small intestinal motility enhancing gastric emptying but causes extrapyramidal side effects and galactorrhea due to central D_2 blockade. Reversible dystonias and tardive dyskinesia can occur after single IV administration. Usually they disappear after cessation of drug or respond to anticholinergics but prolonged therapy can result in irreversible tardive dyskinesia. Children and elderly are more sensitive for this side effect so it is not preferred in them. Metoclopramide is also useful in gastroparesis and GI dysmotility syndromes.

Drug of Choice: Domperidone

RATIONALE

Vomiting center mediated emesis is stimulated by four different pathways. Amygdala mediated pathway that is stimulated by sight, smell and emotion, vestibular pathway, peripheral GIT mediated pathway and through CTZ. Dopamine, serotonin, acetylcholine and histamine are factors that mediate these pathways. **Metoclopramide** has **both central** and **peripheral actions**. As antiemetic it blocks D_2 receptors centrally and also increases lower esophageal tone increasing gastric emptying through stimulation of antral and small intestinal motility. By stimulating $5HT_4$ receptors it promotes gastric motility. Hence, both D_2 blockade and $5HT_4$ agonism favor its prokinetic action. Since it crosses BBB and **antagonizes central D_2 receptors** in vomiting center it causes **extrapyramidal** symptoms. **Children** and **elderly** are **particularly susceptible** to it. Hence, it should be avoided in these age groups. **Domperidone** acts by blocking D_2 receptors **selectively**. Hence, it has only **moderate prokinetic** activity. It acts on CTZ and **does not cross BBB** and so **does not result in extrapyramidal symptoms**. Although it is less effective than metoclopramide domperidone is preferred in children and elderly.

9. *Aprepitant/Fosaprepitant as antiemetic for cancer chemotherapy induced vomiting in combination with ondansetron.*

BACKGROUND

Neurokinin 1 (NK1) receptors are found both in central and peripheral nervous system such as brainstem, neurons, vascular endothelium, GIT, lungs and other tissues. The binding of substance P with neurokinin receptors triggers inflammation, contraction of smooth muscles and also cellular excitability. It stimulates phospholipase mediated calcium release, IL 1 and dopamine release. Chemotherapy induced vomiting occurs due to activation of $5HT_3$ and NK1 receptors. It can be acute starting within minutes to hours after starting chemotherapy or it can have delayed onset and persist up to 7 days after initiation of therapy. Anticipatory nausea and vomiting occur very commonly following chemotherapy. Cisplatin, cyclophosphamide and most other alkylating agents are highly emetogenic. Neurokinin antagonists are effective in controlling both acute and delayed vomiting. So they are combined with $5HT_3$ antagonists in chemotherapy induced emesis. Neurokinin antagonists inhibit broader range of emetic stimuli than $5HT_3$ blockers. Combination of $5HT_3$ antagonists and NK1 antagonists form the first line therapy. Ondansetron and NK1 antagonists are given on first day to inhibit acute phase. This is followed by NK1 antagonists for 3 more days to prevent delayed vomiting.

FOSAPREPITANT

Oral administration may not be always feasible in unconscious or uncooperative patients. It cannot be administered during episodes of vomiting as it results in loss of entire dose. Fosaprepitant is available as IV formulation so bypasses problems of oral administration. It is a prodrug of aprepitant and activated by phosphatase enzymes. It has similar efficacy and toxicity profile of aprepitant with advantage of IV formulation.[141] Both the drugs can cause diarrhea.

APREPITANT

Aprepitant acts centrally and inhibits acute and delayed chemotherapy induced vomiting. It blocks substance P induced activation of NK1 receptors in vomiting center. It has 90% efficacy rate[142] but less preferred as it is available only as oral formulation. It is unsuitable in patients with oral mucositis, the common side effect of anticancer drugs.

Drug of Choice: Fosaprepitant

RATIONALE

Nuerokinin 1 (NK1) receptors are found both in central and peripheral nervous system. Binding of substance P with neurokinin receptor triggers inflammation. **Chemotherapy induced** vomiting occurs due to **activation of 5HT$_3$** and **NK1 receptors.** Hence **combination** of **5HT$_3$ antagonists** and **NK1 antagonists** form **first line therapy. Aprepitant** acts **centrally inhibiting acute** and **delayed** chemotherapy induced **vomiting.** It has **90% efficacy rate but** less preferred as it is **available only** as **oral formulation.** It cannot be administered **during episodes** of **vomiting** and **unsuitable** in patients with oral mucositis, a major side effect of most anticancer drugs. **Fosaprepitant** is available as **intravenous formulation** so avoids problems of oral administration. It has **similar efficacy** and toxicity profile as aprepitant with advantage as IV formulation hence preferred.[143]

Special Systems

59

Obstetric and Gynecological Pharmacology

1. *Combined OCP/Progestins in endometriosis.*

BACKGROUND

Endometriosis is the ectopic presence of endometrium in dependent pelvic parts. It occurs mainly in women of reproductive age and causes infertility. Dysmenorrhea and chronic pelvic pain occur in most individuals. Reduction in hormone levels suppresses hormone mediated stimulation of endometrium. This favors atrophy of endometrium, reduces pain and dysmenorrhea. Hormone therapy for a period of 4 to 9 months ameliorates the symptoms associated with endometriosis and inhibits ovulation.

COMBINED OCP

Low dose combined oral contraceptive pills (OCP) increase the peripheral level of estrogen and progesterone. This causes feedback inhibition of hypothalamus inhibiting release of GnRH, FSH and LH inhibiting endometrial proliferation and ovulation. Ovulation resumes within few months after stopping therapy but prolonged therapy with combined pills can result in atrophy of ectopic endometrium.

PROGESTINS

Depot medroxyprogesterone acetate and norethindrone acetate are the progestins used and are effective in suppressing pain associated with endometriosis. Though they reduce frequency they increase the amplitude of pulsatile GnRH release. This reduces the level of

FSH and LH resulting in inhibition of ovarian steroidogenesis and induces decidual transformation leading to endometrial atrophy on continuous therapy but ovulation fails to resume for prolonged period after stopping progestin therapy. Progestin therapy lowers estrogen levels causing spotting and breakthrough bleeding.

Drug of Choice: Combined OCP

RATIONALE

In women of reproductive age presence of ectopic endometrium outside uterus in dependent pelvic parts causes pain and infertility. Hormone therapy for a period of 4 to 9 months ameliorates symptoms associated with endometriosis inhibiting ovulation and suppressing hormone mediated stimulation of endometrium, relieving the pain associated with endometriosis. **Low dose combined pills** are **very effective** as they suppress ovulation and endometrial proliferation through feedback inhibition of GnRH and **ovulation resumes within few months** on stopping therapy. **Depot medroxyprogesterone acetate** and norethindrone acetate are the progestins used. They **reduce frequency** but **increase** the **amplitude** of **pulsatile GnRH release** reducing the level of FSH and LH inhibiting ovarian steroidogenesis leading to **endometrial atrophy**. Since **ovulation fails to resume** for a **prolonged period** it is not preferred for endometriosis. Even after stopping therapy progestin preparation causes spotting and breakthrough bleeding.

2. *Nifedipine/Magnesium sulfate as tocolytic agent in preterm labor.*

BACKGROUND

Delivery occurring between 24 to 37 weeks of gestation is known as preterm labor. It should be prevented to reduce the adverse manifestations on neonate. Effacement and dilatation of cervix prior to gestational period result in increased frequency of uterine contractions. Preterm infants may develop neurological problems, visual and hearing impairment. β_2 receptor agonist terbutaline causes tachycardia, pulmonary edema and hypotension, so it should be avoided. Ideal tocolytic agent should be inexpensive, acting specifically at myometrium and should be easier to administer with higher efficacy and minimal toxicity. It should not interfere with neonatal outcomes and devoid of long-term side effects.

NIFEDIPINE

Nifedipine the calcium channel blocker inhibits uterine contractions and can be administered parenterally, sublingually or orally in preterm labor. It is cheaper, better tolerated, effective and safe. The efficacy of 20 mg every 6 hours oral or sublingual nifedipine is similar to magnesium sulfate. Nifedipine is associated with significantly lesser maternal side effects but when given in twin gestation with compromised cardiac function it aggravates MI, hypotension and dyspnea.[144] It reduces incidence of respiratory distress syndrome, neonatal jaundice, intraventricular hemorrhage and enterocolitis. It also reduces the rate of neonatal hospitalization.

MAGNESIUM SULFATE

Magnesium sulfate is given as bolus dose of 4 to 6 g followed by continuous infusion of 2 g/hour. It reduces the frequency of uterine contractions, delays labor and reduces incidence of cerebral palsy in neonates but the incidence of maternal adverse effects is higher with magnesium sulfate and neonatal hospitalization is also higher.

Drug of Choice: Nifedipine

RATIONALE

An ideal tocolytic agent should act specifically at myometrium, should be easier to administer, inexpensive, have higher efficacy with minimal toxicity and should not interfere with neonatal outcomes and devoid of long-term side effects. **Nifedipine**, the calcium channel blocker can be administered **orally, sublingually or parenterally**. It has **similar efficacy** to magnesium sulfate but **better tolerated, cheaper** and associated with **infrequent maternal side effects**. It **reduces** incidence of **respiratory distress syndrome, neonatal jaundice, intraventricular hemorrhage, enterocolitis** and **neonatal hospitalization**. If given in twin gestation it causes

MI, hypotension and dyspnea more frequently. **Magnesium sulfate reduces** the **frequency** of **uterine contractions** and delays labor but **increases incidence of maternal** adverse effects and **neonatal hospitalization.**[145] So, magnesium sulfate is not preferred as suitable tocolytic.

3. *Oxytocin/Methylergonovine in postpartum hemorrhage.*

BACKGROUND

Postpartum hemorrhage (PPH) is the leading cause of maternal mortality in developing world and uterine atony or failure of uterus to contract after delivery is the potential cause. Retained placenta, placenta accreta, hypertension and induction of labor are some other causes that result in PPH. Uterine atony causes rapid and severe hemorrhage leading to hypovolemic shock. Relative or absolute over distension due to polyhydramnios, multifetal gestation or fetal macrosomia are the major risk factors for atony. Poor uterine contraction is either due to fatigue of prolonged labor or due to rapid forceful labor. Normally the detachment and expulsion of placenta occurs due to uterine contraction and relaxation. Complete detachment and expulsion of placenta, causes occlusion of blood vessels. The uterine blood vessels traverse through myometrium fibers to supply the placental site and blood vessels are kinked following contraction of muscle fibers to occlude blood flow. The arrangement of uterine muscle is referred to as physiologic sutures or ligatures.

OXYTOCIN

Oxytocin is the first line drug in management of postpartum hemorrhage. Oxytocin increases both frequency and force of uterine contractions besides causing complete relaxation of uterus in between contractions. Uterine contraction compresses blood vessels passing through myometrial muscles. Unlike methylergonovine, oxytocin is given as slow IV infusion as it is short acting and helps for easy monitoring of the intensity of action and to decide about its termination, if necessary. 20 IU of oxytocin is diluted in 1L of IV solution and given at the rate of 10 mL/minute and rate of infusion should slowly be reduced to 1–2 mL/minute till bleeding stops.

METHYLERGONOVINE

Methylergonovine increases the motor activity of uterus and induces sustained contractions thereby increasing the risk of uterine tetany. Hence, it is not preferred. The onset of action is rapid and it can be administered only through IM route. It elevates blood pressure, so should be given only in hemodynamically stable patients. Frequent side effects of methylergonovine are nausea and vomiting.

Drug of Choice: Oxytocin

RATIONALE

Uterine blood vessels traverse through myometrial fibers to supply the placenta and these blood vessels are kinked following contraction of muscle fibers and occlude blood flow. This arrangement of uterine muscle is referred to as physiologic sutures or ligatures. Hence uterine atony causes rapid and severe hemorrhage as well as hypovolemic shock. **Oxytocin** increases both **frequency** and **force of uterine contraction**. It is given as IV infusion permitting for easy monitoring of its action. At therapeutic doses it **does not cause sustained contraction** or uterine atony. **Methylergonovine** causes **sustained powerful contraction** resulting in **tetany,** so not preferred. Besides it **increases blood pressure** and should be administered only to hemodynamically stable patients.[146] The frequent side effects of methylergonovine are nausea and vomiting.

4. *Clomiphene/Metformin in polycystic ovarian syndrome (PCOS).*

BACKGROUND

PCOS is characterized by polycystic ovaries, chronic anovulation and hyperandrogenism and is usually associated with obesity and hirsutism with high risk for diabetes and cardiac problems. Menorrhagia, amenorrhea, infertility, acne, hirsutism and insulin resistance are frequent symptoms. Due to unopposed secretion of estrogen long-term risk of endometrial cancer is high. Weight reduction and exercise is very helpful in obese individuals with PCOS as it reverses metabolic effects and induces ovulation in obese patients.

CLOMIPHENE

The first line therapy in PCOS is the ovulation inducing agent clomiphene as it increases FSH level and improves the chances for ovarian follicular maturation and ovulation. In around 80% of women who take clomiphene it stimulates ovulation up to three menstrual cycles. It causes hot flushes, headache, nausea, abdominal cramps and changes in mood but these symptoms are reversible and resolve once it is discontinued.

METFORMIN

Metformin induces weight loss and increases the rate of ovulation. It is more useful when combined with clomiphene in obese patients with insulin resistance. When compared to clomiphene the efficacy of metformin in improving pregnancy rate is low. Hence, clomiphene is preferred to metformin in the treatment of PCOS.

Drug of Choice: Clomiphene

RATIONALE

PCOS is characterized by polycystic ovaries, chronic anovulation and hyperandrogenism. It is associated with obesity, hirsutism and has high risk for diabetes and cardiac problems. Most common symptoms are menorrhagia, amenorrhea, infertility, acne, hirsutism and insulin resistance. Due to unopposed secretion of estrogen, long term risk of endometrial cancer is high. **Clomiphene** increases FSH level **improving** chances of ovarian **follicular maturation** and **ovulation** in **80%** of women who take this drug up to **three menstrual cycles**. It causes hot flush, headache, nausea, abdominal cramps and changes in mood but these symptoms are reversible on stopping therapy. **Metformin** reduces weight, induces ovulation but when compared to clomiphene, metformin **monotherapy does not increase pregnancy rates**. It is more useful if combined with clomiphene in obese patients with insulin resistance.

5. *Ramipril/Methyldopa as antihypertensive in pregnant women.*

BACKGROUND

Drugs used during pregnancy should not be teratogenic. They should be safe to mother and should not interfere with fetal growth. Maintenance of blood supply is essential for proper fetal circulation. Therefore, blood pressure should be maintained within physiological limits during pregnancy.

METHYLDOPA

Methyldopa, the α_2 agonist is a centrally acting antihypertensive drug. It is a prodrug, and metabolized to α-methyl norepinephrine that acts as a substitute for norepinephrine. α-methyl norepinephrine inhibits the neuronal transmission. The effect of methyldopa is delayed for a period of 6 to 8 hours, time required for the drug to reach CNS. It results in transient sedation, dry mouth and extra pyramidal symptoms but it is not teratogenic. Hence, despite its adverse effects, it is preferred as anti hypertensive drug in pregnancy.

RAMIPRIL

Ramipril and other ACE inhibitors are teratogenic and should be avoided. Ramipril is absorbed quickly, reaches peak plasma concentration within an hour. It belongs to pregnancy category D and is contraindicated in pregnancy. If given during second and third trimesters, it reduces renal function potentiating fetal and neonatal morbidity and mortality. It causes oligohydramnios, skull hypoplasia, hypotension, anuria, fetal lung hypoplasia, skeletal deformities and renal failure. Ramipril should not be used while methyldopa can be used safely during pregnancy.

Drug of Choice: Methyldopa

RATIONALE

Methyldopa is a α_2 **agonist and centrally** acting antihypertensive drug. Its active metabolite α-norepinephrine is as a

pseudotransmitter, competes with neurotransmitter norepine-phrine in CNS and **inhibits** neuronal transmission. In spite of its capacity to induce sedation and hyperprolactinemia, it is preferred as it has a **proven safety profile** in pregnancy. **Ramipril** and other ACE inhibitors belong to **category D** and are contraindicated during pregnancy as they are teratogenic. Ramipril also worsens fetal renal function potentiating fetal morbidity and mortality.

6. *Propylthiouracil/Carbimazole for thyrotoxicosis during **second** and **third** trimester of pregnancy.*

BACKGROUND

Thyrotoxicosis in pregnancy occurs most frequently due to Graves' disease. The peripheral levels of bound T_4 and free T_4 are increased in most women. Serum TSH level is low in 18% of pregnant women. Since radioactive iodine is contraindicated during pregnancy only antithyroid drugs can be given. Graves' disease improves as pregnancy advances, so its dose has to be reduced accordingly. Carbimazole and propylthiouracil cross placenta at almost equal concentrations.

CARBIMAZOLE

Carbimazole should be avoided during first trimester at the time of organogenesis but it is the drug of choice during second and third trimester of pregnancy. It is started at 5 to 15 mg once daily but can be reduced gradually. Dose is split twice for those unable to tolerate once daily dose due to GIT side effects. In 4% of neonates it has resulted in major congenital malformations, such as esophageal atresia, omphalocele and aplasia cutis when given during first trimester.

PROPYLTHIOURACIL

Propylthiouracil significantly increases incidence of hepatic failure during pregnancy. It is preferred only during first trimester because carbimazole should be avoided. It is rarely associated with aplastic anemia, arthritis, hypoprothrombinemia and lupus.

Drug of Choice: Carbimazole

RATIONALE

Incidence of Graves' disease induced hyperthyroidism during pregnancy is high. Radioactive iodine is contraindicated during pregnancy and so only antithyroid drugs are given. **Propylthiouracil** and **carbimazole** can both **cross placenta at equal levels**. **Carbimazole interferes** with **organogenesis** and causes esophageal atresia, omphalocele and aplasia cutis, so **avoided during first trimester but** it is **safe in second and third trimester** as the risk of **hepatotoxicity** is **high with propylthiouracil**. Those unable to tolerate propylthiouracil can still be given carbimazole at low dose even during first trimester.

7. *Insulin/Sulfonylureas in gestational diabetes mellitus.*

BACKGROUND

Complication due to diabetes can affect both fetal and maternal health. Renal dysfunction, pre-eclampsia and retinopathy are frequent maternal complications. Gastroparesis in uncontrolled diabetes increases severity of pregnancy induced nausea. Poor glycemic control during early pregnancy can lead to spontaneous abortion. Congenital malformations are common, if glycemic control is poor in early pregnancy. Fetal macrosomia, preterm labor, still birth and polyhydramnios occur in late pregnancy.

INSULIN

Insulin is preferred to glyburide as it belongs to category B indicating no risk in animal studies. Insulin lispro or aspart, the fast acting insulin analogs are preferred. NPH is safer in pregnancy for basal coverage and glargine is also found to be safer.

SULFONYLUREA

Sulfonylureas are found to be unsafe in diabetes during pregnancy.[147] Glyburide, the second generation sulfonylurea, has been tried in gestational diabetes although it belongs to category C. Since it is administered orally it is convenient to those who refuse to take insulin. Initial reports found it to be safer but current reports indicate lesser safety than Insulin. Glyburide increases incidence of severe neonatal hypoglycemia at the time of delivery. Respiratory distress, jaundice, birth injury, large size neonates, preterm birth and higher risk of hospitalization of neonates in ICU[148] are other risks.

Drug of Choice: Insulin

RATIONALE

Complication due to diabetes can affect both fetal and maternal health. Gastroparesis due to uncontrolled diabetes increases severity of pregnancy induced nausea and vomiting. Renal dysfunction, pre-eclampsia and retinopathy also occur frequently in pregnant women. Poor glycemic control during early pregnancy can lead to spontaneous abortion while fetal macrosomia, preterm labor, still birth and polyhydramnios occur in late pregnancy. **Glyburide** belongs to **category C** but still tried in pregnancy associated with diabetes. It is found to be effective but increases incidence of neonatal hospitalization in ICU compared to insulin as glyburide causes **hypoglycemia, respiratory distress, jaundice, birth injury** and **preterm birth**. **Insulin** belongs to **category B** and much safer than glyburide.[149] Although **glargine** is **safe** NPH is used for basal maintenance while insulin **aspart** and insulin **lispro** are the preferred fast acting analogs.

8. *Betamethasone/Dexamethasone for reducing neonatal pulmonary complications in women at risk of premature labor.*

BACKGROUND

Steroids given to women at risk in preterm labor reduce mortality. They reduce fetal neonatal respiratory distress and cerebroventricular hemorrhage. They also reduce neonatal developmental delay and hyaline membrane disease. It is administered as a single course and not as multiple doses otherwise infants later suffer from adrenal suppression and low birth weight. Antenatal steroids stimulate gene expression that promotes maturation of lung and accelerate the expression of type 1 and 2 pneumocytes in lung that improves the lung volume and compliance through structural and biochemical changes. Increased expression of type 2 lung pneumocytes increases surfactant production because they induce the proteins and enzymes necessary for synthesis of surfactant. They also up regulate sodium channels necessary for absorption of lung fluid after birth. Induction of fetal antioxidants is another important action of pneumocytes. Steroids are administered between 24 to 36 weeks in women at risk for premature labor. The efficacy, safety, availability and cost determine the choice of steroid.

BETAMETHASONE

Betamethasone is long acting steroid with negligible mineralo-corticoid activity. Two doses of intramuscular betamethasone 12 mg twice with a gap of 24 hours are given. It significantly lowers the rate of pulmonary complications due to prematurity. Incidence of respiratory distress is much less with betamethasone than dexamethasone.

DEXAMETHASONE

The clinical efficacy and availability of dexamethasone is similar to betamethasone. It is also long acting agent with negligible mineralocorticoid activity. It has greater capacity to reduce occurrence of neonatal intraventricular hemorrhage but it increases puerperal sepsis and has to be given IM as four doses of 6 mg every 12 hours. Further it increases the occurrence of respiratory distress syndrome in neonates.

Drug of Choice: Betamethasone

RATIONALE

Glucocorticoids are given in antenatal period in women at risk for premature labor to prevent complications such as intraventricular

hemorrhage, respiratory distress and to reduce perinatal mortality. Steroids are administered between 24 to 36 weeks in women
at risk for premature labor. They accelerate the expression of type
1 and 2 pneumocytes in lung thereby **increasing** the **synthesis** of
surfactants. Betamethasone and dexamethasone are long acting
steroids and have greater anti-inflammatory activity with negligible mineralocorticoid activity. **Betamethasone** is preferred as it
reduces complications, such as **respiratory distress** better than
dexamethasone and it **does not cause puerperal sepsis**. Although
few reports indicate that **dexamethasone** reduces the incidence
of intraventricular hemorrhage is yet to be proved. Further, it
increases maternal complications such as **puerperal sepsis**
and does not effectively prevent fetal pulmonary complications.
Hence, betamethasone is preferred[150] to dexamethasone for lung
maturity.

9. *Gentamicin/(Ampicillin + Clavulanic acid) in UTI due to susceptible E. coli in pregnant women.*

BACKGROUND

E. coli is gram negative organism and a common pathogen responsible for majority of uncomplicated UTI. The preferrence of antibiotic
in pregnancy is limited. The safety of the drug is more important
than efficacy during pregnancy. Although effective, drugs with teratogenic potential should not be used. Risk is high, if given between
fourth to seventh weeks of gestation.

AMPICILLIN + CLAVULANIC ACID

Ampicillin is very effective against susceptible *E. coli* infection
as it is bactericidal and effective against rapidly multiplying bacteria. Addition of clavulanic acid improves the efficacy of ampicillin. Ampicillin-clavulanic acid combination is relatively safe in
pregnancy. It belongs to category B indicating no evidence for risk
during pregnancy.

GENTAMICIN

Gentamicin is also bactericidal against gram negative organisms and inhibits even ampicillin resistant strains of *E. coli*. Small amounts of drug are present in urine 10 to 20 days after its discontinuation as it binds to renal tissue resulting in antibacterial activity, improving its efficacy. Action of gentamicin is concentration dependent and in uncomplicated cases even a single injection is effective and attains peak level. Post antibiotic effect of gentamicin potentiates its toxicity. Administration during pregnancy leads to accumulation of drug in fetal plasma. Gentamicin belongs to category D indicating positive fetal risk. Hence, gentamicin should be avoided in UTI treatment during pregnancy.

Drug of Choice: Ampicillin + Clavulanic Acid

RATIONALE

Choice of antibiotic during pregnancy is determined by safety rather than efficacy. Ampicillin is moderately effective, if given alone. Addition of clavulanic acid, the β-lactamase inhibitor augments therapeutic efficacy. **Ampicillin-clavulanic** acid combination belongs to pregnancy category B and is relatively **safe**. **Gentamicin** is very effective against gram negative *E. coli* and even single dose results in adequate therapeutic benefit in uncomplicated UTI. If given during pregnancy, it **accumulates in fetal plasma**. Since it belongs to **category D**, it causes high fetal risk. Besides, it results in **sustained** therapeutic effect and such **post antibiotic effect** can augment the fetal toxicity. Hence, it should be avoided.

10. *Rifampin/Rifabutin as antituberculous drug during pregnancy.*

BACKGROUND

Obstetric complications are common due to tuberculosis during pregnancy. If not managed properly, it causes both maternal and fetal complications. Spontaneous abortion, small for date uterus and preterm labor occur in mothers. Increased incidence of neonatal mortality is the frequent fetal complication. INH, rifampin and ethambutol are the first line drugs. INH is safer although it crosses placenta but should be monitored for hepatotoxicity. Pyridoxine must be definitely supplemented along with INH in pregnancy. Ethambutol can cause reterobulbar neuritis in mothers but does not interfere with ocular development of infants during pregnancy. Hence, these two drugs can safely be given during pregnancy to treat tuberculosis.

RIFABUTIN

Rifabutin is more effective and belongs to first line supplemental drugs. It belongs to pregnancy category B indicating no evidence of risk. Hence, it can be safer alternative for antituberculous regimen during pregnancy.

RIFAMPIN

As a first line drug, rifampin is effective in inhibiting *M. tuberculosis* bacilli but may increase the risk of hemorrhagic disorders in new born. So, vitamin K 10 mg/day supplemented in the last 4 to 8 weeks of pregnancy. However, rifampin belongs to pregnancy category C indicating risk cannot be ruled out and should be avoided during pregnancy.

Drug of Choice: Rifabutin

RATIONALE

To prevent obstetric complications during pregnancy, antituberculous drugs should be given. INH, rifampin and ethambutol belongs to first line drugs used in this condition. Rifampin may increase the **risk of hemorrhagic disorders** in new born hence vitamin K is administered during the last 2 months of pregnancy. However, it belongs to pregnancy **category C** and should better be avoided. **Rifabutin** is **more effective**, requires **lower MIC** for its antituberculous action and belongs to pregnancy **category B** hence, preferred to rifampin.

11. *Zidovudine/Efavirenz for antireteroviral therapy (ART) in pregnancy.*

BACKGROUND

Significant proportion of women requiring ART are in child bearing age group and often HIV is diagnosed for the first time during pregnancy and ART started. Main goal of ART during pregnancy is to prevent transmission of HIV to unborn child. ART helps to maintain *viral load* below the level of detection throughout pregnancy. The drug chosen should be relatively safe, should result in excellent early virological suppression and should have a record of experience during pregnancy. It should not interact with coadministered drugs and should be convenient to patient. Factors such as pharmacokinetic changes during pregnancy, comorbidities, the degree of placental transfer of drugs, potential adverse effects and exaggerated metabolism of drugs during pregnancy should be considered before choosing a drug.

ZIDOVUDINE

Zidovudine is a NRTI undergoing rapid first pass metabolism with 64% bioavailability. The pharmacokinetic profile of zidovudine is not significantly altered in pregnancy and freely crosses placenta attaining good fetal plasma concentration. Its plasma concentration in fetus is on par with maternal concentration. It is one of the oldest antiretroviral drugs with established safety during pregnancy. Zidovudine is approved during pregnancy, to prevent mother to fetus transmission. Even as monotherapy it significantly reduced perinatal transmission. One of the safest regimens used is zidovudine + lamivudine + ritonavir/lopinavir.

EFAVIRENZ

Efavirenz is a NNRTI and does not need intracellular phosphorylation for its action. It is teratogenic, if used within first 8 weeks of first trimester. It causes anencephaly, facial cleft, neural tube defects and microphthalmia. Women of child-bearing age group taking efavirenz should avoid conception and it should not be started for pregnant women diagnosed for first time during pregnancy.

Drug of Choice: Zidovudine

RATIONALE

The main goal of ART during pregnancy is to prevent transmission of HIV to unborn child. It also helps to maintain *viral load* below the level of detection throughout pregnancy. Antenatal drug administration reduces *viral load* in blood as well as genital secretions. **Efavirenz** should not be used in early pregnancy as it is toxic to fetus. It is **contraindicated** especially during **first trimester** as it is highly **teratogenic** during this period. **Zidovudine** is one of the oldest drugs but **well-tolerated** with consistent reports of **safety** during **pregnancy**. Although it crosses placenta and attains **plasma concentration on par** with **maternal** level it is not teratogenic. So it is included in all regimens used during pregnancy.

12. *Sodium valproate/Levetiracetam as a safer antiepileptic drug during pregnancy.*

BACKGROUND

Proper and efficient control of seizures during pregnancy is very important but higher incidence of teratogenic effects by anti epileptic drugs is reported so care should be taken to avoid drugs that are teratogenic. Phenytoin, carbamazepine and lamotrigine are also unsafe. These drugs are included in pregnancy category D. Gabapentin, pregabalin and oxcarbazepine are not given as monotherapy as they are ineffective in most seizures and little is known about their safety in pregnancy.[151] Conflicting reports are available about the use of topiramate.[152] Some reports claim that it causes cleft lip while few other reports claim its safety.

LEVETIRACETAM

Monotherapy of levetiracetam is reported to be safe and has minimal risk.[153] When given as monotherapy, it does not cause major congenital abnormalities (category C). The risk is found to be higher, if it is combined with other drugs. Mechanism of levetiracetam is not clearly understood. It is used routinely as an adjunctive with other antiepileptic drugs. It is used in partial, generalized and myoclonic seizures. Very low concentration of levetiracetam is excreted in milk. It is a safer alternative as an antiepileptic drug.[154] It is preferred in women of reproductive age group and during pregnancy.

SODIUM VALPROATE

Risk of teratogenicity is very high for sodium valproate. So it should be avoided in women of reproductive age group and during pregnancy. Spina bifida and neural tube defects are most common teratogenic effects.

Drug of Choice: Levetiracetam

RATIONALE

Epidemiological evidence points to higher incidence of teratogenic effects by antiepileptic drugs. Polytherapy in pregnancy poses more threat to fetus as most of the antiepileptic drugs are unsafe and belong to category D. **Sodium valproate**, the **broad spectrum** antiepileptic, belongs to **high risk category** and should be avoided in pregnancy. Most of the newer drugs are given only as adjuncts because they are not effective as monotherapy. **Levetiracetam** is reasonably **safe** has only minimal risk for developing major congenital anomalies. Besides it is effective as monotherapy in partial, generalized and myoclonic seizures. Hence, it is preferred to sodium valproate as monotherapy in pregnancy.

13. *Sucralfate/Proton Pump Inhibitors (PPI) for mild GERD in pregnancy.*

BACKGROUND

GERD especially heart burn is a frequent occurrence in 80% of pregnant women. These symptoms worsen as pregnancy advances requiring therapy. Hormone induced relaxation of lower esophageal sphincter causes acid reflux as maternal estrogen and progesterone reduces lower esophageal sphincter pressure. This causes laxity of the sphincter resulting in acid regurgitation into esophagus. Pepsin mediates hydrolysis of mucosal proteins causing mucosal erosions. These mucosal ulcerations can be inhibited by sulfated polysaccharides.

SUCRALFATE

Sucralfate is the combination of aluminum hydroxide and octasulfate of sucrose. It undergoes enormous cross-linking in acid environment at pH less than 4. The sticky viscous polymer adheres to ulcer crater and epithelial cells for about 6 hours. It also stimulates epidermal growth factor and prostaglandins promoting ulcer healing. Since conservative measure is needed during pregnancy, sucralfate is the drug of choice. It does not get absorbed and has local action, so is preferred during pregnancy. Sucralfate is also useful in other conditions like nosocomial pneumonia. Since alkaline medium favors growth of nosocomial pneumonia in critically ill-patients, PPI or H_2 blockers which increase pH, are ineffective in preventing organism growth. Sucralfate does not increase pH, so effective in preventing nosocomial pneumonia.

PROTON PUMP INHIBITORS

PPIs are found to be safer during pregnancy but should be avoided when symptoms are minimal. Except omeprazole that belongs to category C all other PPIs belong to category B, but still are reserved only for severe symptoms of GERD during pregnancy. If sucralfate fails, famotidine (category B) is given as it reduces nocturnal acid.

Drug of Choice: Sucralfate

RATIONALE

GERD especially heart burn is a frequent occurrence in 80% of pregnant women and worsens as pregnancy advances necessitating therapy. Maternal estrogen and progesterone reduces lower esophageal sphincter pressure causing laxity of sphincter, resulting in acid regurgitation into esophagus. **Although PPIs except omeprazole** belong to **category B** and are found to be safer and very effective during pregnancy they are **avoided,** if symptoms are mild, as conservative measures are more favored. **Sucralfate** is ulcer protective agent. It polymerizes extensively, cross-linking in acid environment at pH less than 4 covering ulcer crater. It also **secretes prostaglandins** and favors **ulcer healing** by stimulating epidermal growth factor. Hence, it is first line drug in GERD with mild symptoms during pregnancy as it **does not get absorbed** and has local action. PPI is reserved only for severe symptoms like erosive esophagitis.

14. *Statins/Bile acid sequestrants for treating hypercholesterolemia during pregnancy.*

BACKGROUND

Lipoproteins undergo qualitative modification during pregnancy and hypertriglyceridemia is more common than hypercholesterolemia during this period. Incidence of gestational pancreatitis is reported to be around 25%. It is due to estrogen mediated suppression of lipoprotein lipase reducing the clearance of triglycerides. The levels of LDL-C and VLDL-C increase during first and third trimester and triglycerides increase during the third trimester of pregnancy.

BILE ACID SEQUESTRANTS

Bile acid sequestrants are the only hypolipidemic agents safe during pregnancy. The positively charged bile acid sequestrants bind with negatively charged bile acids forming an insoluble complex in the intestine. The insoluble complex is not absorbed as it is large and gets excreted. This action promotes depletion of bile acids reducing their plasma level. The hepatic synthesis of bile acids increases as its plasma level declines stimulating synthesis of LDL receptors necessary for clearance of LDL-C. These agents can increase serum triglyceride levels and should be monitored. They are unpalatable and result in bloating, dyspepsia as well as constipation. Bile acid sequestrants are not absorbed and do not cause systemic side effects. Colesevelam is preferred to cholestyramine or colestipol in pregnancy. Since their plasma level is negligible, they do not cross- placenta. Hence, they are safely given in pregnancy.

STATINS

Statins belong to pregnancy X category and should not be given during pregnancy. Women in childbearing age, on therapy with statins should use proper contraception. Since statins are teratogenic, it is necessary to avoid pregnancy.

Drug of Choice: Bile Acid Sequestrants

RATIONALE

Statins are absolutely **contraindicated** during pregnancy. The only safer hypolipidemic agents during pregnancy are bile acid sequestrants. **Bile acid sequestrants act locally** in GIT by forming complexes with bile acids preventing their enterohepatic circulation. Secondary to this effect they reduce LDL-C and increase HDL-C. They can increase serum triglycerides level, cause bloating, dyspepsia and constipation.

15. *Tinidazole/Paromomycin in giardiasis during pregnancy.*

BACKGROUND

Ten percent become carriers and 25 to 50% develop acute diarrhea if infected with *Giardia lamblia*. Acute diarrhea is usually self-limiting but generally progresses to chronic state but the duration of cyst excretion is often prolonged for weeks to months. Chronic disease results in malabsorption and vitamin deficiencies.

PAROMOMYCIN

Paromomycin is preferred for giardiasis in pregnancy during first trimester. It is also effective against metronidazole resistant strains of *Giardia lamblia*. It is given in the dose of 500 mg three times a day for 10 days. The cure rate of paromomycin against *Giardia lamblia* is around 55 to 90%. When given orally it is not well-absorbed and its actions are confined to intestinal lumen. Since it is not absorbed systemically, it does not cause teratogenicity. It is an aminoglycoside but does not cause ototoxicity or nephrotoxicity through oral route as it is not absorbed.

TINIDAZOLE

Tinidazole is very effective and has higher cure rate in giardiasis. It is well-tolerated and given as a single large dose of 2G but it is carcinogenic and teratogenic in animal studies. It belongs to pregnancy category C and contraindicated during pregnancy. It is mainly avoided during first trimester due to its potential for embryo toxicity.

Drug of Choice: Paromomycin

RATIONALE

Tinidazole is **very effective** in *Giardia lamblia* infections resulting in **high cure rate**. It is highly **teratogenic** in animal studies and therefore **contraindicated** especially during first trimester as it is toxic to embryo. The **efficacy** of **paromomycin** is **variable** from **moderate** 55% to **high** 90% cure rate. It is also effective against metronidazole resistant strains. It is safe, **not absorbed** from GIT so **not teratogenic** and preferred during pregnancy.

16. *Chloroquine/Quinine as chemoprophylaxis during pregnancy for malaria due to susceptible strains of P. vivax.*

BACKGROUND

As far as possible, pregnant women should avoid journeys to endemic areas and benefits should outweigh risks while selecting an antimalarial during pregnancy. Safety data for atovaquone + proguanil and artemether + lumefantrine is insufficient. Mefloquine, doxycycline and primaquine are unsafe and so contraindicated. Chloroquine and quinine are found to be safe during first trimester of pregnancy.

CHLOROQUINE

Chloroquine is 100% effective against susceptible strains of *Plasmodium vivax*. It is safe during the entire period of pregnancy and so preferred. It is a weak base and accumulates in acidic digestive vacuoles of *Plasmodium* generating free radicals inducing oxidative damage killing the organisms. It is highly effective against asexual erythrocytic forms of *Plasmodium vivax*. It is contraindicated in G6PD deficiency as it can cause hemolysis.

QUININE

Quinine also has similar mechanism and inhibits asexual erythrocytic forms. It is safe only during first trimester and not during second or third trimester. It causes severe hypoglycemia frequently in pregnant women and so not preferred. During pregnancy regular intake of food and consuming an antimalarial agent after food has reduced the frequency of hypoglycemia.

Drug of Choice: Chloroquine

RATIONALE

Chloroquine and quinine can both be safely used during first trimester of pregnancy.[155] While chloroquine is safe during the entire period of pregnancy quinine is unsafe during second and third trimesters of pregnancy. **Chloroquine** is **more effective** on **susceptible strains** of *P. vivax*. It is less toxic and **does not induce hypoglycemia** but it can **cause hemolysis** in persons with **G6PD deficiency**. **Quinine** is **equieffective**, but **more toxic** and **increases** the frequency of **hypoglycemia**. Hence, chloroquine is preferred to quinine for *P. vivax* infection during pregnancy.

17. *Chloroquine/Quinine as chemoprophylaxis during first trimester of pregnancy in malaria due to P. falciparum.*

BACKGROUND

Chemoprophylaxis is necessary for pregnant women traveling to endemic areas. Chloroquine and quinine are relatively safe during the first trimester of pregnancy. They do not increase the incidence of congenital anomalies, still birth or low birth weight.

QUININE

In India, quinine is very effective against malaria due to *Plasmodium falciparum*. It is devoid of teratogenicity during the first trimester of pregnancy but the frequency of hypoglycemia is high. This may be due to its powerful stimulation of pancreatic beta cells which results in hyperinsulinism leading to severe hypoglycemia. It can be reduced by frequent administration of fluids and taking tablets along with food.

CHLOROQUINE

The safety of chloroquine during entire pregnancy is established. Chloroquine is very effective on all susceptible strains of *Plasmodium*, but in India *Plasmodium falciparum* has developed resistance to chloroquine. It is high in North Eastern States, AP, MP, Orissa, Chhattisgarh and Jharkhand. Hence, chloroquine is unsuitable for chemoprophylaxis of *P. falciparum* malaria.

Drug of Choice: Quinine

RATIONALE

Most strains of *P. falciparum* in India have developed resistance to chloroquine. The resistance is very high in North Eastern States like Assam and other states like AP, MP, Orissa, Goa, Chhattisgarh and Jharkhand. Resistance is also prevalent in larger areas in other states except Tamil Nadu and Kerala. Only small areas of TN and Kerala are resistant to chloroquine. Hence, chloroquine is not suitable for chemoprophylaxis in *P. falciparum* malaria. **Quinine** is highly **effective against *P. falciparum* malaria in India**. It does **not** result in **teratogenicity,** if given in first trimester but can cause hypoglycemia in pregnant women. The incidence of hypoglycemia can be reduced through proper food intake and taking the drug on full stomach.

18. *Quinine/Artemisinin combined therapy (ACT) for chemoprophy-laxis of P. falciparum in pregnancy during second and third trimester.*

BACKGROUND

P. falciparum affects all stages of erythrocytes resulting in high parasitemias in blood provoking severe constitutional symptoms. Cytoadherence proteins assembled by *P. falciparum* produce 'knobs' in erythrocytes which cling to vascular endothelium and escape splenic destruction. The growth of parasites occurs in unfavorable conditions like low O_2 and high CO_2. It causes blockade of microvasculature in brain or organs and releases cytokines and nitric oxide. Placental malaria occurs as a consequence of vascu-lar blockade during pregnancy. Hence, it is imperative to institute chemoprophylaxis during pregnancy.

ARTEMISININ COMBINED THERAPY (ACT)

Limited data is available regarding safety of artemisinin derivatives in early pregnancy and its embryo/fetal toxicity has been reported in animal studies. Skeletal and visceral abnormalities have been primarily noted in animals. They are therefore not recommended as first line drugs by WHO during first trimester but they are proved to be safer during second and third trimester. Artemisinins have a very short half-life and lead to high recrudescence rates hence they are not suitable as monotherapy for chemoprophy-laxis. Coadministration of either lumefantrine or sulfadoxine-pyrimethamine is preferred. Artemether-lumefantrine is preferred for *P. falciparum* prophylaxis in NE states. Artesunate-sulfadoxine-pyrimethamine combination is preferred in other states.

QUININE

Quinine is very efficient in suppressing *P. falciparum* malaria but its safety in second and third trimester is not well-established. It causes hyperinsulinemia leading to hypoglycemia during pregnancy. In spite of glucose infusions it can still be life-threatening during later months of pregnancy. As pregnancy advances susceptibility for quinine induced hypoglycemia is high. Hence, it is not preferred for prophylaxis in second and third trimester of pregnancy.

Drug of Choice: Artemisinin Combined Therapy (ACT)

RATIONALE

Plasmodium falciparum can cause placental malaria. Therefore, chemoprophylaxis is required for pregnant women who travel to endemic areas. **Quinine** is **unsafe** during second and third trimester of pregnancy. **Artemisinin** derivatives are **not safe** during **first trimester** but are relatively safe during **rest of pregnancy**. They cannot be given alone due to their short half-life resulting in higher rate of relapse. Hence, ACT or artemisinin combined therapy is given. Artesunate-sulfadoxine-pyrimethamine is preferred to all states in India except North Eastern states as *P. falciparum* has developed resistance to sulfadoxine-pyrimethamine combination in those states. Instead artemether-lumefantrine is preferred for NE states. Primaquine should never be given during pregnancy.

19. *GnRH agonists/GnRH antagonists to inhibit premature luteinization in assisted reproductive technologies.*

BACKGROUND

In vitro fertilization (IVF) benefits those who do not respond to traditional methods. Administration of high doses FSH induces maturation of at least 5 to 20 oocytes that are retrieved for this purpose during *in vitro* fertilization. Eggs fertilized *in vitro* are transferred back into uterus as embryos. Premature LH surge causes premature luteinization of ovarian follicles, gonadotropins with GnRH agonists or antagonists suppress this LH surge.

GnRH ANTAGONISTS

GnRH antagonists such as ganirelix and cetrorelix suppress the LH surge that is required to induce ovulation and hypothalamic mediated pituitary FSH and LH secretion. Hence, they are used in assisted reproduction technology to increase pregnancy rate. GnRH antagonists inhibit premature increase in LH at a much shorter time. They cause competitive and immediate suppression of GnRH receptors, in ovary. They are used along with gonadotropins in assisted reproduction. Being antagonists they do not cause transient increase in gonadotropin release. Unlike GnRH agonists they do not result in biosynthesis of sex steroids. Hence, they are more effective than GnRH agonists for assisted reproduction. GnRH antagonists cause dose related suppression of gonadotropins. Optimal therapeutic benefit can be obtained through once daily subcutaneous administration of GnRH agonists and this helps for significant reduction in the duration of treatment schedules. They cause mild hypersensitivity reactions but rare anaphylaxis has also been reported. They do not result in hot flushes and other symptoms of estrogen withdrawal.

GnRH AGONISTS

Exogenous gonadotropin and GnRH agonists such as leuprolide, goserelin, histrelin, nafarelin and triptorelin result in high pregnancy rates. They suppress pituitary FSH and LH more effectively compared to gonadotropin alone. They prevent premature LH surge and luteinization enhancing follicular recruitment. In a long protocol, GnRH agonist is started on 21st day in luteal phase of earlier cycle and continued till gonadotropin injection is given to induce ovulation. In a short protocol the agonist is given on day 2, a day prior to gonadotropin injection. Short protocol permits recovery of many oocytes, if started in follicle or luteal phase. Synthetic GnRH agonists have longer half-lives, so they suppress GnRH receptors in ovary. They cause desensitization, hot flushes, headache and hyperstimulation of ovary.

Drug of Choice: GnRH Antagonists

RATIONALE

Administration of high doses of FSH induces maturation of at least 5 to 20 oocytes. Premature LH surge causes premature luteinization of ovarian follicles. Gonadotropins with GnRH agonists or antagonists suppress this LH surge. **GnRH agonists** are given either as a long protocol or short protocol. In long protocol, GnRH agonist is started on 21st day in luteal phase of the previous cycle. It is continued till gonadotropin injection is given to induce ovulation. In short protocol the agonist is given on day 2, a day prior to gonadotropin injection but these long acting preparations cause **hot flushes, headache, desensitization of ovarian GnRH receptors** and hyper stimulation of ovary. Unlike GnRH agonists, **GnRH antagonists do not cause estrogen withdrawal symptoms** such as hot flushes. They have **higher efficacy** but do not cause transient increase in gonadotropin level, quicker acting and bring about significant reduction in treatment period.[156] Hence, GnRH antagonists are preferred.

20. *Clomiphene/Tamoxifen in infertility.*

BACKGROUND

The incidence of infertility in developed nations is slowly increasing and is around 10 to 15%. The cause is attributed to one-third in women, one-third in men and one-third in both. Anovulation is the primary cause of infertility in 50% of women, so ovulation inducing drugs are useful. Diagnosis of anovulation is confirmed through luteal phase progesterone and luteinizing hormone levels.

CLOMIPHENE

Clomiphene is antiestrogen and stimulates ovulation in women with intact HPA axis. It inhibits estrogen mediated negative feedback on hypothalamic pituitary axis. So, it enhances maturation of ovarian follicles by increasing FSH levels. It is started between 2nd and 5th day of menstrual cycle at 50 mg daily and continued for 5 days. If ovulation does not occur the dose is increased to 100 mg then to 150 and 200 mg. The adverse effects of clomiphene is called ovarian hyper stimulation syndrome characterized by ovarian cyst, multifetal gestation, hot flushes and headache.

TAMOXIFEN

Tamoxifen belongs to the selective estrogen receptor modulator group. Similar to clomiphene it is also a very effective ovulation inducing agent. It is used off-label in those who are unable to tolerate the adverse effects of clomiphene but it is not approved as ovulation inducing drug by FDA in the treatment of infertility. It induces proliferation of endometrium increasing the risk of endometrial carcinoma.

Drug of Choice: Clomiphene

RATIONALE

Infertility is on raising trend and cause is attributed to one-third in women, one-third in male and one-third in both. **Clomiphene** is **ovulation inducing** drug. It is an agonist-antagonist and inhibits estrogen mediated negative feedback on hypothalamic-pituitary axis. It increases FSH levels enhancing follicular maturation but **can cause ovarian hyper stimulation syndrome**. It increases the incidence of multifetal pregnancy, ovarian cysts and blurring of vision. Although **not approved by FDA, off-label use of tamoxifen** is to induce ovulation but it can **increase the risk of endometrial carcinoma** through stimulation of endometrial proliferation. Hence, it is not preferred.

21. *Mifepristone/Medroxyprogesterone acetate for termination of early pregnancy.*

BACKGROUND

For maintenance of pregnancy, progesterone is very essential. It is secreted by corpus luteum and suppresses uterine contraction. Progesterone deficiency often results in spontaneous abortion. Mifepristone is a competitive antagonist of progesterone receptors. Medroxyprogesterone acetate is a progesterone compound.

MIFEPRISTONE

By blocking uterine progesterone receptors mifepristone causes decidual breakdown. This detaches the blastocyst, reducing production of human chorionic gonadotropin and progesterone secretion from corpus luteum causing further decidual breakdown. By blocking progesterone receptors and by reducing progesterone secretion it causes abortion. Focal hemorrhage and inhibition of stomal tissue factor also contribute to its actions. Mifepristone causes cervical softening facilitating the expulsion of fetus. It causes infection and vaginal bleeding that can continue for a period of 8 to 17 days. **Black box FDA** warning is added to the product label regarding this risk. It causes prostaglandin induced uterine cramps, abdominal pain, vomiting and diarrhea. Antiglucocorticoid activity of mifepristone can cause adrenal insufficiency.

MEDROXYPROGESTERONE ACETATE

Medroxyprogesterone acetate is essential for maintenance of pregnancy. Being progesterone it suppresses uterine contractility and prolongs luteal phase inducing decidual changes similar to early pregnancy. Progesterone is used to prevent threatened abortion and to continue pregnancy. Hence, instead of inducing abortion it helps to prolong pregnancy, so not preferred.

Drug of Choice: Mifepristone

RATIONALE

Progesterone is useful in prolongation of luteal phase and to maintain pregnancy. Progesterone antagonists block the facilitatory action of progesterone in maintenance of pregnancy and cause abortion. **Mifepristone** is **antiprogesterone**, binds to progesterone receptors and **inhibits progesterone competitively**. By blocking progesterone receptors it causes **decidual breakdown, detaches blastocyst** and reduces production of HCG. It also causes **cervical softening** and **facilitates expulsion** of fetus. A **black box** warning is added to its product label regarding its capacity to induce the **risk of vaginal bleeding** and infection. **Medroxyprogesterone acetate** is **essential** for **maintenance** of pregnancy by prolonging the luteal phase. Hence, it **cannot** be used for **inducing abortion**.

Dermatological Pharmacology

1. *Finasteride/Minoxidil for androgenic alopecia in women.*

BACKGROUND

Alopecia is either due to abnormal cyclical hair growth or due to damaged hair follicle. Most common cause of hair loss in women is androgenic alopecia. Other causes are alopecia aerata, telogen effluvium, traumatic and cicatrical alopecia. Each hair follicle continuously goes through three phases namely anagen, telogen and catagen. Anagen is growth phase, telogen the rest phase and catagen the involution or transition phase. Telogen effluvium is temporary increase in resting or telogen phase for many hairs and it occurs due to fever, stress, malnutrition, surgery, postdelivery period or shock and is often self-limiting. Androgenic alopecia the common cause is a genetically inherited trait where dihydro-testosterone activates genes on binding to androgen receptor in hair follicles. This genetic activation transforms larger hair follicles into small vellus follicles.

MINOXIDIL

Hypertrichosis, the adverse effect of minoxidil is exploited for treatment of alopecia. It is used as topical solution of 2 and 5% in the treatment of alopecia. It is useful for smaller areas of alopecia which has an onset of less than 5 years. It stimulates and prolongs growth or anagen phase increasing number and length of hair. It also increases follicular size and thickness of hair shafts as long as it is used. Hair growth stops if it is discontinued and it can cause allergic or contact dermatitis.

FINASTERIDE

Type II 5α reductase is found in prostate, seminal vesicles, hair follicles and epididymis. Finasteride is competitive and specific inhibitor of type II 5α reductase enzyme in hair with 100 fold more selectivity to type II than to type I isoenzyme. Type II 5α reductase enzyme converts testosterone to dihydrotestosterone (DHT) and is responsible for two thirds of circulating dihydrotestosterone. Turnover of this enzyme is slow and takes about 30 days so inhibition by finasteride is prolonged causing significant reduction in peripheral conversion of testosterone to DHT. In androgenic alopecia balding areas have miniature hair follicles and increased DHT. Finasteride decreases both serum and scalp dihydrotestosterone in these men. Finasteride at the dose of 1mg/day if given for 2 years increases the hair growth and the amount of hair growth over frontal scalp and vertex is increased. Continuous treatment is required otherwise growth of new hair is lost. It causes erectile dysfunction, decreased libido and disorders of ejaculation. It is not approved for use in women and can be given only in men. It is teratogenic, so contraindicated in pregnancy and women in reproductive age group. Postmenopausal women with androgenic alopecia do not benefit from finasteride. Therapy even up to 12 months does not result in clinical improvement or hair counts in them.

Drug of Choice: Minoxidil

RATIONALE

Each hair follicle continuously grows through a cyclical growth pattern consisting of three phases namely anagen, telogen and catagen phase. Androgenic alopecia is the common cause and a genetically inherited trait. Finasteride is competitive and specific inhibitor of type II 5α reductase enzyme in hair follicles and has 100 fold more affinity to type II when compared to type I. **Finasteride increases** the amount of **hair growth** over frontal scalp and vertex but it is **not approved** for use **in women**. It is teratogenic so **contraindicated** in **pregnancy** and in women of **reproductive age** group. In postmenopausal women with androgenic alopecia, therapy even up to 12 months does not result in clinical improvement or hair counts. The **side effect** of **minoxidil** is **hypertrichosis** and that is **exploited** for **treatment** of alopecia. It is effective as topical solution of 2 and 5% only for **smaller areas** of alopecia with an **onset** of **less than 5 years**. It **stimulates** and **prolongs** growth or **anagen phase** increasing the number and length of hair, follicular size and **thickness** of hair shafts as long as it is used. Hair growth stops if it is discontinued and it can cause allergic or contact dermatitis. Minoxidil is effective and approved for use in women. Hence, it is preferred.

2. *Hydroquinone/Monobenzone in treatment of hyperpigmentation.*

BACKGROUND

Hyperpigmentation is mainly caused by excess production of melanin. Increased melanin in epidermis tends to be more brownish appearance. High melanin between upper dermis and epidermis causes brown, grey or blue lesion. It appears grey or blue when it is due to increased melanin concentration in dermis. Drugs can cause secondary hyperpigmentation that may appear as bluish grey. Melasma, drugs and cancers are few causes of widespread hyperpigmentation. It also occurs in hemochromatosis, biliary cirrhosis or Addison disease. Inflammation, photo dermatitis and acanthosis nigricans cause focal hyperpigmentation. Amiodarone, zidovudine, clofazimine and many anticancer drugs can cause hyperpigmentation.

HYDROQUINONE

The first line agent in the treatment of hyperpigmentation is hydroquinone. It inhibits tyrosinase suppressing the conversion of dopa to melanin pigment thereby reducing the production of melanin pigment by melanocytes. It inhibits synthesis of DNA, RNA, promotes degradation of melanosomes and destruction of melanocytes. Monitoring is required as it causes ochronosis, the yellow discoloration and dermatitis. Ochronosis occurs due to accumulation of homogentisic acid in connective tissues. Pruritus, erythema, desquamation, dryness and burning sensation are other side effects. Since it does not cause permanent depigmentation it is preferred for therapy.

MONOBENZONE

Monobenzone is the monobenzylether of hydroquinone and insoluble in water. When applied pigmented skin fades rapidly than normal skin and exposure to sun reduces its action. Monobenzone may cause destruction of melanocytes and permanent depigmentation. Its action is erratic and may take up to 4 months to occur for existing melanin to be lost due to normal sloughing of stratum corneum. It causes depigmentation of areas of normal skin distant to sites of application. It can result in irregular, excessive and frequently permanent depigmentation. It causes mild transient irritation, skin sensitization and eczematous lesions.

Drug of Choice: Hydroquinone

RATIONALE

Melasma, drugs, hemochromatosis, biliary cirrhosis, Addison disease and cancer are few causes of widespread hyperpigmentation. Inflammation, photo dermatitis and acanthosis nigricans cause focal hyperpigmentation. Amiodarone, zidovudine, clofazimine and most anticancer drugs cause hyperpigmentation. Hydroquinone and monobenzone are effective only in sun light induced or hormonally induced hyperpigmentation and not in inflammation or other types of hyperpigmentation. **Hydroquinone**, the first line agent **inhibits** enzyme tyrosinase suppressing conversion of dopa to **melanin** reducing its **production** by melanocytes. It promotes degradation of melanosomes and destruction of melanocytes. It causes **ochronosis**, due to accumulation of **homogentisic acid in connective tissues** resulting in **yellowish** discoloration. Hence, regular monitoring is required but it **does not cause permanent depigmentation** so preferred for therapy. **Monobenzone** the monobenzylether of hydroquinone causes destruction of melanocytes and **permanent depigmentation**. Although it takes up to 4 months for permanent depigmentation, the period required for loss of existing melanin due to normal sloughing of stratum corneum, it can cause irregular, excessive and frequently permanent depigmentation. Therefore, it is not preferred.

3. *First generation retinoids/Third generation retinoids for topical use in acne.*

BACKGROUND

Topical retinoids are drugs of choice for comedonal non-inflammatory acne. In inflammatory acne, they are given in combination with other anti-acne agents. Retinoids are both synthetic and natural and have vitamin-A like activity. They activate retinoid X receptors (RXR) and retinoic acid receptors (RAR). The three isoforms α, β and γ of both receptors are expressed in cells and tissues. The binding of retinoid with RAR causes cellular differentiation and proliferation. Drugs binding with retinoid receptor RXR induce apoptosis. So, they are used in acne.

THIRD GENERATION RETINOIDS

Third generation retinoids are formed as molecular modifications of 1st generation agents. These agents have a common property of selective binding to nuclear retinoid receptors. Third generation retinoids such as adapalene, tazarotene and bexarotene bind to RXR and so are more effective in acne. They are well tolerated, have better efficacy, reduce overall disease severity and result in significant reduction in postinflammatory hyperpigmentation.

FIRST GENERATION RETINOIDS

First generation retinoids bind to retinoid receptors in both cytosol and nucleus and also bind to RAR and cause cellular proliferation and differentiation. They reduce cohesiveness of follicular epithelial cells and decrease microcomedo formation. First generation retinoids such as tretinoin, isotretinoin and alitretinoin are irritants causing dry skin, peeling of skin, erythema and pruritus. Since they have minimal safety profile they are less preferred.

Drug of Choice: Third Generation Retinoids

RATIONALE

Retinoids activate retinoid X receptors (RXR) and retinoic acid receptors (RAR). The three isoforms α, β and γ of both receptors are expressed in cells and tissues and are activated when retinoids bind to their receptors. Binding of retinoids with RAR causes cellular differentiation and proliferation. Since drugs binding with retinoid receptor RXR induce apoptosis, they are useful in acne. **First generation retinoids bind** to **retinoid receptors** in both **cytosol** and **nucleus** but are **not selective** and bind to RAR causing cellular **proliferation** and **differentiation**. Although they are effective in reducing cohesiveness of follicular epithelial cells and decrease microcomedo formation they are not preferred as they are not selective in action and have **minimal safety profile**. **Third generation retinoids** are more selective and bind to only RXR. They are **well tolerated**, have **better efficacy, reduce overall severity** and so preferred.

4. *Adapalene/Tazarotene as topical application in acne.*

BACKGROUND

Hyperplasia of sebaceous glands and hyperkeratotic follicles form acne. It is caused due to colonization of *Propionibacterium acnes* leading to inflammation. Closed or open comedones, pustules, papules and cysts occur in acne. Acne vulgaris is more common in young persons and more severe in males. Pathophysiology includes plugging of infundibulum of follicles and retention of sebum. Overgrowth of *P. acnes* causes release of sebum and irritation due to accumulation of fatty acids. Retinoids modulate cellular proliferation, immunity, cause tumor suppression and improve vision. Adapalene and tazarotene bind to RXR and used in treatment of acne. They also improve photo aging manifested as dyspigmentation and wrinkles.

TAZAROTENE

Tazarotene is the most potent third generation topical retinoid used in acne. One percent of tazarotene ameliorates wrinkling, facial hypo and hyperpigmentation. It undergoes hydrolysis by esterases to its active metabolite tazarotenic acid. It has better efficacy in reducing overall severity of the condition. It causes significant reduction in postinflammatory hyperpigmentation. Although infrequent it results in mild irritation in few patients and rarely causes desquamation, erythema, dry skin, contact dermatitis, pruritus and rash.

ADAPALENE

Adapalene is chemically stable retinoid-like third generation retinoid. It modulates cellular differentiation, keratinization and inflammatory process. Adapalene binds to specific nuclear receptor but not to cytosolic receptor. It normalizes differentiation of follicular epithelial cells and reduces microcomedone formation. Absorption of adapalene through human skin is very low even on chronic administration. It is less effective in reducing post inflammatory hyperpigmentation. It causes pruritus, erythema, scaling, irritation, stinging and burning sensation. It can cause acne flares in first month but these lesions decrease in frequency and severity.

Drug of Choice: Tazarotene

RATIONALE

Acne is characterized by closed or open comedones, pustules, papules as well as cysts and caused by colonization of ***Propionibacterium acnes***. Adapalene and tazarotene are third generation retinoids and bind to RXR so, used in treatment of acne. **Adapalene modulates** cellular **differentiation**, keratinization and inflammatory process but is **less effective** in reducing **postinflammatory hyperpigmentation. Tazarotene** is **more potent, has better efficacy** in reducing overall severity of the condition and causes greater and significant reduction in postinflammatory hyperpigmentation.[157] Hence, it is preferred to adapalene.

61

Ocular Pharmacology

1. *Tear solutions/Ointments in dry eye (keratoconjunctivitis sicca).*

BACKGROUND

Dry eye is a multifactorial disorder of tear film and ocular surface causing discomfort, visual disturbance and damage to ocular surface. Women particularly at peri- and postmenopausal age groups are more susceptible. Tear secretion, meibomian gland and conjunctival goblet cell functions are impaired. Meibomian gland dysfunction is associated with chronic androgen deficiency. It has a higher prevalence in postmenopausal women using estrogen containing HRT. Other causes are laser-assisted *in situ* keratomileusis or photorefractive keratectomy. Dry eye is provoked by long-term use of contact lens and extended visual tasking like watching TV. Humid conditions, extreme heat or cold and vitamin A deficiency can worsen dry eye. Stevens-Johnson syndrome, Sjogren's syndrome and trachoma are few other causes.

TEAR SOLUTIONS

Tear solutions are preferred to ophthalmic lubricants for management of dry eye. Tear substitutes include isotonic or hypotonic solutions used for supplemental lubrication. They contain surfactants, electrolytes, preservatives and various types of viscosity agents which increase residence time of drops in precorneal tear film and *cul-de-sac*. Preservative-free and preservative-containing tear drops are available. However, ocular inflammation can be exacerbated by preservatives. The frequently used preservative in tear drops is benzalkonium chloride which de-stabilizes precorneal tear film damaging epithelial cells. Carboxymethyl cellulose, methyl cellulose, hydroxypropylmethyl cellulose, hydroxyethyl and propyl-cellulose are some of the preparations.

OINTMENTS

Lubricating ointments contain white petrolatum, mineral oil, or alcohol lanolin. They are highly viscous and lead to blurring of vision so, used only at bed time. They may lubricate and protect eye from epithelial erosion but they are highly uncomfortable and never should be used with contact lenses. Hence, they are only second line drugs in severe dry eye or in critically ill patients.

Drug of Choice: Tear Solutions

RATIONALE

Dry eye is a multifactorial disorder of tear film and ocular sur-face causing discomfort, visual disturbance and damage to ocu-lar surface. Women particularly at peri- and postmenopausal age groups are more susceptible. Hot humid conditions, extreme heat or cold, vitamin A deficiency, Stevens-Johnson syndrome, Sjogren's syndrome and trachoma are some of the causes of conjunctivitis sicca. **Tear substitutes** are **isotonic or hypotonic** solutions used for supplemental lubrication. They **contain** surfactants, electrolytes, preservatives and various types of **viscosity agents** that **increase residence time** of drops in **precorneal tear film** and *cul-de-sac*. Since ocular inflammation can be exacerbated by preservatives, **preservative-free tear drops** are **preferred**. Lubricating **oint-ments** are **highly viscous** lead to **blurring** of vision. They are highly **uncomfortable** and **can never** be **used** with **contact lenses**. They can be used only at bed time so are second line drugs in severe dry eye or in critically ill patients.

2. *Proparacaine/Pramoxine as ocular anesthetic.*

BACKGROUND

Anesthesia of cornea and conjunctiva occurs when topical anes-thetics are applied. Only a few local anesthetics qualify for this purpose as most local anesthetics are irritants to eye. Ocular anesthesia is required for performing tonometry, for removal of foreign bodies from cornea as well as conjunctiva and for nasolacrimal canalicular manipulation. Corneal anesthesia is necessary in laser refractive surgery. It is also used for placing corneal rings intrastromally. Generally vascularity of the applied area determines the duration of action of local anesthetics. Since cornea is avascular, the duration is prolonged in a normal cornea but the effect of the local anesthetic is short in inflamed conjunctiva. Hence, repeated instillations may be required for effective anesthetic action but it can lead to pitting and sloughing of corneal epithelium and damage of corneal epithelium interferes with healing process.

PROPARACAINE

Proparacaine is rapid acting local anesthetic suitable for ophthalmic use. Its action starts within 30 seconds and lasts for a short period. It is used in tonometry for measurement of intraocular pressure. It is also useful in procedures such as removal of foreign bodies and sutures in cornea, in conjunctival scrapings and can be used as topical anesthetic prior to cataract surgery. Proparacaine causes either minimal or nil corneal irritation, stinging, burning or redness. It is also less antigenic when compared to other local anesthetics. Individuals sensitive to other benzoate local anesthetics can still tolerate it better.

PRAMOXINE

Pramoxine is an effective surface anesthetic for skin and mucous membrane. It is devoid of cross sensitivity allergic reactions. It can be used as surface anesthetic in individuals sensitive to other local anesthetics but it is a severe irritant to the eye. Hence, it should never be used as local anesthetic for ocular procedures.

Drug of Choice: Proparacaine

RATIONALE

Ocular anesthesia using surface anesthetics is required for conducting various procedures. Proparacaine is rapid acting local anesthetic. Its action starts within 30 seconds and lasts for a short period. It is used for various purposes such as tonometry, removal of foreign bodies as well as sutures in cornea and during conjunctival scraping. It is also used frequently as topical anesthetic prior to cataract surgery. **Proparacaine** is **less antigenic** and so is **better tolerated even by individuals sensitive to other benzoate** local **anesthetics**. It causes **minimal** corneal **irritation, stinging, burning or redness** hence, preferred for ocular anesthesia. Unlike proparacaine, **pramoxine** is not a benzoate ester, devoid of cross sensitivity but **irritant** to eye. Hence, it **cannot be used** for ocular anesthesia.

3. *Bevacizumab/Ranibizumab for age-related macular degeneration (ARMD).*

BACKGROUND

Leading cause of permanent visual loss in old people is ARMD. It is classified as atrophic, dry or geographic and neovascular, exudative or wet. Gradually progressive bilateral visual loss occurs in atrophic degeneration due to degeneration of retinal epithelium and outer retina. Growth of new choroidal blood vessels occurs in neovascular degeneration. New blood vessels form between retinal pigment epithelium and Bruch membrane resulting in accumulation of serous fluid, hemorrhage and fibrosis. Ninety percent of ARMD are mainly due to neovascular degeneration causing loss of central vision.

RANIBIZUMAB

VEGF-A causes neovascularization and leakage associated with ocular angiogenesis and contributes to progression of neovascular or vascular type of ARMD. Ranibizumab binds to VEGF-A preventing its interaction with $VEGFR_1$ and $VEGFR_2$ present on the surface of vascular endothelial cells. This interaction inhibits endothelial proliferation, angiogenesis and vascular leakage. It reduces foveal retinal thickness and choroidal neovascularization. Ranibizumab is a variable and not a full length IgG with anti-angiogenic action.

It is an altered version of bevacizumab with deletion of Fc segment. Hence, it cannot bind to FcRn receptor in tissues and other blood vessels. Besides, systemic bioavailability is minimal following intravitreal administration. Hence, the systemic side effects of ranibizumab are lower than bevacizumab.

BEVACIZUMAB

Bevacizumab inhibits binding of VEGF to its receptors on endothelial cell surface preventing endothelial cellular proliferation and new vessel formation or angiogenesis. It is full length IgG and interacts with FcRn receptors in blood and other tissues. This nonselective action causes severe nonocular adverse effects of bevacizumab. Even intravitreal administration of bevacizumab causes higher systemic concentration. Adverse effects such as vessel injury, bleeding, epistaxis and poor wound healing, hypertension, proteinuria, GI perforation and thromboembolism can occur. It is cheaper among VEGF antagonists but not preferred due to its toxicity profile.

Drug of Choice: Ranibizumab

RATIONALE

Leading cause of permanent visual loss in old people is ARMD. It is classified as atrophic, dry or geographic and neovascular, exudative or wet. Ninety percent incidence is due to neovascular degeneration causing loss of central vision. Bevacizumab prevents binding of VEGF to its receptors on endothelial cell surface preventing endothelial cell proliferation and angiogenesis. **Intravitreal administration** of **bevacizumab** causes **higher systemic concentration**. Since it is a **full length IgG** interaction with FcRn receptors in blood and other tissues increases the severe **nonocular adverse effects.**[158] **Ranibizumab** is **a variable and not a full length IgG** with deletion of Fc segment. So it **does not bind to FcRn receptor** in tissues and other blood and its **systemic bioavailability** is **minimal** following intravitreal administration.[159] Hence, systemic side effects of ranibizumab are lower than bevacizumab.

References

1. Hanwella R, Senanayake M, de Silva V. Comparative efficacy and acceptability of methylphenidate and atomoxetine in treatment of attention deficit hyperactivity disorder in children and adolescents. BMC Psychiatry. 2011;11:176.
2. Gibson AP, Bettinger TL, Patel NC, et al. Atomoxetine versus stimulants for treatment of attention deficit hyperactivity disorder. Ann Pharmacotherapy. 2006;6:1134-6.
3. Panda S, Hazra A, Kundu AK. Evaluation of Silodosin in comparison with Tamsulosin in Benign Prostatic Hyperplasia: A randomised control trial. Ind J Pharmacol. 2014;46(6):601-7.
4. Syed M Nurulain. Efficacious oxime for organophosphate poisoning—A mini review. Trop J Phar Res. 2011;10(3):341-9.
5. Eddleston M, Buckley NA, Eyer P, et al. Management of acute organophosphorus compound poisoning. Lancet. 2008;371(9612): 597-607.
6. Gitanjali B, "Valethamate bromide - Is there any proof of efficacy and safety for its use in labor". Journal of Pharmacology and Pharmacotherapeutics. 2010;1(1):2-3.
7. Madhu C, Mahavarkar S, Bhave S. A Randomised controlled study comparing Drotaverine hydrochloride and Valethamate bromide in augmentation of labor. Arch Gynecol Obstet. 2010;282(1):11-5.
8. Marsch SC, Steiner L, Bucher E, et al. Succinyl choline versus Rocuronium for rapid sequence intubation in intensive care: A prospective randomised controlled trial. Critical Care. 2011;15(4):R1999.
9. Barbosa RM, da Silva CMG, Bella TS, et al. Cytotoxicity of solid lipid nanoparticles and nanostructured lipid carriers containing the local anesthetic Dibucaine designed for topical application. J Phys. Conference Series 2013;429:012035.
10. Weaver LC, Richards AB, Abreu BE. Central nervous system effects of a local anesthetic dyclonine. Toxicology and Applied Pharmacology. 1960;2(6):616-27.
11. Gethin G. The significance of surface pH in chronic wounds. Wounds UK. 2007;3(2):52-7.

12. Kar S, Krishnan A, Preetha K, et al. A review of antihistamines used during pregnancy. J Pharmacol Pharmacother. 2012;3(2):105-8.

13. Weber-Schoendorfer C, Schaefer C. The safety of Cetirizine during pregnancy: A prospective observational cohort study. Reprod Toxicol. 2008;26(1):19-23.

14. Ornstein M, Einarson A, Koren G. Benedictin/Dilectin for morning sickness: A Canadian follow up of an American tragedy. Reprod Toxicol. 1995;9(1):1-6.

15. Koren G, Clark. S, Hankins GDY, et al. Effectiveness of delayed release Doxylamine and Pyridoxine for nausea and vomiting: A randomised placebo controlled trial. Am J Obstet Gynecol. 2010;203(6):571.

16. Uchio E. Treatment of allergic conjunctivitis with Olapatadine hydrochloride eye drops. 2008;2(3):525-31.

17. Visser WH, Terwindt GM, Reines SA, et al. Rizatriptan vs Sumatriptan in the acute treatment of migraine: A placebo controlled dose ranging study. Dutch/US Rizatriptan study group. Arch Neurol. 1996;53(11):1132-7.

18. Schmidt R, Oestreich W. Flunarizine in migraine prophylaxis: the clinical experience. J Cardiovas Pharmacol. 19918;suppl 8:S21-6.

19. Kovacs G, Wachtel AE, Basharova EV, et al. Palonosetron vs Ondansetron of chemotherapy–induced nausea and vomiting in pediatric patients with cancer receiving moderately or highly emetogenic chemotherapy: A randomised, phase 3, double blind, double dummy, non-inferiority study. Lancet Oncol. 2016;7(3):332-44.

20. Papanikolaou EG, Pluchouras N, Drougia A, et al. Comparison of Misoprostol and Dinoprostone for elective induction of labor in nulliparous women at full term: A randomised prospective study. Reprod Biol Endocrinol. 2004;2:70.

21. Sueiman YM, Krdoghli NF, Ahmad AJ. Comparison of Ketorolac tromethamine and Prednisolone acetate in preventing surgically induced miosis during cataract surgery. Sultan Qaboos Univ Med J. 2010;10(1):57-63.

22. Kessel L, Tendal B, Jorgensen KJ, et al. Post Cataract Prevention of Inflammation and Macular edema by Steroid and Non-steroidal anti-inflammatory eye drops–A Systematic Review. Am Acad Ophthalmol. 2014:1915-24.

23. Simone JN, Pandeltron RA, Jenkins JE. Comparison of the efficacy and safety of Ketorolac tromethamine 0.5% and Prednisolone acetate 1% after cataract surgery. J Cataract Refract Surg. 1999;25(5): 699-704.

24. Becker MA, Schumacher HR, Wortmann RL, et al. Febuxostat compared with Allopurinol in patients with hyperuricemia and Gout. N Engl J of Med. 2005;353:2450-61.

25. Mattson RH, Cramer JA, Collins JF. A comparison of Valproate with Carbamazepine for the treatment of complex partial seizures and secondarily generalised tonic-clonic seizures in adults. N Engl J Med. 1992;327:765-71.

26. Koch MW, Polman SKL. Oxcarbazepine verses Carbamazepine monotherapy for partial onset seizures. Cochrane Database Sys Rev. 2009;(4):CD 006453.

27. Zakrzewska JM, Linskey ME. Trigeminal neuralgia. Br Med J Clin Evid. 2009;1207.

28. Snodgrass SR. Felbamate therapy in Lennox-Gastaut syndrome. N Engl J Med. 1993;328:1641.

29. Stafstrom CE. Update on the management of Lennox-Gastaut syndrome with a focus on rufinamide. Neuropsychiatr Dis Treat. 2009; 5:547-51.

30. Garza I, Swanson JW. Prophylaxis of migraine. Neuropschychiatr Dis Treat. 2006;2(3):281-91.

31. Corey D, Fogleman MD. Gabapentin for the prophylaxis of episodic migraine in adults. Am Fam Phy. 2014;89(9):714-5.

32. Knake S, Hamer HM, Schomberg U, et al. Tiagabine induced absence status in idiopathic generalised epilepsy. Seizure. 1999;8(5):314-7.

33. Faugh E. Topiramate in the treatment of partial and generalised epilepsy. Neuropsychiatr Dis Treat. 2007;3(6):811-21.

34. Constantin IM. Neuronal T type calcium channels: what is new? J Med Life. 2011;4(2):126-38.

35. Genton P, Gelisse P, Thomas P, et al. Do Carbamazepine and Phenytoin aggravate juvenile myoclonic epilepsy. Neurol. 2000;55(8): 1106-9.

36. Aranto K, Mattila MJ, Seppala T. Development of tolerance and cross tolerance to the psychomotor actions of Lorazepam and Diazepam. Br J Clin Pharmacol. 1983;15(5):545-52.

37. Aldridge BK, Gelb AM, Issacs SM, et al. A comparison of Lorazepam, Diazepam and Placebo for the treatment of out of hospital status epilepticus. N Engl J Med. 2001;345:631-7.

38. Fernandez Guisasola J, Gomez-Arnau J, Cabrera Y, et al. Association between nitrous oxide and the incidence of postoperative nausea and vomiting in adults—a systematic review and meta-analysis. Anaesth. 2010;65(4):379-87.

39. Lacrox G, Lessard MR, Trepanier CA. Treatment of postoperative nausea and vomiting—Comparison of Propofol, Droperidol and Metoclopramide. Can J Anaesth. 1994;43(2):115-20.

40. Swami SS, Keniya VM, Dhadi S, et al. Comparison of Dexmedetomidine and Clonidine ($\alpha 2$ agonistic drugs) as an adjuvant to

local anaesthesia in supraclavicular brachial plexus block; A double blind prospective study. Ind J Anaesth. 2012;56(3):243-9.

41. Mahendru V, Tewari A, Katyal S, et al. A comparison of intrathecal Dexmedetomidine, Clonidine and Fentanyl as adjuvants to hyperbaric Bupuvcaine for lower limb surgery—A double blind controlled study. J Anaesth Clin Pharma. 2013;29(4):496-502.

42. Jun-Chi H, Naoyuki F, Noriaki K, et al. Bronchospasm induced by Propofol in a patient with sick house syndrome. Anaesth Analges. 2003;96(1):163-4.

43. Nishiyama T. Propofol results in higher incidence of bronchoconstriction in allergic patients. Med Arch. 2013;67(3):168-70.

44. Dave VB, Chokshi JM, Bandopadhyaya AK. Ketamine and intraocular pressure. Ind J Ophthalmol. 1996;24(2):5-8.

45. Fameevo CE, Odugbersan CO, Osuntokun OO. Effect of Etomidate on intraocular pressure. Can Anaesth Soc J. 1977;24(6):712-6.

46. Moss E, Powell D, Gibson RM, et al. Effect of Etomidate on intracranial pressure. Br J Anaesth. 1979;51(4):347-52.

47. Landoni G, Biondi-Zoccai G, Zangrillo A, et al. Desflurane and Isoflurane in cardiac surgery; A meta-analysis of randomized clinical trials. J Cardiothorac Vasc Anaesth. 2007;21(4):502-11.

48. Rooks JP. Safety and risks of Nitrous oxide labor analgesia: A review. J Midwifery Women's Health. 2011;56(6):557-65.

49. Bhatia V, Tandon RK. Stress and gastrointestinal tract. J Gastroenterol Hepatol. 2005;20(3):332-9.

50. Williams SH. Medications for treatment of alcohol abuse. Am Fam Phys. 2005,71(1):1775-80.

51. Morley KC, Teesson M, Reid SC, et al. Naltrexone versus Acamprosate in the treatment of alcohol dependence: A multicenter randomised double-blind placebo controlled study. Addict. 2006;101(10); 1451-62.

52. Bonza C, Angles M, Munoz A, et al. Efficacy and safety of Naltrexone and Acamprosate in the treatment of alcohol dependence: a systematic review. Addict. 2004;99(7):811-28.

53. Brent J, Martin KM, Phillips S, et al. Safe and effective antidote for use in the treatment of Methanol poisoning. N Engl J Med. 2001; 344:434-29.

54. Beetty L, Green R, Magee K, et al. A systematic review of Ethanol and Fomepizole use in toxic alcohol ingestions. Em Med Inter Vol 2013;2013:1-14. Article ID 638057.

55. Fernandez NH, Freidman JH, Jacques C, et al. Quetiapine in the treatment of drug induced psychosis in Parkinson's disease. Mov Discard. 1999;14(3):484-7.

56. Merims D, Balas M, Peretz C, et al. Rater-blinded, prospective comparison: Quetiapine versus Clozapine for Parkinson's disease psychosis. Clin Neuropharmacol. 2006;29(6):331-7.

57. Mamo DC, Sweet RA, Keshavan MS. Managing antipsychotic-induced Parkinsonism. Drug Saf. 1999;20(3):269-75.

58. Bullock R, Touchon J, Bergman H, et al. Rivastigmine and Donepezil treatment in mild to moderately severe Alzheimer's disease over a period of 2 years. Curr Med Res Opin. 2005;21(8):1317-27.

59. Levine TD, Bowser R, Hank N, et al. A pilot trial of Memantine and Riluzole in ALS: Correlation of CSF biomarkers. Amyotroph Lateral Scler. 2010;11(6):514-9.

60. Mossaheb N, Kaufmann RM. Role of Aripiprazole in treatment resistant Schizophrenia. Neuropsychiatr Dis Treat. 2012;8:235-44.

61. Eduardo J, Samuel A, Siris G, et al. Can Atypical antipsychotics reduce suicidal risk in patients with Schizophrenia. Psychiatr Tim. 2008.

62. Owen RT. Olanzapine: a review of rapid and long acting potential formulations. Drug Today. 2010;46(3):173-81.

63. Lorenzo RD, Brogli A. Profile of Olanzapine long acting injection for the maintenance treatment of adult patients with Schizophrenia. Neuropsychiatr Disease Treat. 2010;6:573-81.

64. Thase ME. Quetiapine monotherapy for Bipolar disorder. Neuropsychiatr Dis Treat. 2008;4(1):21-31.

65. Bender KJ. Olanzapine/Fluoxetine combination affirmed for Bipolar depression. Psychiatr Times. 2013.

66. Manning S. Effective treatment of Bipolar depression: Monotherapy and combination strategies. J Clinical Psychiatr. 2015;76(11):e1481.

67. Alexander W. Pharmacotherapy for Posttraumatic Stress Disorder in combat veterans. Pharma Therapeutic. 2012;31(1):32-8.

68. Bergeron R, Ravindran AV, Chaput Y, et al. Sertraline and Fluoxetine treatment of Obsessive Compulsive Disorder. J Psychopharmacol. 2002;22(2):148-54.

69. Irons J. Fluvoxamine in the treatment of anxiety disorders. Neuropsychiatr Dis Treat. 2005;1(4):289-99.

70. Handley AP, Williams M. The efficacy and tolerability of SSRI/SNRI in the treatment of vasomotor symptoms in menopausal women: A systematic review. J Am Assoc Nur Prac. 2015;27(1):54-61.

71. Wright CL, Mist SD, Ross RL, et al. Duloxetine for the treatment of fibromyalgia. Exp Rev Clin Immunol. 2010;6(5):745-56.

72. Osmidon MK, Sarmas I, Kyritsis A. Patient compliance with SSRI and Gabapentin in painful diabetic neuropathy. Clin J Pain. 2007; 23(3):267-9.

73. Barney P, Halpein D, Tango R, et al. A major change of prescribing pattern in absence of adequate evidence: Benzodiazepines versus

newer anti-depressants in anxiety disorders. Psychopharmacol Bullet. 2008;41(3):39-47.

74. Liebouttz MR, Gelenberg AJ, Munjack D. Venlafaxine extended release versus placebo and Paroxetine in Social Anxiety Disorder. JAMA Psychiatr. 2005;62(2):190-8.

75. Allqulander C, Mangano R, Zhang J, et al. Efficacy of Venlafaxine ER in patients with Social Anxiety Disorder: A double blind placebo controlled, parallel–group compared with Paroxetine. Psychopharmacol. 2004;19(6):387-96.

76. Amanta F, Lanari A, Mignini F, et al. Nicardipine use in cerebrovascular disease: A review of controlled clinical studies. J Neurosci. 2009;283(1-2):219-23.

77. Bucci C, Mamdani MM, Juurlink DN, et al. Dihydropyridine Calcium channel blockers and cardiovascular outcomes in elderly patients: A population based study. Can J Cardiol. 2008;24(8):629-32.

78. Hermandez AF, Harrington RA. Comparative Effectiveness of Angiotensin Converting Enzyme Inhibitors. Is an ACE always an ace? JAMC. 2008;178(10):1316-9.

79. Noto H, Goto A, Tscijimato T, et al. Effect of Calcium channel blockers on incidence of Diabetes: A Meta-analysis. Diabetes Metab Syndr Obes. 2013;6:251-61.

80. Norris G, Rhoney DH. A comparison of Nicardipine and Labetolol for acute hypertension management following stroke. Neurocritical care. 2008;9(2):167-76.

81. Lofdahl CG. Antihypertensive drugs and airway function with special reference to Calcium channel blockade. J Cardiovasc Pharmacol. 1989;14(10):S40-51.

82. Talwar D, Jindal SK. Effects of Enalapril, an angiotensin converting enzyme inhibitor on bronchial hyper-responsiveness in asthmatics. Ind J Physiol Pharmacol. 1993;37(3):217-20.

83. Myon S, Fujimara M, Kamio Y, et al. Effect of Losartan, a type I Angiotensin II blocker on bronchial hyper-responsiveness to Methacholine in patients with bronchial asthma. Am J Respir Crit Care Med. 2000;162(1):40-4.

84. Houston MC. Treatment of hypertensive emergencies and urgencies with oral clonidine loading and titration: A review. Arch Intern Med. 1996;146(3):586-9.

85. Magee LA, Cham C, Waterman EJ, et al. Hydralazine for treatment of severe hypertension in pregnancy: A meta-analysis. BMJ. 2003;327(7421):955-60.

86. Vernon J, Marik PE. Perioperative hypertension management, Vascular health and risk management; 2008;4(3):615-25.

87. Connolly SJ, Ezekonitz MD, Yusuf S, et al. Dabigatran versus Warfarin in patients with atrial fibrillation. N Engl J Med. 2009;361:1139-51.

88. Norgard NB, Dinicolantonia J. Clopidogrel, Prasugrel or Ticagrelor? A practical guide to use of antiplatelet agents in patients with acute coronary syndrome. Postgrad Med. 2013;125(4):91-102.

89. Payne DJ, Cramp R, Winstanley DJ, et al. Comparative activities of Clavulanic acid, Sulbactum, Tezobactum against clinically important β-lactamases. 1994;38(4):767-72.

90. World Health Organization. Background document: the diagnosis, treatment and prevention of typhoid fever; Communicable Disease Surveillance and Response. Geneva: World Health Organization; 2003. pp. 1-48.

91. Nicholas RO, Berry V, Hunter PA, et al. Antifungal activity of Mupirocin. J Antimicrob Chemother. 1998;63(4):579-82.

92. Guidelines for Diagnosis and Treatment of malaria in India; 2014; National Institute of Malaria Research; Govt of India. New Delhi.

93. Martin MV. The use of Fluconazole and Itraconazole in the treatment of Candida albicans infection: a review. J Antimicrob Chemother. 1999;44(4):429-36.

94. Pappas PG, Rothstein CM, Betts RF, et al. Micafungin versus Caspofungin for treatment of Candidemia and other forms of invasive Candidiasis. Clin Infect Dis. 2007;45(7): 883-93.

95. de Naurosis J, Gill MJ, Marti FM, et al. Management of Febrile neutropenia: ESMO Clinical practical guideline. Ann Oncol. 2010;27(5):v252-6.

96. Pagano L, Caira M, Cuenca-Estrella M. The management of febrile neutropenia in the Posaconazole era: a new challenge. Haematologica. 2012;97 (7):963-5.

97. Malik IA, Moid I, Aziz Z, et al. A randomized comparison of Fluconazole with Amphoteracin B as Empiric antifungal agents in cancer patients with prolonged neutropenia. Am J Med. 1998;105 (6):478-83.

98. Winston DJ, Hawthorn JW, Schuster MG, et al. A multicenter randomized trial of Fluconazole versus Amphoteracin B for antifungal therapy of Febrile neutropenic patients with cancer. Am J Med. 2000;108(4):282-9.

99. Roberts DJ, Taylor WD, Boyle J. Guidelines for treatment of Onchomycosis. Br J Dermatol. 2003;148:402-10.

100. Westerberg DP, Voyack MJ. Onchomycosis: Current trends in diagnosis and treatment. Am Fam Physician. 2013;88(11):762-70.

101. Anderlini P, Benjamin RS, Wong FC, et al. Idarubicin cardiotoxicity: a retrospective study in Acute Myeloid Leukemia and Myelodysplasia. J Clin Oncol. 1995;13(11):2827-34.

102. Mandelli F, Vignetti M, Sueiu S, et al. Daunorubicin versus Mitoxantrone versus Idarubicin as induction and consolidation

chemotherapy for adults with Acute Myeloid Leukemia. J Clin Oncol. 2009;27(32):5397-403.

103. Vogelzang NJ, Bhor M, Liu Z, et al. Everolimus versus Temsirolimus for advanced renal cell carcinoma. Clin Genitourin Cancer. 2013;11(2):115-20.

104. Patel SB, Stenehjem DD, Gill DM, et al. Everolimus versus Temsirolimus in metastatic renal cell carcinoma after progression with previous systemic therapies. Clin Genitourin Cancer. 2016;14 (2):153-9.

105. Pyrhonen S, Valavaara R, Modig H, et al. Comparison of Toremifene and Tamoxifen in post-menopausal patients with advanced breast cancer: a randomized double-blind, the 'Nordic' phase III study. B J Cancer. 1997;76(2):270-4.

106. Gheitti OA, Bakr MA, Shokair MA, et al. Comparative analysis of Azathioprine versus Cyclosporine based therapy in primary haplo-identical live-donar kidney transplantation: A 20 year experience. 2008;19(4):564-71.

107. Janknegt R, Boone N, ErdKamp F, et al. GnRH agonists and antagonists in prostate cancer. GaBI J. 2014;3(3):133-42.

108. Chanson P, Boerlin V, Ajzenberg C, et al. Comparison of Octreotide acetate LAR and Lanreotide SR in patients with acromegaly. Clin Endocrinol. 2000;53(5):577-86.

109. Kauschansky MG. Preoperative treatment of intractable hyperthyroidism with acute Lithium administration. Eur J Paediatr Surg. 1996;6(5):301-2.

110. Dampetla S, Malik M. Lithium in the acute pre-operative preparation of thyrotoxicosis: a case series. Endocr Abstracts. 2011;26:410.

111. Tsunoda T, Mochinaga N, Eto T, et al. Lithium carbonate in the preoperative preparation of Graves disease. Japanese J Surg. 1991; 21(3):292-6.

112. Buttgereit F, Straub RH, Wehling M, et al. Glucocorticoid in the therapy of Rheumatic diseases: An update on mechanism of action. Arthritis Rheumatol. 2004;50(11):3408-17.

113. Verhoef C, Van Roon JAG, Vianan M, et al. The immunosuppressive effect of Dexamethasone in Rheumatoid arthritis is accompanied by upregulation of IL-10, and by differential changes in interferon-γ and interlukin-4 production. Ann Rheumat Dis. 1999;58(1):49-54.

114. Smith MD, Ahern MJ, Roberts-Thomson PJ. Pulse steroid therapy in Rheumatoid arthritis: can equivalent doses of oral Prednisolone give similar clinical results to IV methyl Prednisolone. Ann Rheumat Dis. 1988;47:28-33.

115. Sadra V, Kbabbazi A, Kolahi S, et al. Randomized double-blind study on the effects of Dexamethasone and Methyl Prednisolone pulse in

the control of Rheumatoid arthritis flare up: A preliminary study. Int J Rheumat Dis. 2014;17(4):389-93.

116. Ference JD, Last AR. Choosing topical corticosteroids. Am Fam Physician. 2009;179(2):135-40.

117. Daily G, Strange P. Lower severe hypoglycemia risk: Insulin Glargine versus NPH insulin in type 2 Diabetes. Am J Manag Care. 2008; 14(1):25-30.

118. Rosenstock J, Fonseca V, Schinzel S, et al. Reduced risk of hypoglycemia with once daily Glargine versus twice daily NPH and number needed to harm with NPH to demonstrate the risk of one additional hypoglycemic event in type 2 Diabetes: Evidence from a long-term controlled trial. J Diabetes Complications. 2014;28(5):742-9.

119. Kamatani N, Katoh T, Sawai Y, et al. Comparison between the clinical efficacy of Linagliptin and Sitagliptin. J Diabetes Endocrinol. 2013;4(4):51-4.

120. Umpires GE, Jones S, Smiley D, et al. Insulin analogs versus human insulin in the treatment of patients with Diabetic ketoacidosis: A randomized controlled trial. Diabetes care. 2009;32(7):1164-9.

121. Davidson JA, Brett J, Falahati A, et al. Mild renal impairment and the efficacy and safety of Liraglutide. Endocr Pract. 2011;17(3):345-55.

122. Minnemann T, Schubert M, Freude S, et al. Comparison of a new long-acting testosterone undecanoate formulation vs testosterone enanthate for intramuscular androgen therapy in male hypogonadism. J Endocrinol Investigations. 2008;31(8):718-23.

123. Reid DM, Hosking D, Kendler D, et al. A comparison of the effect of Alendronate and Risedronate on bone mineral density in postmenopausal women with osteoporosis: 24-month results from FACTS-International. Int J Clin Pract. 2008;62(4):575-84.

124. Rosen LS, Gordon D, Kaminski M, et al. Long-Term Efficacy and Safety of Zoledronic Acid compared with Pamidronate Disodium in the treatment of Skeletal Complications in Patients with advanced Multiple Myeloma or Breast Carcinoma: A Randomized, Double-Blind, Multicenter, Comparative Trial. Cancer. 2003;98(8):735-44.

125. Major P, Lortholary A, Hon J, et al. Zoledronic acid is superior to Pamidronate in the treatment of hypercalcemia of malignancy: a pooled analysis of randomized, controlled clinical trials. J Clin Oncol. 2001;17(2):558-67.

126. Swaran J, Flora S, Pachauri V. Chelation in metal intoxication. Int J Environ Res Public Health. 2010;7(7):2745-88.

127. Daley-Yates PT, Price AC, Sisson JR, et al. Beclomethasone dipropionate: absolute bioavailability, pharmacokinetics and metabolism following intravenous, oral, intranasal and inhaled administration in man. BrJ Clin Pharmacol. 2001;51(5):400-9.

128. Fabbri L, Burge PS, Goonenborgh L, et al. Comparison of Fluticasone Propionate with Beclomethasone dipropionate in moderate to severe asthma treatment for one year: International study group. Thorax. 1993;48:817-23.

129. Nathan RA. Beta 2 agonist therapy: Oral versus Inhaled delivery. J Asthma.1992;29 (1):49-54.

130. Goldstein MF, Chervinsky P.Efficacy and safety of Doxofylline compared to Theophylline in chronic reversible asthma- a double-blind randomized placebo-controlled multicentre clinical trial. Med Sci Monit. 2002;8(4): CR297-304.

131. Margay SM, Farhat S, Kaur S, et al To study the efficacy and safety of Doxofylline and Theophylline in Bronchial asthma. J Clin Diagn Res. 2015;9(4):FC05-8.

132. Verstraeten JM. Mucolytic treatment in chronic obstructive lung disease: double-blind comparative clinical trial with N-Acetylcysteine, Bromhexine and placebo. Acta tuberc Pneumol Belg. 1978;70(1): 71-80.

133. Seagrave JC, Albrecht HH, Hill DB, et al. Effects of Guaifenacin, N-Acetylcysteine and Ambroxol on MUC5AC and mucociliary transport in primary differentiated human tracheal-bronchial cells. Resp Res. 2012;13:98.

134. Augestad KM, Delaney CP.Postoperative ileus: Impact of pharmacological treatment, laproscopic surgery and enhanced recovery pathways. World J Gastroenterol. 2010;16(17):2067-74.

135. Mehta S, Khandelwal PD, Jain VK, et al. A comparative study of Racecadotril and single dose Octreotide as an anti-secretory agent in acute infective diarrhea. J Assoc Physicians India. 2012;60:12-5.

136. Talley NJ. Evaluation of drug treatment in irritable bowel syndrome. Br J Clin Pharmacol. 2003;56(4):362-9.

137. Adeyemo MA, Chang L. New treatments for irritable bowel syndrome in women. Womens Health. 2008;4(6):605-23.

138. Rahimi R, Nikfar S, Rezaie A, et al. Efficacy of Tricyclic antidepressants in Irritable bowel syndrome: A meta-analysis. World J Gastroenterol. 2009;15(13):1548-53.

139. Thayalasekeran S, Ali H, Her-Hsin T. Novel therapies for constipation.World J Gastroenterol. 2013;19(45):8247-51.

140. Bassari R, Koea JB. Jaundice associated pruritus: A review of pathophysiology and treatment. World J Gastroenterol. 2015;21(5): 1404-13.

141. Grunberg S, Chua D, Maru A, et al. Single dose Fosaprepitant for the prevention of chemotherapy-induced nausea and vomiting associated with Cisplatin therapy: randomized, double-blind study protocol—EASE. J Clin Oncol. 2011;29(11):1495-501.

142. Hargreaves R, Ferreira JC, Hughes D, et al. Development of Aprepitant, the first Neurokinin-1 receptor antagonist for the prevention of chemotherapy-induced nausea and vomiting. Ann NY Acad Sci. 2011;1222:40-8.

143. Langford P, Chrisp P. Fosaprepitant and Aprepitant: an update of the evidence for their place in the prevention of chemotherapy induced nausea and vomiting. Core Evidence. 2010;5:77-90.

144. Conde-Agudelo A, Romero R, Pedro J, et al. Nifedipine for the management of preterm labor: A systematic review and met analysis. Am J Obstet Gynecol. 2011;4(2):134.e1-20.

145. Lyell DJ, Pullen K, Campbell L, et al. Magnesium sulfate compared with Nifedipine for acute tocolysis of preterm labor: A randomized controlled trial. Obstet Gynecol. 2007;110(1):61-7.

146. Anderson J. Prevention and management of postpartum hemorrhage. Am Fam Physician. 2007;75(6):875-82.

147. Gaal Z, Klupa T, Kantor I, et al. Sulfonylurea use during entire pregnancy in Diabetes because of KCNJ11 mutation: A report of two cases. Diabetes care. 2012;35(6):e40.

148. Wise J. Use of Glyburide to treat gestational Diabetes is linked to adverse outcomes in babies, study finds. Br Med J. 2015;350:h1709.

149. Castillo WC, Boggess K, Sturmer T, et al. Association of adverse pregnancy outcomes with Glyburide vs Insulin in women with Gestational Diabetes. JAMA Pediatrics. 2015;169(5):452-8.

150. Feldman DM, Carbone J, Belden L, et al. Betamethasone versus Dexamethasone for prevention of morbidity in low birth weight neonates. Am J Obstet Gynecol. 2007;197(3):284.

151. Lander CM. Antiepileptic drugs in pregnancy and lactation. Austral Prescrib. 2008;31:70-2.

152. Hunt S, Russel A, Smithson WH, et al. Topiramate in pregnancy. Neurol. 2008;71(4);272-6.

153. Mawhinney E, Craig J, Morrow J, et al. Levitiracetam in pregnancy; results from Ireland epilepsy and pregnancy registers. Neurol. 2013; 80(4):400-5.

154. Koubeissi M. Levitiracetam: More evidence of safety in pregnancy. Epilepsy Curr-Rev Crit Anal. 2013;13(6):271-81.

155. McGready R, Thwai KL, Samuel CT. Effect of Quinine and Chloroquine antimalarial treatments in the first trimester of pregnancy. Trans R Soc Trop Med Hyg. 2002;96(2):180-4.

156. Depalo R, Jayakrishnan K, Garrutti G. GnRH agonists versus GnRH antagonists in invitro fertilization and embryo transfer. Reprod Biol Endocrinol.2012;13:10-26.

157. Tanghetti E, Dhawan SG, Rosso JD, et al. Randomized comparison of the safety and efficacy of Tazarotene 0.1% cream and Adapalene 0.3% gel in the treatment of patients with moderate facial acne vulgaris. J Drug Dermatol. 2010;9(5):549-58.

158. Moja L, Lucenteforte E, Kwag KH, et al. Systemic safety of Bevacizumab versus Ranibizumab for neo-vascular age-related macular degeneration. Cochrane Database Syst Rev. 2014;15(9):CD011230.

159. Azana Perea JR, Layana AG. Ranibizumab versus Bevacizumab: pharmacological considerations. Arch Soc Esp Oftal. 2012;87(1):3-9.

FURTHER READING

1. Brunton LL, Chabner B, Knollman BC. Goodman and Gilman's The Pharmacological Basis of Therapeutics,, 12th edition. USA: McGraw Hill; 2011.

2. Fauci A, Kasper D, Hauser S, Longo D, Jameson L, Loscalzo J. Harrison's Principles of Internal Medicine, 19th edition. USA: McGraw Hill; 2015.

3. Katzung BG,. Masters SB, Trevor AJ. Basic and Clinical pharmacology, 12th edition. USA: McGraw Hill; 2012.

4. Papadakis MA, McPhee SJ. Current Medical Diagnosis and Treatment, 54th edition. USA: McGraw Hill; 2015.

Index